Human Anatomy and Physiology

Inner Ear Development and Hearing Loss

HUMAN ANATOMY AND PHYSIOLOGY

Additional books in this series can be found on Nova's website
under the Series tab.

Additional e-books in this series can be found on Nova's website
under the e-book tab.

HUMAN ANATOMY AND PHYSIOLOGY

INNER EAR DEVELOPMENT AND HEARING LOSS

SAIMA RIAZUDDIN
AND
ZUBAIR AHMED
EDITORS

NOVA BIOMEDICAL
New York

For permission to use material from this book please contact us:
Telephone 631-231-7269; Fax 631-231-8175
Web Site: http://www.novapublishers.com

NOTICE TO THE READER

Additional color graphics may be available in the e-book version of this book.

Library of Congress Cataloging-in-Publication Data

ISBN: 978-1-62417-011-9

Library of Congress Control Number: 2012949632

Published by Nova Science Publishers, Inc. † New York

CONTENTS

PREFACE

Inner Ear Development and Hearing Loss is a user-friendly book focused on understanding the inner ear structure and genetics of hearing loss. It has been designed to be a source of succinct information for practicing general otolaryngologists, developmental biologist, geneticists and medical students, graduate students and researchers. The book, authored by 23 international otolaryngologist and researchers, is both comprehensive and easy to follow. Each chapter is short, informative and self-contained. It will provide an overview of four main topics related to inner ear development, hearing loss and clinical remedies, and the genetics of deafness in a post-genomic era.

The overall objective of this book is to bring together noted otolaryngologists and scientists from the perspectives of disciplines complementary to the science of inner ear development and hearing loss, in order to create a thorough review of the current state of knowledge and the available clinical therapies for hearing loss in humans. In the last fifteen years, we have witnessed tremendous progress in understanding the basic biology and genetics of the physiological processes involved in hearing. Many molecular components necessary for the development, function and maintenance of inner ear sensory epithelium have been discovered as a result of identifying the genes for nonsyndromic and syndromic forms of hearing loss in humans and in mice. We know have an unprecedented understanding of the molecular pathways involved in sound transduction, the molecular epidemiology of deafness, and we have reached a new capacity for genetic diagnosis and counseling. With such improvements in clinical practices, the development of novel therapeutic interventions is imminent.

The first section presents an overview of inner ear development. Chapter 1 discussed briefly the development of inner ear structure and signaling molecules that trigger the differentiation of sensory and non-sensory epithelium in the organ of Corti. Chapter 2 is focused on tight junction proteins and their role in maintaining the integrity of the hearing organ. In this chapter, we also describe the clinical manifestations of losing function of tight junction proteins, as seen in humans, and we discuss various phenotypes observed in mutant mouse models. Finally, we examine the recent evidence suggesting the role tight junction proteins play in regulating gene expression. Chapter 3 reviews the emerging evidence around the roles of known Usher and Bardet-Biedl syndrome proteins in orchestrating inner ear sensory epithelium through the planar cell polarity (PCP) pathway, as the inner ear is an ideal system by which to observe PCP in mammals.

The next section focuses on two clinical disorders involving inner ear dysfunction and cochlear implantation as an available remedy of hearing loss. In Chapter 4, Roberto Bovo and Chiara Faccioli provide an overview of autoimmune inner ear disease and available medical treatments. Autoimmune inner ear disease (AIED) accounts for less than 1% all cases of hearing impairment or dizziness, though incidence might be underestimated due to a lack of specific diagnostic testing, Therefore, in this chapter, the authors provide a practical tool for the diagnosis and treatment of AIED. In Chapter 5, the clinical and genetic presentations of Labyrinthine Aplasia, Microtia and Microdontia (LAMM) syndrome are reviewed. Since the initial description in 2007 by Mustafa Tekin and co-authors, 56 individuals with LAMM syndrome from 13 unrelated families have been reported. Kumarie Latchman and Mustafa Tekin discuss the variability observed in the clinical presentation of LAMM syndrome and its association with missense, nonsense and small deletions leading to the loss of FGF3 function. In Chapter 6, Daniel Choo discusses cochlear implantation, which has transformed the lives of deaf individuals and has provided a powerful tool for otolaryngologists. He also, however, describes some of the associated negative social ramifications, such as the response from the Deaf community around cochlear implantation and the financial costs of widespread cochlear implantation. Chapter 7 is a review of the literature on incidences of cochlear implantation in families exhibiting genetic deafness, to determine if there were any characteristic findings regarding performance outcome. Viet Pham, Dayton Young and Tomoko Makishima reviewed reports in the literature (from 1994 to 2012) on patients with definitive diagnoses of genetic hearing loss who underwent cochlear implantation (total of 104 reports). They concluded that cochlear implantation is capable of providing significant rehabilitation to patients with severe to profound hereditary and non-hereditary forms of sensorineural hearing loss.

The third section discusses the accelerating discovery of genes and gene variants, and the role of emerging sequencing technologies in improving our understanding of molecular components of the inner ear. In Chapter 8, Tal Elkan-Miller and Karen B. Avraham review the discovery of the deafness gene in the genomic era. According to the authors, since the completion of the Human Genome Project (HGP) and the creation of massively parallel sequencing (MPS) technologies, rapid high-throughput identification of new deafness genes has been greatly streamlined. In addition, in Chapter 9, Regie Lyn P. Santos-Cortez and Suzanne M. Leal discuss the utility of extended and consanguineous families in the identification of genes, variants and description of genotype-phenotype correlations. They conclude that despite advanced technologies, families with linkage information, paired with deep sequencing, are the most powerful tool in the identification of deafness genes.

Genetic screening, the last section of the book, presents an overview of population-specific screening strategies and their interpretations. Chapter 10 describes the interpretation of variants of uncertain clinical significance (VUCS) in individuals with Usher syndrome, a deaf-blindness disorder. Since the inception of the personalized molecular genetics era, the chance of identifying VUCS has massively increased. Proper assessment of these variants has become a major issue in many human diseases, including Usher syndrome, cystic fibrosis and breast cancer. In this chapter, authors point out relevant clinical and genetic features and the range and type of mutations found. They focus on a simple methodology that has been designed to assess the potential clinical impact of VUCS identified in Usher genes. In Chapter 11, Soo-Young Choi, Kyu Yup Lee and Un-Kyung Kim describe the molecular genetic studies conducted on the *GJB2* gene in the Korean population. The gap junction beta 2

(*GJB2*) gene encoding the connexin26 (Cx26) protein is one of the main causative genes of nonsyndromic hearing loss in many populations. Screening of 324 Korean subjects with nonsyndromic hearing loss revealed that mutations in *GJB2* are a less common cause of hearing loss they are in East Asian populations. The c.235delC mutation accounts for more than half of the mutations in the Korean population. Similarly, in Chapter 12, Koji Nishimura and Shin-ichiro Kitajiri review the frequency of GJB2 in the Japanese population and conclude that genetic variants of hereditary hearing loss in the Asian population are different from those found in the Caucasian population group. Therefore, population-specific genetic screening strategies for mutation detection would be feasible and cost-efficient genetic test for deafness.

We would like to extend our thanks to the many authors who have devoted an extensive amount of time to the development of this book. Our thanks to our team members – Arnaud Giese, Thomas Jaworek, Rizwan Yousaf, Gowri Nayak and Elodie Richard – for their help in making this book a reality. We would also like to thank Nova Science Publishers for their commitment to publishing texts that report on the most current and emerging scientific knowledge available. This book would have remained an unfulfilled dream if not for the support of our daughter, Mariya R. Ahmed who allowed us the many weekends spent writing and editing this book.

Disclaimer

Statements and opinions expressed in the chapters are these of the individual contributors and not necessarily those of the editors or publisher. No responsibility is accepted for the accuracy of information contained in the published chapters.

Saima Riazuddin
Cincinnati, Ohio

Zubair M. Ahmed
Cincinnati, Ohio

In: Inner Ear Development and Hearing Loss
Editors: Saima Riazuddin and Zubair Ahmed
ISBN: 978-1-62417-011-9

Chapter 1

THE BIRTH OF A MECHANOSENSOR: DEVELOPMENT OF VERTEBRATE HAIR CELLS

Tomoko Kita,
Stephen D. Freeman
and Raj K. Ladher*
Lab for Sensory Development,
RIKEN Center for Developmental Biology,
Chuo-ku, Kobe, Japan

ABSTRACT

The vertebrate inner ear hair cell can be considered as the apogee of cellular differentiation. It possesses apical modifications, the stereocilia and the kinocilia, that show remarkable sensitivity to the mechanical stimulation generated in the course of hearing or balance sensation. Understanding how these specializations occur would thus be a prerequisite to designing any cellular therapies to repair inner ear damage. In this chapter we describe the developmental decisions that a progenitor needs to make to become a hair cell and how these choices provide the context within which the mechanisms that lead to hair cell specialization can operate.

INTRODUCTION

The origin of vertebrate inner ear hair cells can be traced back to the otic placode, a thickened epithelium found on either side of the caudal part of the hindbrain, early in the life of the embryo. The purpose of this chapter is to describe how an undifferentiated population of cells becomes differentiated. This daunting task is undertaken in steps, and we use these milestones as the headings for this chapter, going from otic placode induction, through to hair cell specialization. In general, development uses recursive processes and concepts, such as

* Email: raj-ladher@cdb.riken.jp:

induction (the process by which one cell type changes a property of another) or competence (the ability of a cell type to respond appropriately to a given inductive cue) to make hierarchical lineage decisions that direct the fate of cells, and these are based on tools that are reused throughout differentiation. Understanding the process through which hair cells develop, has of course, a direct bearing on our ability to produce inner ear hair cells in a dish, a feat that would have a tremendous impact on the potential to design therapies and conduct research, and one that has hitherto proven difficult.

INDUCTION OF THE INNER EAR

Cranial Placodes

Any discussion on the induction of the inner ear needs to introduce the placode. Indeed, most vertebrate sensory systems, and the nerves that transmit their information, have their origin in disks of thickened epithelia known as cranial placodes [1]. The most anterior of these placodes is the olfactory placode, which will produce the olfactory epithelium as well as the first cranial nerve, the olfactory nerve. The otic placode, is more caudally located, and forms the inner ear as well as the eighth cranial nerve, the cochleovestibular nerve. There are also placodes that are exclusively neurogenic, and do not produce any sensory structures per se. The trigeminal placode, split into the ophthalmic and maxillo-mandibular lobes, forms the sensory components of the fifth cranial nerve and mediates pain, touch and temperature sensation in the skin of the head, as well as the eyes and jaw muscles. In addition, three epibranchial placodes lie around the otic placode. Their introduction is important as they are induced in a common progenitor region with the inner ear. The most anterior, the geniculate, forms the sensory component of the seventh nerve, the facial nerve, innervating the taste buds as well as transmitting information from the ear lobes. The second epibranchial placode, the petrosal, forms part of the ninth cranial nerve (the glossopharyngeal nerve) and also provides some innervation to the tongue as well as the carotid sinus, regulating blood pressure, and the carotid body, which senses blood oxygen. The most caudal epibranchial placode is the nodose, contributing to the tenth cranial nerve, the vagus, which conveys sensory information from almost every organ in the body.

Cranial placodes form from the ectoderm, the outer-most of the three germ layers in the early embryo. In the head region of the embryo, the ectoderm can be thought of as being of two types, the neural ectoderm that will give rise to the central nervous system (CNS) and the non-neural ectoderm, that forms the epidermis. The boundary of these two territories forms a region of competence. While on the neural-side it is endowed with the ability to generate neural crest cells, a migratory population that forms in the head, the skeletal structures and the glia of the peripheral nervous system (PNS), on the non-neural side, the neural-non-neural border is competent to form sensory placodes [2]. It is this region, known as the pre-placodal region that will give rise to all of the cranial placodes described above [3, 4]. The mechanism of how individual placodes are generated from the pre-placodal region is not relevant to this chapter; instead in the next section we restrict our focus to the otic placode.

Otic Specification

Identifying the source and nature of the inductive signals that trigger the development of the otic placode has been a fascination for many developmental biologists. These studies implicate the necessity of the tissues that surround the site of the future otic placode for its induction. Furthermore, they point to a particular class of growth factor signaling molecules, known as fibroblast growth factors (FGFs), as the causative molecules that impart the pre-placodal region with the ability to form the otic placode.

However it is necessary to introduce a caveat; recent findings have revealed that the question "how to induce an inner ear" is not strictly correct. Instead, an emerging concept is that the otic placode is not specified alone, rather it is jointly induced with the epibranchial placodes [5-8]. This region, known variously as the posterior placodal area (PPA), the otic-epibranchial progenitor region (OEPD) or the pre-otic field (POF), was first postulated based on gene expression patterns, particularly that of the transcription factor Pax2, but was later confirmed by lineage labeling. Streit used a lipophilic dye to mark patches of cells that fell within the Pax2 territory, and found that these cells contribute to the inner ear and the epibranchial placodes [9]. This is supported by data in which the Pax2 postive cells were genetically marked, and again their progeny were found in both the inner ear and the epibranchial placodes [10]. The expression of Pax2, in the chick, appears after around 1 day of development, soon after the neural folds are formed [11]. Similarly in mouse, expression of Pax2 and the closely related Pax8 commences at embryonic day (E) 9, soon after the neural folds form [12]. It is found in an ectodermal domain, lateral to the caudal hindbrain and rostral to the first somite. In both chick and mouse, Pax2 marks a morphologically distinct region of the ectoderm, that is, the entire Pax2 expressing ectoderm is thicker than the surrounding non-expressing ectoderm [1]. Thus, it is apparent that the first step to making an inner ear is the induction of a progenitor domain for both inner ear and epibranchial placodes. However, the nature of the PPA still needs to be elucidated: is it a region of equivalence, that is, are all cells in the PPA equally competent to form either inner ear or epibranchial placodes, or are the two lineages already specified as the PPA itself forms.

A number of experiments have suggested that the source of the PPA-inducing signal is the mesoderm that underlies it and the adjacent neural ectoderm (reviewed by [13]). Studies in the chick show that removal of the mesoderm underlying the PPA cause a loss of Pax2 expression [14]. Conversely, transplanting the sub-PPA mesoderm to ectopic locations cause an ectopic domain of Pax2 expression thatshows sufficiency of the mesoderm [14]. Support for this role of the mesoderm comes from the genetic removal of paraxial mesoderm (mesoderm that lies on either side of the midline) but not the axial, midline, mesoderm in zebrafish [15]. Again, ablation results in the failure to induce Pax2 or Pax8 in the PPA. While these studies do suggest that the mesoderm itself is sufficient to induce the PPA, recombination experiments argue against it [16]. In these experiments, pure populations of tissues that are microdissected and placed together in culture are assessed for a variety of markers. Using this paradigm, it was found that the mesoderm needs the inclusion of the neural ectoderm to induce Pax2 in non-neural ectoderm [16]. Thus, the induction of the PPA is under the control of signals from the mesoderm and the adjacent hindbrain.

Signals Inducing the PPA

The FGF family of secreted growth factors has long been thought to be involved in the induction of the PPA. A number of FGF ligands are expressed in either the sub-otic paraxial mesoderm or in the adjacent hindbrain in the correct temporal pattern to suggest a role in PPA induction [17]. However, gene knockout or knockdown studies do not implicate any one particular FGF in this process. Instead, it is likely that the embryo compensates for the absence of one FGF by altering the expression of another, and that at least two FGF ligands are involved in PPA induction. Fgf3 is common amongst all vertebrate species thus far investigated. In fish, both Fgf3 and Fgf8 need to be downregulated for PPA formation to be affected [18-21]. In mice, Fgf3 together with either Fgf10 or Fgf8 are responsible for PPA induction [22-24], and in chick, Fgf3 and Fgf19 need to be downregulated [8], although blocking only Fgf8 also inhibits the formation of the PPA [23]. This rather complicated scheme can be simplified by thinking of Fgf3 and Fgf8 as basal components of the PPA induction pathway, with an additional Fgf being necessary in terrestrial vertebrates. It is still unclear why this additional Fgf is required in amniotes. The role of Fgf8 in this process has come under considerable scrutiny. In chick, Fgf8 acts from the endoderm, triggering the overlying mesoderm to express Fgf19, and thus induces the PPA [23]. In mouse, tissue specific ablations suggest that removing Fgf8 in either mesoderm or endoderm, in combination with a global loss of Fgf3, results in a loss of the PPA [24].

Segregation of the PPA

The inner ear and epibranchial placodes emerge from the PPA under the control of signals emanating from the hindbrain and the pharyngeal endoderm. The expression of a member of the Wnt family of secreted factors, Wnt8a, strongly suggests its role in imparting otic identity on the PPA [16, 25, 26]. This idea finds strong support from functional experiments. Firstly, it was found that Fgf signaling can only induce otic fate in tissue in combination with Wnt8a [16]. Secondly, over-expressing the activated down-stream components of the Wnt signaling pathway, in both the chick and the mouse causes an expansion of the otic territory at the expense of the epibranchial domain [8, 25]. Importantly, ectopic Wnt signaling can only expand the otic territory within the PPA. The converse experiment, where Wnt signals are repressed causes an expansion of the epibranchial domain and represses otic formation [8]. While Wnt signals are required for otic specification within the PPA, chick experiments suggest that continued Fgf signaling is inhibitory to otic specification [8]. FGF signaling must be attenuated for the PPA to be able to respond to Wnt signals. While the exact mechanism through which this happens is unclear, one hypothesis is that continued FGF signaling maintains the PPA cells in a otic refractory state, restricting the population to be large enough to then be acted on by Wnt signals to shift their fate. Thus, through the action of FGF and then Wnt, non-neural ectoderm is given an inner ear fate, establishing the correct environment in which hair cells can be generated.

Morphogenesis of the Otic Placode

While specification events alter the patterns of gene expression, more visible events in the ontogeny of the inner ear can also be observed. The otic placode is induced as a thickened patch of epithelium that is located superficially within the ectoderm, however, the inner ear is found embedded within the mesenchyme of the head. The mechanisms that transform the flat otic placode into essentially a spherical otocyst have recently begun to be elucidated. The initial indication of morphogenesis is a deformation of the epithelium such that it begins to sink into the ectoderm, forming a small pit [27, 28]. This process, termed invagination, can be thought of as a composite of several cell behaviors, which result from alterations in the cytoskeletal architecture of the otic placode [29]. The main components of the cytoskeleton are actin filaments, myosin motors and microtubules. Actin filaments (which are sometimes called F-actin) are polymers made up of actin monomers. These can slide against each other using myosin motors, in particular myosinII. This in effect causes constriction although in rare cases depolymerization can also occur. MyosinII is a heteromeric protein made up of 4 subunits, two units of myosin heavy chain (MHC) and two of myosin light chain (MLC). MLC phosphorylation leads to conformational changes in the protein complex, which allows myosinII to "walk" along an actin filament. Microtubules are rigid struts made up of monomers of tubulin. They provide tracks that aid in the reorganization of organelles and vesicular structures within the cell. All three structures are involved in the morphogenesis of the otic placode.

The initial step in otic invagination is basal expansion, and a hallmark of this step is the emergence of apically-polarized actin [29, 30]. Thus, to understand the control of basal expansion is to understand the generation of this polarity. This has been investigated and has been found to be controlled by FGF signaling, the very same signaling system that induces the PPA, the progenitor region of the otic placode. FGF signaling, acting on the basal face of the otic placode cells, causes the activation of the regulatory sub-unit of the motor protein myosin-II, the MLC. Phosphorylated MLC in turn exerts a non-canonical activity, causing the depletion of actin filaments from the basal side of the otic placode together with an enrichment of apical actin [30]. These two activities result in the expansion of the basal side of the cell, and also establish the necessary conditions for the next phase, apical constriction. The mechanisms of apical constriction are less clear. This step in invagination is characterized by the apical re-localization of phosphorylated MLC. By analogy with other systems, in particular the lens placode, it is likely that small GTPases such as RhoA, Rac1 or cdc42 participate in the constriction of actin filaments, resulting in a tightening of junctional actin that encircles the apices of each otic cell [31, 32]. Apical constriction drives the pit (formed by basal expansion) into a progressively deepening cup, which then pinches off from the surrounding non-neural ectoderm, to form a hollowed sphere, known as the otocyst [27, 28].

The formation of the otocyst is merely the first step in the elaboration of the final inner ear form. The mechanisms of this transformation are quite unclear, but again it is a composite of several different processes that act together to shape the inner ear. As we will show in the subsequent section, these processes are linked to the establishment of the axes of the inner ear that is necessary for its subsequent differentiation.

Patterning the Otocyst

The inner ear is patterned along all three axes – the dorsal-ventral, anterior-posterior and the medial-lateral axes. This is clearly seen in the placement of the vestibular apparatus, dorsally and the auditory portions ventrally, the generation of neurons from the anterior-ventral regions of the otocyst or the formation of the endolymphatic duct from the medial otocyst. Experiments in which the otocyst is rotated with respect to its surrounding tissues suggest that the patterning signals come from the latter [33-35]. These rotation experiments suggest that the first axis to be fixed is the anterior-posterior axis. In chick, and probably in mammals as well, recent data suggests that this axis is dependant on signals from the surrounding non-neural ectoderm [36]. If the otocyst is rotated in isolation from other tissues, the ear is relatively normal. However, if some adjacent ectoderm is also included, a higher proportion of the resulting inner ears have a reversed polarity. Enzymes that generate the powerful patterning molecule retinoic acid are found posterior to the otocyst in both mouse and chick. Furthermore, inhibition of retinoic acid after the otic placode has been induced leads to a loss of posterior otocyst characters and an expansion of the anterior [36]. In fish and frogs, the generation of the anterior-posterior axis is different, and instead relies on localized signals emanating from the hindbrain [37]. This is superficially not conserved in amniotes (birds, reptiles and mammals), where hindbrain signals are involved in patterning the dorsal-ventral axis [38].

The involvement of the hindbrain in dorsal-ventral patterning in amniotes has long been suspected [39]. Classical embryological studies suggest a role for the hindbrain in dorsal-ventral patterning of the otocyst [13]. More recently, the hindbrain has been shown to be necessary for a marker of the dorsal otocyst, Lmx1 [40]. Moreover, genetic perturbations of the hindbrain also provide further support for this idea. Kreisler mutants show perturbed hindbrain development and also show defects in dorsal derivatives of the otocyst [41, 42]. Tissue ablation or rotation experiments suggest that the ventral otocyst is also under active specification, in this case from the notochord and the ventral neural tube [35, 43]. This system is reminiscent of dorsal-ventral patterning of the neural tube [44]. In fact, the same molecule used in ventral patterning of the neural tube is used in ventral patterning of the otocyst. Sonic hedgehog (shh) is expressed in the notochord and the floor-plate of the neural tube. Analysis of mutant mice reveal that in the absence of shh signaling, the cochlea fails to develop, leading to the suggestion that the notochord and ventral neural tube are sources of shh that impart ventral identity on to the otocyst [45]. This idea is supported by the expression of downstream effectors of shh signaling; both the transcription factor that mediates its signaling (Gli transcription factors) and a downstream response element of shh signaling, the Patched receptor (ptc), are expressed in gradients, with highest expression observed ventrally and lower levels seen dorsally [46, 47]. However, a number of observations suggest that a ventral gradient is not sufficient to impart full patterning on the otocyst. The shh receptor, smoothened (smo), can be inactivated in localized domains and this renders that tissue "blind" to shh [48]. If smo is inactivated in the otocyst, the ventral components of the inner ear, the saccule and the cochlea, are absent, but the dorsal portion of the inner ear remains unaffected [48]. This suggests that other signals, located dorsally and acting as a counterpoint to the shh gradient, regulate dorsal otocyst development. Wnt and possibly Fgf family members provide these patterning cues. At least 4 Wnt family members are expressed dorsally, Wnt1, Wnt3a,

Wnt6 and Wnt8a [26, 49, 50], although knockout of just two of them, Wnt1 and Wnt3a results in a dramatic inner ear defect in mice [49]. Here, the dorsal derivatives of the inner ear, that is the endolymphatic duct, the semi-circular canals, the cristae and the utricle, are missing, and the cochlea is severely hypoplastic. In addition to Wnt signals, Fgf signaling, particularly that of Fgf3, also plays a role in dorsal otocyst determination, although it may serve to facilitate Wnt signal reception [51]. Finally, signaling from the bone morphogenetic protein (Bmp) family, Bmp4 in particular, has also been postulated to play a role in the dorsal patterning of the otocyst [52]. Vestibular development is sensitive to changes in the levels of BMP signals, as shown by treatment of the chick otocyst with noggin, an inhibitor of BMP signaling. Furthermore, in mice in which the otocyst is devoid of Bmp4, the sensory cristae and semi-circular canals fail to form. Whether Fgf3, Bmp4 and Wnt signals operate independently to specify different portions of the dorsal otocyst, or are in fact hierarchically organized so that the activity of one leads to the expression of the other, is not clear.

Shaping the Inner Ear

The translation of signaling activity into a morphogenetic mechanism that shapes the otocyst is not clear. Probably best understood is the formation of the vestibular apparatus. Here, one of the first events is a rapid expansion of the dorsolateral wall of the otocyst as a necessary first step in forming the vestibular chamber [52]. Recent studies have shown that otocyst cells in the dorsolateral region transform from a quite thick columnar epithelia, into a more squamous cell type. Inhibition and suppression of BMP signaling reveals that it is this signaling system that controls the change in cellular activity, however it is not clear what the underlying mechanism is [52]. Fgf signaling is involved in the elaboration of the vestibular chamber into what will become the semi-circular canal and the cristae [53]. One possible model is that the Fgf activity induces two pouches to grow out of the vestibular chamber, a horizontal pouch that will form the lateral semi-circular canal and the vertical pouch that will form both the anterior and posterior canals, joined by the common crus. Outgrowth of the pouch ultimately causes the faces of the more proximal parts to fuse, which triggers the resorption of this part of the pouch. The net effect is to leave behind the parts of the pouch where the faces are not apposed [46]. These are the more distal parts of the pouch, and after the resorption process, the remaining structure is a tube.

While this model is conceptually quite simple, there are regions of the pouches where in addition to physical constraints, molecular mechanisms operate that are necessary for apposition. In mice mutant for Fgf9 and Netrin1, there is a failure in apposition, and consequently a failure in resorption [54-56]. This in effect, prevents the formation of the common crus.

The cochlea depends very much on its final form to transduce tonal information about the auditory environment. In both birds and mice, the cochlear duct grows out from within the ventral half of the otocyst (in fact from a postero-lateral region). While in birds, the cochlea (more properly called the basilar papilla) has a slight curve, the curvature of the mammalian cochlea is extreme and it adopts a coiled configuration. The number of coils varies from species to species; mice have 1.75 whereas humans have 2.5 turns. Thus, we can consider at least two types of movement; outgrowth and, in mammals, coiling.

Analysis of a number of mutants that affect a process called planar cell polarity (PCP), suggests one mechanism that partially explains outgrowth. PCP provides cells in an epithelium (such as in the cochlear primordia) with a polarity. As we discuss later, PCP is especially important in orienting the stereocilia of inner ear hair cells, but the polarity information also provides important guidance for cellular rearrangements known as convergent extension [57]. Here, cells within an epithelial sheet reorganize, intercalating radially such that the sheet goes from being wide and short to narrow and long [57]. In the cochlear duct this occurs in the proximal-distal axis, and the information on how to intercalate is provided by the PCP pathway genes. In mutants of these genes, the cochlea is shorter [57-59]. Furthermore, while the organ of Corti normally has an invariant number of hair cell rows (1 row of inner hair cells and 3 rows of outer hair cells), in PCP mutants there are extra rows of hair cells. Yet more evidence for this mode of cochlear extension comes from organotypic cultures of the cochlea. Cochlear explants can be cultured on filter paper, and while this supports good cellular differentiation it prevents the radial intercalation of progenitor cells as they undergo convergent extension. Similar to the PCP mutants, extra rows of hair cells form, even though the hair bundles are well-oriented [57].

Thus far, PCP and convergent extension has only been described for the sensory portions of the cochlear duct, however there are more non-sensory than sensory cells in the cochlea and it is unclear if the non-sensory cells can undergo convergent extension in the same way. Thus, other mechanisms must exist that regulate the outgrowth of the cochlear duct. There have been several suggestions that the peri-otic mesenchyme provides a proliferative signal which may regulate cochlear outgrowth. Indeed, the ablation of Tbx1 in just the mesoderm surrounding the cochlear duct results in a dramatically shortened and poorly coiled cochlea [60], perhaps through the regulation of retinoic acid pathway genes[61].

Inner Ear Neurogenesis

The afferent innervation of the inner ear is produced by the inner ear itself, primarily within the anterior-ventral quadrant of the otocyst. The mechanisms that pattern the otocyst have been described above, however, it is clear that a separate mechanism overlays this with a field of competence to form otic-derived neurons. Like neurogenesis in the CNS, the starting point for PNS neurogenesis is with the expression of a member of the HMG-domain SoxB1 transcription factor, in this case Sox3. Sox3 is initially expressed in a swathe of cells [62]. Its expression is controlled by FGF signaling, but its induction seems to be separate from the induction of the PPA [63]. Indeed, otic specification is super-imposed onto Sox3 expression such that the otic placode now retains a portion of Sox3, which is destined to become neurogenic [63]. It is probable that the otocyst patterning cues trigger a neurogenic response in the Sox3 positive cells, initiating a molecular cascade of pro-neurogenic basic helix-loop-helix (bHLH) transcription factors including Neurod1 and neurogenin [1, 64].

In the course of specification, the neuronal precursors exit the inner ear epithelium. The mechanism of how this is achieved is not clear, but data from the closely related epibranchial placodes suggest a mechanism. This does not seem to be a typical epithelial-mesenchymal transition. Instead, neural progenitors change their behavior during the course of division. Usually cells in a thick epithelium (such as the inner ear), divide using a mode of division called interkinetic nuclear migration, where nuclei move to the apex of the epithelium, away from the basal lamina, divide and then the daughter cells move back [65]. During neuronal delamination from the inner ear, after they have divided, neural precursors cause local degradation of the basal lamina, which enables the cells to exit the epithelium. Once out, neuroblasts aggregate in knots of cells called the acoustico-vestibular ganglia (AVG: alternative names include the cochleovestibular ganglion or the stato-acoustic ganglion), and from there send out both peripheral and central axonal processes [66]. As this is not the primary focus of this chapter, the interested reader is directed to other excellent reviews on inner ear neurogenesis and innervation [64, 66, 67].

Specification of Mechanosensory Hair Cells

The formation of the sensory epithelia, and thus the mechanosensory hair cells which reside within them, can be viewed as a two-step process. The first step requires the generation of a pool of progenitors, residing within the sensory patch, that are primed to acquire sensory identity. As they become more committed, they exit the cell cycle to become prosensory cells. Then, in the second step, these populations of prosensory cells are further patterned to produce the distinct architecture of mechanosensory hair cells and non-sensory supporting cells that is present in all vertebrate inner ears. The aim of this section is to describe the morphological and molecular changes that occur during these two steps, and to introduce the main signaling pathways that underpin their regulation.

As we have described already, soon after it has vesiculated and separated from the surface ectoderm, the otic vesicle undergoes a series of rapid morphological changes that set up the morphology of the mature inner ear. Firstly, neuroblasts that will give rise to the AVG delaminate from the ventral side of the otocyst. Following on from this is a dorso-medial extension that will form the endolymphatic duct, and a ventral extension that will become the cochlear duct. Finally, as the inner ear matures, six individual regions become specified to form the sensory patches containing both mechanosensory hair cells and non-sensory supporting cells. These patches are responsible for the arbitration of the different aspects of hearing and balance. They include the organ of Corti in mammals and the basilar papilla in non-mammals that detect auditory stimuli, the utricular and saccular maculae that detect linear acceleration due to gravity, and the three cristae that detect angular acceleration in response to the flow of fluid in the three semi-circular canals.

Local cell-cell communication in combination with cellular responses to wider-ranging secreted signaling molecules appear critical in establishing first the prosensory domains, their boundaries, and then the ordered cellular patterning within them. Recent studies have revealed that members of the Notch, BMP, and FGF signaling families all exhibit regional expression at key stages of the development of the vertebrate inner ear. Genetic manipulation studies further suggest the importance of, and interactions between, these families during both prosensory specification and subsequent hair cell differentiation.

Although our knowledge of these processes is far from complete, key recurring themes emerge from the data currently available. Firstly, it is likely that each signaling family that patterns the inner ear does not work in isolation. Cross talk and interaction between families, whether in the form of transcriptional activation or repression, or protein-protein interaction, is widespread during the development of the embryo. And the inner ear is no different. Key genes, often termed "master regulators" of sensory epithelia development have been identified, but recent experiments suggest that even these can only confer sensory identity in a spatially and temporally dependent manner. Secondly, the same set of signaling families appear key to both steps of mechanosensory hair cell development – that is the acquisition of prosensory identity, and the patterning of prosensory patches into sensory hair cells and non-sensory supporting cells. The fact that these same molecules can fulfil vastly different roles highlights the importance of spatial and temporal context.

Changes in both the epigenetic and transcriptional states of cells during inner ear development are translated into different cellular interpretations of these signals. It is useful to keep these ideas at the forefront of your mind when considering the mechanisms that govern the progression towards hair cell differentiation.

Specification of the Sensory Patches

The specification of an initial pool of sensory progenitors represents the first step in the development of the sensory epithelia. The precise timing of sensory specification is unclear, however, the expression of two sensory markers, BMP4 and Jagged1, suggest that specification begins relatively early in the development of the inner ear [68-73]. In chick, it begins approximately three days post-fertilization, whereas in mice its onset is approximately ten days post-fertilization. Current models remain split on whether the prosensory patches are all derived from a single, posterior-ventral domain that rapidly subdivides, or if two separate domains, one anterior and one posterior, are specified separately. What is clear, however, is that these initial prosensory progenitors eventually resolve down to form the six distinct sensory epithelia of the inner ear.

Local Cell-Cell Communication: Notch Signals

Establishing defined groups of cells with a common identity is a key part of forming all six of the inner ear sensory epithelia. One way of achieving such populations is via a community-effect positive feedback loop, in which gene expression in one cell promotes expression of the same gene in its neighbours. The Notch signaling pathway has been identified as a regulator of such a positive feedback loop, termed lateral induction, in the inner ear. Notch communication only occurs between neighbouring cells, as both the receptors and ligands are transmembrane proteins. Signaling, thus, depends on direct cell-cell contact. Feedback is a critical feature of the Notch signaling mechanism. The strength of the signal a cell receives affects the strength of the signal it then produces, and this facilitates the generation of highly-controlled spatial and temporal patterns of gene expression. This, in turn, is translated into differences in cell morphology.

In mammals, the Notch signaling pathway consists of four receptors (Notch 1-4) and five ligands (Delta-like [DLL] 1, 3, and 4, and Jagged1 and 2) [71-73]. At the time of prosensory specification, the Notch1 receptor is expressed almost ubiquitously throughout the avian and mammalian otocyst [74]. Jagged1 is the earliest expressed Notch ligand in the mammalian inner ear and its expression marks the prosensory patches [71, 75]. In humans, Alagille syndrome is an autosomal-dominant disorder caused by mutations in Jagged 1, the symptoms of which include deafness, suggesting an important role for the Jagged1-Notch interaction in sensory patch development. Indeed, experiments in a number of model systems have confirmed the idea that Notch1-Jagged1 binding plays a role in specifying the sensory patches, via lateral induction, within the inner ear [76]. Genetic manipulation of Notch signaling results in increases to both size and number of sensory patches, and conversely loss or reduction of sensory patch size, depending on the manipulation performed. Kiernan and co-workers used the Jagged1 mouse mutant headturner (*htu*) to show that a loss of Jagged1 results in the formation of sensory patches that are severely reduced in size [71]. Conversely, *Cre-/loxP* conditional activation of the Notch pathway results in the expansion of sensory patch size. Perhaps most tellingly, conditional activation of Notch in non-sensory regions of the early otocyst results in an upregulation of Jagged1 that begins within the Notch-activated cell and then spreads to its immediate neighbours, laterally inducing prosensory character on cells several cell-diameters from the original source [77].

The importance of lateral induction to prosensory specification is not limited to mammals. Daudet and co-workers used Notch inhibitors to show that a loss of notch activation causes loss of Jagged 1 expression (serrate) and impairs the development of the avian sensory epithelia [78]. Interestingly, they noted that the initial expression of Jagged 1 in the prosensory domains was not hindered by notch inhibition, whereas its subsequent maintenance was. This raises a question as to whether Notch activation truly does specify prosensory identity in the inner ear, or simply acts to maintain it once it has been acquired. Nevertheless, both mammalian and avian studies confirm that lateral induction is a key regulator of prosensory identity during the early stages of inner ear morphogenesis.

Sox2

Jagged1 likely regulates prosensory specification via regulation of Sox2 expression. Sox2, a high-mobility-group transcription factor, is initially expressed broadly in prosensory and proneural regions of the otocyst, but is refined to overlap with the expression of Jagged1. As we will discuss later, Sox2 is at the top of a transcriptional hierarchy that leads to the differentiation of hair cells. Indeed, Kiernan and co-workers have demonstrated that mutations in an otocyst-specific promoter of Sox2 in mice leads to a failure of prosensory domain formation and a complete absence of hair cells and support cells [79]. The expression of Sox2 is reduced in Jagged1-deficient cochleae and is upregulated in response to ectopic expression of the constitutively-active Notch intracellular domain [77, 80]. Together these experiments suggest that Jagged1 activation of Notch acts to induce prosensory identity through the maintenance of Sox2 [81].

The Role of BMPs in Prosensory Domain Specification

As introduced earlier, secreted signaling molecules that can exert an influence over long cellular distances are also key to the production of the mature sensory epithelia. BMPs are one such family of molecules, and the expression of a number of BMPs in the otic vesicles of fish, birds and mammals identify BMP signaling as a candidate regulator of sensory patch specification in the inner ear. Of particular focus has been BMP4 expression, which in the chick is initially observed in an anterior-ventral stripe and a posterior-ventral spot. From here it is localized to each of the developing sensory epithelia [70]. A similar early expression pattern is observed in the mouse, with BMP4 eventually located in the sensory epithelia of the three cristae, and in a region adjacent to the developing sensory domain in the cochlea at later stages [82]. Early experiments focused upon a morphological analysis of the inner ear in response to large changes in BMP concentration. The use of blanket inhibitors and activators of BMP signaling have helped to show that both positive and negative changes in BMP signal intensity cause widespread disruption of sensory patch formation in the chick [83, 84].

Analysis of BMP mouse mutants has further added weight to the importance of BMP signalling to prosensory specification. In the organ of Corti, only a subset of the rather large Sox2 positive sensory patch is destined to form hair cells. This region is not only characterized by the expression of particular genes, but also by the cessation of cell division, as the sensory progenitors drop out of mitosis [85]. The knockout of two BMP receptors in mammalian inner ear results in a loss of cochlear structures at E12.5, a time at which the prosensory domain is established. Importantly, the expression of Sox2 is not affected [86]. An opposing experiment, in which the expression of a BMP antagonist, Noggin, is repressed reveals large increases in hair cell numbers [87]. This suggests an increase in prosensory patch size. A particularly elegant piece of work from Ohyama and co-workers recently highlighted the importance of precise morphogen concentrations for correct prosensory specification. Here, experiments on E11.5 cochlear explants reveal that the size of the prosensory domain depends on the concentration of the BMP signal. Thus, while low and high concentrations of the BMP signal reduce the size of the prosensory domain, intermediate concentrations expand it [86]. The mechanisms that regulate BMP signal intensity are unknown, however, its expression in the inner ear is often accompanied by that of its antagonist, noggin, which may facilitate fine control of local BMP concentration levels within the prosensory domains. Thus, the conceptual model now is that BMP signaling works to refine the sensory patch established by Notch-mediated lateral induction, and is required for prosensory specification. As BMP4 is expressed abneurally adjacent to the developing auditory prosensory domain, it seems intuitive that BMP4 signaling activity acts as a morphogen in the organ of Corti, helping to sub-divide the Sox2-positive sensory patch into more committed, post-mitotic, precursors. Importantly, in the cochlea, the generation of this post-mitotic domain occurs first in the apical region at E12.5 and spreads basally by E14.5 [88]. This runs counter to the actual wave of differentiation, where the first hair cells to be generated form basally at E14.5 and extend apically by E17.5 [89].

Cell Differentiation within the Sensory Patch: Becoming a Hair Cell

Once a prosensory domain is specified, individual cells within the domain must make a choice to develop as either a mechanosensory hair cell or a non-sensory supporting cell. Contrary to its role in prosensory specification, Notch-mediated hair cell differentiation is governed by a negative feedback system termed lateral inhibition. Its hallmark is the negative regulation of Notch-ligand expression by Notch activity. This creates a feedback loop that is translated into fine-grained mixtures of cells expressing either high or low levels of the Notch ligand. Early studies identify two Notch ligands, Delta1 (Delta-like1 in mammals) and

Jagged2, as regulators of the choice between hair cell and supporting cell fates within the sensory patches [71-73].

Beyond forcing a differential transcriptional output amongst neighbouring cells, the precise downstream effectors through which Notch-mediated lateral inhibition controls hair cell differentiation are not clear. One potential mechanism is by regulating the expression of the basic helix-loop-helix transcription factor Atoh1. Atoh1 expression is a common feature of all hair cells, and represents the earliest definitive marker of hair cell fate [90]. Overexpression and gene transfer experiments have shown that Atoh1 is necessary and sufficient to induce hair cell fate [91, 92]. *In vivo* gene transfer of Atoh1 into otocyst cells of the embryonic mouse elegantly reveal that its expression is enough to produce functional hair cells with mechanosensitive properties comparable with endogenous hair cells [92]. Thus, Atoh1 is regarded as a master gene of hair cell differentiation. Atoh1 expression is upregulated in presumptive hair cells of both the mammalian and avian inner ear at the same time as the lateral inhibition-inducing ligands, Delta1 and Jagged2, and the downstream components of the Notch signaling pathway are upregulated [93, 94].

Sox2 expression, although essential for prosensory specification, must be subsequently downregulated in cells that become hair cells, similar to the dual but contrasting roles played by Notch signaling. Dabdoub and colleagues have shown that forced expression of Sox2 acts to inhibit prosensory cells from differentiating into hair cells [95]. Together with the observation that ectopic expression of Sox2 in non-sensory regions promotes prosensory identity but not Atoh1 expression, has led to the hypothesis that Sox2 and Atoh1 antagonise each other [95]. Evidence for this has been presented in overexpression experiments that have shown that Sox2 is sufficient to directly antagonise Atoh1-driven hair cell fate, as can the Sox2 target gene, Prox1. Given the additional evidence that Notch activation is crucial to the maintenance of Sox2 expression earlier in ear development, all this points towards a model of mutual antagonism between Atoh1 and Sox2. Thus, Atoh1 and Sox2 counteract each other within the prosensory patches during the generation of hair cells, with lateral inhibition regulating the local levels of Sox2 expression [80].

The role of Sox2 has recently become more controversial, however. A study into the upstream regulators of Atoh1 expression suggests that Sox2, in conjunction with two other transcription factors, Eya1 and Six1, cooperatively interacts to activate Atoh1. A series of biochemical binding assays suggest that Sox2, Eya1, and Six1 directly interact to form a multiprotein complex which efficiently upregulates the expression of Atoh1 [96]. Perhaps the most striking finding is that Eya1 and Six1 are able to induce hair cell formation independent of Atoh1 function. The notion of this "Atoh1 independent" pathway is new, and it remains unclear whether it operates in normal hair cell differentiation [96]. Hints that it may occur *in vivo* are seen in the cochleae of conditional Pax2-Cre/Atoh1 mutants. In these mutants, Atoh1 is presumably deleted very early, but some hair cell-specific markers are still expressed [97].

FGFs have also been implicated in the formation of hair cells within the cochlea. Again, genetic abrogation experiments have offered clues as to its precise role. Mice with a conditional, otocyst-specific deletion of the FGF receptor, FGFR1, are characterised by mispatterned sensory patches that lack outer hair cells and infrequently, inner hair cells. Importantly, prosensory markers are still present in these mutants, but Atoh1 is downregulated, implying that signaling through FGFR1 acts downstream of prosensory specification yet upstream of Atoh1 induction (RKL, unpublished observations).

FGFs represent a particularly interesting class of molecules in the context of cell fate decisions in the prosensory patches, as they appear crucial for the specification of both hair cells and support cells. The hair cell is considered the default cell type in the sensory epithelia, and it acts through lateral inhibition to prevent its neighbours from following its lead, thus forcing them into a supporting cell fate. FGF signaling, via FGFR3, is a key player in this process, specifically in the specification of inner pillar cells, a unique cell type found adjacent to inner hair cells in the mammalian cochlea. Pillar cell progenitors express FGFR3 prior to morphological differentiation. Deletion of FGFR3 results in the loss of pillar cells in exchange for additional outer hair cells [98-101].

The formation of additional outer hair cells in FGFR3 mutant mice can be rescued via inhibition of BMP4 [101]. This suggests that reciprocal interactions between FGF and BMP signaling define the number of cells that develop as either inner or outer hair cells. This observation highlights one of the most striking aspects of the mammalian cochlear sensory epithelium – its lateral cellular asymmetry. A single row of inner hair cells and two rows of pillar cells are located medially, while three rows of outer hair cells are located more laterally. Fgf10 and Bmp4 are expressed on opposing flanks of the developing cochlear duct [38], which suggests that morphogen gradients emanating from each flank are key contributors to specifying the different types of hair cells. However, data from the Fgf20 mouse mutant argue against this. The phenotype of this knockout mouse shows aberrant differentiation of the outer hair cells, while the inner hair cells are relatively normal [102, 103]. Fgf20 signals through Fgfr1, and it is entirely possible that the Fgfr1 action is downstream of Bmp signaling to specify the abneural compartment, while Fgf8 and Fgf10 signaling through Fgfr3, signal the neural compartment of the mouse organ of Corti.

From Progenitor to a Mechanosensory Hair Cell

Mechanosensation depends on the hair bundles of the inner ear hair cells. Each bundle comprises of a single true cilium, referred to as the kinocilium, and between 50 and 200 modified microvilli, referred to as stereocilia [104]. The processes described above thus far have steered a non-neural ectodermal cell to a point at which it is poised to perform a function. In this section, we review what is known about the mechanisms that underlie the formation of the hair bundle of an inner ear hair cell as it transforms from an epithelial progenitor into a cell that is capable of transducing mechanical stimuli.

The formation of the hair bundle has been described in some depth [105, 106]. One important point to stress is that the hair cell progenitor, like most other epithelial cells, has a cilium and microvilli on its apical surface. In this respect, the formation of the hair bundle can be viewed as a modification and elaboration of pre-existing sub-cellular structures, and that the earliest developmental cues put in place the machinery that allows this modification. In the mouse, the onset of hair bundle morphogenesis is between E12.5 and E17.5, with vestibular hair cells beginning their differentiation before the cochlear hair cells. In the cochlea, differentiation is presaged by the expression of Atoh1 and occurs from a basal to apical gradient, running counter to the apical to basal gradient of cell cycle exit of hair cell progenitors described above.

The first evidence of specialization is the lengthening of the non-motile cilia, located at the center of the apical surface of the developing hair cell [107, 108]. This can be readily visualized as antibody staining shows an accumulation of tubulin, the component of the microtubule protofilaments found in the cilium, when compared with the primary cilia of the support cells. The kinocilium subsequently moves to the cell periphery. The PCP pathway (described below) coordinates this displacement of the kinocilia and ensures that all hair cells are in register and face the same direction. The displacement of the kinocilium causes the microvilli immediately adjacent to it to begin to elongate, which subsequently become thestereocilia, and induce the elongation of adjacent rows of micovilli to make a staircase configuration [108]. As they grow, the stereocilia also increase in width by adding actin filaments, although the filaments in the central core extend basally to form rootlets. Subsequently, the basal ends of the stereocilia, where they are inserted into the apical membrane adopt a tapered shape.

The Role of the Kinocilium in Hair Bundle Development

As the first sub-cellular structure that shows a hair-cell specific specialization, the kinocilium is likely to play the lead role in organizing the development of the hair bundle. However, a number of features distinguish it from other primary cilia. As already mentioned, the kinocilium is longer than most primary cilia. In addition, vertebrate kinocilia have a slightly unusual axoneme structure, the internal microtubule skeleton of the cilia. Non-motile primary cilia are made up of an array of 9 pairs of protofilament doublets arranged peripherally surrounding an empty core, in contrast withmotile cilia, where the 9 doublets surround a 2 non-doublet of protofilaments [109]. However, transmission electron microscopy data suggest that the vertebrate kinocilium has a typical non-motile ciliary axoneme (9X2+0) close to its base, but further away from the cell one of the doublets drifts towards the core and the kinocilium is left with 8 doublets arranged around a central doublet (8X2+1X2) [110]. The mechanisms that control the transition of both length and axoneme structure are not clear.

The hair bundles also show a polarity within the epithelium, such that the hair bundles all face the same direction. Mutations in genes that are involved in cilia development implicate the kinocilia itself in the generation of a consistently polarized hair bundle. In particular, a study using conditional KO mice for the intraflagellar transport protein (IFT) 88, an essential component of the IFT complex required for ciliogenesis, shows that in the absence of the kinocilia, hair cells are mis-oriented or completely lose their innate polarity [58, 111]. Similarly, mutants of the Bardet-Biedl syndrome protein or the IFT motor, Kif3a, also have mis-oriented hair bundles [58, 112, 113] although the localization of PCP components (see below) is unchanged.

Polarization of the hair bundle is mediated through the PCP pathway. This was first identified in the fruit fly, where it plays a role in orienting the photoreceptors of the fly eye, and organizing bristle pattern. The common feature of these tissues is that polarity must be encoded across the plane of the epithelium. Several recent studies have examined the roles of vertebrate homologs of Drosophila planar cell polarization (PCP) genes, Celsr1, Dishevelled (Dvl), Frizzled (Fzd) scribble (Scrb1) and Vangl2, in the regulation of hair bundle orientation [59, 114-122]. For example, Montcouquiol and collegues [115] demonstrated significant defects in hair bundle orientation in the ears of mice that carry a mutation in Vangl2, although the normal stepped pattern of the stereocilia remains unaffected. The first sign of bundle orientation is the centrifugal movement of the developing kinocilium from the center of the cell towards the periphery. Normally this movement is coordinated such that all the hair bundles are oriented in one direction, however in Vangl2 mutants, while the centrifugal movement still occurs, its direction is randomized. Other mutants in the PCP pathway show similar results. Importantly, only the hair bundles of the inner ear hair cells show polarity problems, while the primary cilia found on the supporting cells are not subject to PCP instructions.

Development of the Stereocilia

After the establishment of planar polarity, hair cell stereocilia elongate to form rows of graded height. Similar to filopodia and microvilli, stereocilia are supported by bundles of uniformly polarized actin filaments with the barbed (plus) ends pointing toward the stereociliary tips [108]. The filaments contain β- and γ-actin and are cross-linked by espin, plastin1, and T-plastin [123-127]. However, unlike filopodia and microvilli, stereocilia are maintained at a constant length throughout life. While β-actin, γ-actin, and espin are expressed in a number of tissues, mutations in their genes predominantly affect hair bundles [125, 128-130]. One feature of stereocilia that distinguish them from microvilli is their dense core of actin filaments. This is relatively uniform along the length of the stereocilia, except at the base, where they taper just prior to insertion into the lumenal surface of the hair cell [131, 132]. The cuticular plate forms underneath the existing stereocilia to stabilize the staircase pattern further. The thick actin core, along with the taper, results in a relatively stiff structure with a hinge point at its base. The actin-filled stereocilia deflect in response to sound by pivoting around rootlets at their insertion points at the hair cell surface. Kitajiri et al. show that the actin-binding protein TRIOBP tightly bundles the actin filaments into rootlets, endowing these stereocilia "pivots" with unique elasticity and robustness [133].

Recent studies indicate that myosin motor proteins transport components of the actin assembly machinery to the tips of stereocilia to regulate their length. Myosin 15a (Myo15a) is thought to regulate stereociliary growth by cooperating with the adaptor protein whirlin. This interaction is suggested by genetic studies, where Myo15a and whirlin mutations lead to shortened stereocilia in mice and hearing loss in humans [134-136]. Myo15a binds whirlin and both show stereocilia tip localization [137-140]. However, whirlin does not localize to the stereocilia tips in Myo15a mutant mice suggesting that the latter transports whirlin and perhaps other hair bundle components to stereociliary tips [138]. Furthermore, whirlin binds the MAGUK protein p55, and protein 4.1R, which are expressed in outer hair cells; and a 4.1R homologue, 4.1B, that is expressed in inner hair cells [141]. Some of these proteins have been shown to regulate actin assembly in erythrocytes and neurons and it is thus tempting to speculate that they may have a similar role in stereocilia of hair cells [142, 143].

Making Links

The morphology and function of the hair bundle depends on the fine filamentous links between the kinocilia and stereocilia and between adjacent stereocilia, termed kinociliary-links and stereociliary links, respectively. For the purpose of this chapter we will focus on the kinociliary links, as they have recently been found to play an important role in the generation of the hair bundle polarity. Kinociliary links form bridges between the kinocilia and the tallest stereocilia, which are adjacent to it. They comprise of adhesion complexes made up of a homodimer of protocadherin15 (Pcdh15) on the kinocilia attached to a homodimer of cadherin 23 (Cdh23) on the stereocilia. Tip-links, one of the stereociliary link types, also comprise the same adhesion complex. However, Cdh23 is on the flank of the taller stereocilia, while pcdh15 is seen at the tip of the neighboring shorter stereocilia [144]. The tip-links have been postulated to gate the presumptive mechanotransduction channel [145].

In mice with mutations in an isoform of Pcdh15 that is specific to the kinocilia, the polarity of the hair bundle and the coupling of the kinocilia to the stereocilia are affected. Moreover, these mutants are profoundly deaf [146]. Pcdh15 is on the kinocilia, and not in other primary cilia, and thus one can speculate that some specific machinery exists within the hair cell, that transports Pcdh15 into kinocilia. From here, the kinocilia can direct both polarization and morphology of the stereocilia. The nature of this machinery is still unclear, but it appears likely that one role for the developmental cues is to establish the conditions and cellular context necessary for the function of this hair cell- specific machinary, which provides the final cues to produce a functional mechanosensory hair cell.

References

[1] Ladher, R.K., P. O'Neill, and J. Begbie, From shared lineage to distinct functions: the development of the inner ear and epibranchial placodes. *Development,* 2010. 137(11): p. 1777-85.

[2] Patthey, C. and L. Gunhaga, Specification and regionalisation of the neural plate border. *Eur. J. Neurosci.*, 2011. 34(10): p. 1516-28.

[3] Baker, C.V. and M. Bronner-Fraser, Vertebrate cranial placodes I. Embryonic induction. Dev. Biol., 2001. 232(1): p. 1-61.

[4] Schlosser, G., Induction and specification of cranial placodes. *Dev. Biol.*, 2006. 294: p. 303-51.

[5] Sun, S.K., et al., Epibranchial and otic placodes are induced by a common Fgf signal, but their subsequent development is independent. *Dev. Biol.*, 2007. 303(2): p. 675-86.

[6] Nikaido, M., et al., Initial specification of the epibranchial placode in zebrafish embryos depends on the fibroblast growth factor signal. *Dev. Dyn.*, 2007. 236(2): p. 564-71.

[7] Nechiporuk, A., et al., Specification of epibranchial placodes in zebrafish. *Development,* 2007. 134(3): p. 611-23.

[8] Freter, S., et al., Progressive restriction of otic fate: the role of FGF and Wnt in resolving inner ear potential. *Development*, 2008. 135(20): p. 3415-24.

[9] Streit, A., Extensive cell movements accompany formation of the otic placode. *Dev. Biol.*, 2002. 249(2): p. 237-54.

[10] Ohyama, T. and A.K. Groves, Generation of Pax2-Cre mice by modification of a Pax2 bacterial artificial chromosome. *Genesis*, 2004. 38: p. 195-9.

[11] Groves, A.K. and M. Bronner-Fraser, Competence, specification and commitment in otic placode induction. *Development*, 2000. 127(16): p. 3489-99.

[12] Wright, T.J. and S.L. Mansour, Fgf3 and Fgf10 are required for mouse otic placode induction. *Development,* 2003. 130(15): p. 3379-90.

[13] Groves, A.K., The induction of the otic placode, in Development of the Inner Ear, M.W. Kelley, et al., Editors. 2005, Springer: new York. p. 10-42.

[14] Kil, S.H., et al., Distinct roles for hindbrain and paraxial mesoderm in the induction and patterning of the inner ear revealed by a study of vitamin-A-deficient quail. *Dev. Biol.*, 2005. 285(1): p. 252-71.

[15] Mendonsa, E.S. and B.B. Riley, Genetic analysis of tissue interactions required for otic placode induction in the zebrafish. *Dev. Biol.*, 1999. 206(1): p. 100-12.

[16] Ladher, R.K., et al., Identification of synergistic signals initiating inner ear development. *Science,* 2000. 290: p. 1965-7.

[17] Schimmang, T., Expression and functions of FGF ligands during early otic development. *Int. J. Dev. Biol.*, 2007. 51(6-7): p. 473-81.

[18] Phillips, B.T., K. Bolding, and B.B. Riley, Zebrafish fgf3 and fgf8 encode redundant functions required for otic placode induction. *Dev. Biol.*, 2001. 235(2): p. 351-65.

[19] Maroon, H., et al., Fgf3 and Fgf8 are required together for formation of the otic placode and vesicle. *Development,* 2002. 129(9): p. 2099-108.

[20] Leger, S. and M. Brand, Fgf8 and Fgf3 are required for zebrafish ear placode induction, maintenance and inner ear patterning. *Mech. Dev.,* 2002. 119(1): p. 91-108.

[21] Liu, D., et al., Fgf3 and Fgf8 dependent and independent transcription factors are required for otic placode specification. *Development,* 2003. 130(10): p. 2213-24.

[22] Wright, T.J., et al., Expression of mouse fibroblast growth factor and fibroblast growth factor receptor genes during early inner ear development. *Dev. Dyn.*, 2003. 228: p. 267-72.

[23] Ladher, R., et al., FGF8 initiates inner ear induction in chick and mouse. *Genes Dev.*, 2005. 19.

[24] Zelarayan, L.C., et al., Differential requirements for FGF3, FGF8 and FGF10 during inner ear development. *Dev. Biol.*, 2007. 308(2): p. 379-91.

[25] Ohyama, T., et al., Wnt signals mediate a fate decision between otic placode and epidermis. *Development,* 2006. 133: p. 865-75.

[26] Urness, L.D., et al., FGF signaling regulates otic placode induction and refinement by controlling both ectodermal target genes and hindbrain Wnt8a. *Dev. Biol.*, 2010. 340(2): p. 595-604.

[27] Meier, S., Development of the embryonic chick otic placode. II. Electron microscopic analysis. *Anat. Rec.,* 1978. 191(4): p. 459-77.

[28] Meier, S., Development of the embryonic chick otic placode. I. Light microscopic analysis. *Anat. Rec.*, 1978. 191(4): p. 447-58.

[29] Alvarez, I.S. and J. Navascués, Shaping, invagination, and closure of the chick embryo otic vesicle: scanning electron microscopic and quantitative study. *Anat. Rec.*, 1990. 228: p. 315-26.

[30] Sai, X. and R.K. Ladher, FGF signaling regulates cytoskeletal remodeling during epithelial morphogenesis. *Curr. Biol.*, 2008. 18(13): p. 976-81.

[31] Chauhan, B.K., et al., Balanced Rac1 and RhoA activities regulate cell shape and drive invagination morphogenesis in epithelia. *Proc. Natl. Acad. Sci. USA*, 2011. 108(45): p. 18289-94.
[32] Plageman, T.F., Jr., et al., A Trio-RhoA-Shroom3 pathway is required for apical constriction and epithelial invagination. *Development*, 2011. 138(23): p. 5177-88.
[33] Harrison, R.G., Relations of symmetry in the developing ear of Amblystoma punctatum. *Proc. Natl. Acad. Sci. USA*, 1936. 22: p. 238-247.
[34] Wu, D.K., F.D. Nunes, and D. Choo, Axial specification for sensory organs versus non-sensory structures of the chicken inner ear. *Development,* 1998. 125(1): p. 11-20.
[35] Bok, J., M. Bronner-Fraser, and D.K. Wu, Role of the hindbrain in dorsoventral but not anteroposterior axial specification of the inner ear. *Development*, 2005. 132: p. 2115-24.
[36] Bok, J., et al., Transient retinoic acid signaling confers anterior-posterior polarity to the inner ear. *Proc. Natl. Acad. Sci. USA*, 2011. 108(1): p. 161-6.
[37] Whitfield, T.T., et al., Development of the zebrafish inner ear. *Dev. Dyn.*, 2002. 223(4): p. 427-58.
[38] Groves, A.K. and D.M. Fekete, Shaping sound in space: the regulation of inner ear patterning. *Development*, 2012. 139(2): p. 245-57.
[39] Fekete, D.M., Cell fate specification in the inner ear. *Curr Opin Neurobiol*, 1996. 6(4): p. 533-41.
[40] Giraldez, F., Regionalized organizing activity of the neural tube revealed by the regulation of lmx1 in the otic vesicle. *Dev. Biol.,* 1998. 203(1): p. 189-200.
[41] McKay, I.J., J. Lewis, and A. Lumsden, The role of FGF-3 in early inner ear development: an analysis in normal and kreisler mutant mice. *Dev. Biol.,* 1996. 174(2): p. 370-8.
[42] Choo, D., et al., Molecular mechanisms underlying inner ear patterning defects in kreisler mutants. *Dev. Biol.*, 2006. 289(2): p. 308-17.
[43] Liang, J.K., J. Bok, and D.K. Wu, Distinct contributions from the hindbrain and mesenchyme to inner ear morphogenesis. *Dev. Biol.*, 2010. 337(2): p. 324-34.
[44] Ulloa, F. and E. Marti, Wnt won the war: antagonistic role of Wnt over Shh controls dorso-ventral patterning of the vertebrate neural tube. *Dev. Dyn.*, 2010. 239(1): p. 69-76.
[45] Riccomagno, M.M., et al., Specification of the mammalian cochlea is dependent on Sonic hedgehog. *Genes Dev*, 2002. 16: p. 2365-78.
[46] Bok, J., W. Chang, and D.K. Wu, Patterning and morphogenesis of the vertebrate inner ear. *Int. J. Dev. Biol.*, 2007. 51(6-7): p. 521-33.
[47] Bok, J., et al., Opposing gradients of Gli repressor and activators mediate Shh signaling along the dorsoventral axis of the inner ear. *Development*, 2007. 134(9): p. 1713-22.
[48] Brown, A.S. and D.J. Epstein, Otic ablation of smoothened reveals direct and indirect requirements for Hedgehog signaling in inner ear development. *Development,* 2011. 138(18): p. 3967-76.
[49] Riccomagno, M.M., S. Takada, and D.J. Epstein, Wnt-dependent regulation of inner ear morphogenesis is balanced by the opposing and supporting roles of Shh. *Genes Dev.*, 2005. 19: p. 1612-23.
[50] Jayasena, C.S., et al., Notch signaling augments the canonical Wnt pathway to specify the size of the otic placode. *Development*, 2008.

[51] Hatch, E.P., et al., Fgf3 is required for dorsal patterning and morphogenesis of the inner ear epithelium. *Development*, 2007. 134(20): p. 3615-25.
[52] Ohta, S., S.L. Mansour, and G.C. Schoenwolf, BMP/SMAD signaling regulates the cell behaviors that drive the initial dorsal-specific regional morphogenesis of the otocyst. *Dev. Biol.*, 2010. 347(2): p. 369-81.
[53] Chang, W., et al., The development of semicircular canals in the inner ear: role of FGFs in sensory cristae. *Development*, 2004. 131(17): p. 4201-11.
[54] Pirvola, U., et al., Fgf9 signaling regulates inner ear morphogenesis through epithelial-mesenchymal interactions. *Dev. Biol.*, 2004. 273(2): p. 350-60.
[55] Salminen, M., et al., Netrin 1 is required for semicircular canal formation in the mouse inner ear. *Development*, 2000. 127(1): p. 13-22.
[56] Abraira, V.E., et al., Cross-repressive interactions between Lrig3 and netrin 1 shape the architecture of the inner ear. *Development*, 2008. 135(24): p. 4091-9.
[57] McKenzie, E., A. Krupin, and M.W. Kelley, Cellular growth and rearrangement during the development of the mammalian organ of Corti. *Dev. Dyn.*, 2004. 229(4): p. 802-12.
[58] Jones, C. and P. Chen, Primary cilia in planar cell polarity regulation of the inner ear. *Curr. Top Dev. Biol.*, 2008. 85: p. 197-224.
[59] Wang, J., et al., Regulation of polarized extension and planar cell polarity in the cochlea by the vertebrate PCP pathway. *Nat. Genet.*, 2005. 37(9): p. 980-5.
[60] Xu, H., L. Chen, and A. Baldini, In vivo genetic ablation of the periotic mesoderm affects cell proliferation survival and differentiation in the cochlea. *Dev. Biol.*, 2007. 310(2): p. 329-40.
[61] Braunstein, E.M., et al., Tbx1 and Brn4 regulate retinoic acid metabolic genes during cochlear morphogenesis. *BMC Dev. Biol.*, 2009. 9: p. 31.
[62] Tripathi, V.B., et al., The surface ectoderm of the chick embryo exhibits dynamic variation in its response to neurogenic signals. *Int. J. Dev. Biol.*, 2009. 53: p. 1023-33.
[63] Abello, G., et al., Independent regulation of Sox3 and Lmx1b by FGF and BMP signaling influences the neurogenic and non-neurogenic domains in the chick otic placode. *Dev. Biol.*, 2010.
[64] Sanchez-Calderon, H., et al., A network of growth and transcription factors controls neuronal differentation and survival in the developing ear. *Int. J. Dev. Biol.*, 2007. 51(6-7): p. 557-70.
[65] Graham, A., et al., Delamination of cells from neurogenic placodes does not involve an epithelial-to-mesenchymal transition. *Development,* 2007. 134(23): p. 4141-5.
[66] Appler, J.M. and L.V. Goodrich, Connecting the ear to the brain: Molecular mechanisms of auditory circuit assembly. *Prog. Neurobiol.*, 2011. 93(4): p. 488-508.
[67] Yang, T., et al., The molecular basis of making spiral ganglion neurons and connecting them to hair cells of the organ of Corti. *Hear Res.*, 2011. 278(1-2): p. 21-33.
[68] Cole, L.K., et al., Sensory organ generation in the chicken inner ear: contributions of bone morphogenetic protein 4, serrate1, and lunatic fringe. *J. Comp. Neurol.*, 2000. 424: p. 509-20.
[69] Wu, D.K. and S.H. Oh, Sensory organ generation in the chick inner ear. *J. Neurosci.*, 1996. 16(20): p. 6454-62.
[70] Oh, S.H., R. Johnson, and D.K. Wu, Differential expression of bone morphogenetic proteins in the developing vestibular and auditory sensory organs. *J. Neurosci.*, 1996. 16(20): p. 6463-75.

[71] Kiernan, A.E., et al., The Notch ligand Jagged1 is required for inner ear sensory development. *Proc. Natl. Acad. Sci. USA*, 2001. 98: p. 3873-8.
[72] Morrison, A., et al., Expression of Delta1 and Serrate1 (Jagged1) in the mouse inner ear. *Mech. Dev.*, 1999. 84: p. 169-72.
[73] Adam, J., et al., Cell fate choices and the expression of Notch, Delta and Serrate homologues in the chick inner ear: parallels with Drosophila sense-organ development. *Development*, 1998. 125: p. 4645-54.
[74] Eddison, M., I. Le Roux, and J. Lewis, Notch signaling in the development of the inner ear: lessons from Drosophila. *Proc. Natl. Acad. Sci. USA*, 2000. 97(22): p. 11692-9.
[75] Kiernan, A.E., J. Xu, and T. Gridley, The Notch ligand JAG1 is required for sensory progenitor development in the mammalian inner ear. *PLoS Genet*, 2006. 2: p. e4.
[76] Brooker, R., K. Hozumi, and J. Lewis, Notch ligands with contrasting functions: Jagged1 and Delta1 in the mouse inner ear. *Development,* 2006. 133: p. 1277-86.
[77] Hartman, B.H., T.A. Reh, and O. Bermingham-McDonogh, Notch signaling specifies prosensory domains via lateral induction in the developing mammalian inner ear. *Proc. Natl. Acad. Sci. USA*, 2010. 107(36): p. 15792-7.
[78] Daudet, N. and J. Lewis, Two contrasting roles for Notch activity in chick inner ear development: specification of prosensory patches and lateral inhibition of hair-cell differentiation. *Development*, 2005. 132(3): p. 541-51.
[79] Kiernan, A.E., et al., Sox2 is required for sensory organ development in the mammalian inner ear. *Nature*, 2005. 434(7036): p. 1031-5.
[80] Liu, Z., et al., In vivo Notch reactivation in differentiating cochlear hair cells induces Sox2 and Prox1 expression but does not disrupt hair cell maturation. *Dev. Dyn.*, 2012. 241(4): p. 684-96.
[81] Neves, J., et al., Jagged 1 regulates the restriction of Sox2 expression in the developing chicken inner ear: a mechanism for sensory organ specification. *Development*, 2011. 138(4): p. 735-44.
[82] Morsli, H., et al., Development of the mouse inner ear and origin of its sensory organs. *J. Neurosci.*, 1998. 18(9): p. 3327-35.
[83] Gerlach, L.M., et al., Addition of the BMP4 antagonist, noggin, disrupts avian inner ear development. *Development,* 2000. 127(1): p. 45-54.
[84] Chang, W., et al., Ectopic noggin blocks sensory and nonsensory organ morphogenesis in the chicken inner ear. *Dev. Biol.,* 1999. 216(1): p. 369-81.
[85] Chen, P. and N. Segil, p27(Kip1) links cell proliferation to morphogenesis in the developing organ of Corti. *Development*, 1999. 126: p. 1581-90.
[86] Ohyama, T., et al., BMP signaling is necessary for patterning the sensory and nonsensory regions of the developing mammalian cochlea. *J. Neurosci.*, 2010. 30(45): p. 15044-51.
[87] Hwang, C.H., et al., Role of bone morphogenetic proteins on cochlear hair cell formation: analyses of Noggin and Bmp2 mutant mice. *Dev. Dyn.*, 2010. 239(2): p. 505-13.
[88] Lee, Y.S., F. Liu, and N. Segil, A morphogenetic wave of p27Kip1 transcription directs cell cycle exit during organ of Corti development. *Development*, 2006. (null): p. (null).
[89] Chen, P., et al., The role of Math1 in inner ear development: Uncoupling the establishment of the sensory primordium from hair cell fate determination. *Development*, 2002. 129(10): p. 2495-505.

[90] Bermingham, N.A., et al., Math1: an essential gene for the generation of inner ear hair cells. *Science*, 1999. 284(5421): p. 1837-41.

[91] Kawamoto, K., et al., Math1 gene transfer generates new cochlear hair cells in mature guinea pigs in vivo. *J. Neurosci.*, 2003. 23(11): p. 4395-400.

[92] Gubbels, S.P., et al., Functional auditory hair cells produced in the mammalian cochlea by in utero gene transfer. *Nature*, 2008. 455(7212): p. 537-41.

[93] Hayashi, T., et al., Hesr1 and Hesr2 may act as early effectors of Notch signaling in the developing cochlea. *Dev. Biol.*, 2008. 316(1): p. 87-99.

[94] Tateya, T., et al., Cooperative functions of Hes/Hey genes in auditory hair cell and supporting cell development. *Dev. Biol.*, 2011. 352(2): p. 329-40.

[95] Dabdoub, A., et al., Sox2 signaling in prosensory domain specification and subsequent hair cell differentiation in the developing cochlea. *Proc. Natl. Acad. Sci. USA*, 2008. 105(47): p. 18396-401.

[96] Ahmed, M., et al., Eya1-Six1 interaction is sufficient to induce hair cell fate in the cochlea by activating Atoh1 expression in cooperation with Sox2. *Dev. Cell*, 2012. 22(2): p. 377-90.

[97] Pan, N., et al., Conditional deletion of Atoh1 using Pax2-Cre results in viable mice without differentiated cochlear hair cells that have lost most of the organ of Corti. *Hear Res.*, 2011. 275(1-2): p. 66-80.

[98] Hayashi, T., D. Cunningham, and O. Bermingham-McDonogh, Loss of Fgfr3 leads to excess hair cell development in the mouse organ of Corti. *Dev. Dyn.*, 2007. 236(2): p. 525-33.

[99] Jacques, B.E., et al., Fgf8 induces pillar cell fate and regulates cellular patterning in the mammalian cochlea. *Development*, 2007. 134(16): p. 3021-9.

[100] Mueller, K.L., B.E. Jacques, and M.W. Kelley, Fibroblast growth factor signaling regulates pillar cell development in the organ of Corti. *J. Neurosci.*, 2002. 22: p. 9368-77.

[101] Puligilla, C., et al., Disruption of fibroblast growth factor receptor 3 signaling results in defects in cellular differentiation, neuronal patterning, and hearing impairment. *Dev. Dyn.*, 2007. 236(7): p. 1905-17.

[102] Hayashi, T., C.A. Ray, and O. Bermingham-McDonogh, Fgf20 is required for sensory epithelial specification in the developing cochlea. *J. Neurosci.*, 2008. 28(23): p. 5991-9.

[103] Huh, S.H., et al., Differentiation of the lateral compartment of the cochlea requires a temporally restricted FGF20 signal. *PLoS Biol.*, 2011. 10(1): p. e1001231.

[104] Hackney, C.M. and D.N. Furness, Mechanotransduction in vertebrate hair cells: structure and function of the stereociliary bundle. *Am. J. Physiol.*, 1995. 268(1 Pt 1): p. C1-13.

[105] Schwander, M., B. Kachar, and U. Muller, Review series: The cell biology of hearing. *J. Cell Biol.*, 2010. 190(1): p. 9-20.

[106] Petit, C. and G.P. Richardson, Linking genes underlying deafness to hair-bundle development and function. *Nat. Neurosci.*, 2009. 12(6): p. 703-10.

[107] Tilney, L.G., et al., Actin filaments, stereocilia, and hair cells of the bird cochlea. III. The development and differentiation of hair cells and stereocilia. *Dev. Biol.*, 1986. 116(1): p. 100-18.

[108] Tilney, L.G., M.S. Tilney, and D.J. DeRosier, Actin filaments, stereocilia, and hair cells: how cells count and measure. *Annu Rev Cell Biol*, 1992. 8: p. 257-74.

[109] Eggenschwiler, J.T. and K.V. Anderson, Cilia and developmental signaling. *Annu. Rev. Cell Dev. Biol.*, 2007. 23: p. 345-73.
[110] Sobkowicz, H.M., S.M. Slapnick, and B.K. August, The kinocilium of auditory hair cells and evidence for its morphogenetic role during the regeneration of stereocilia and cuticular plates. *J. Neurocytol.*, 1995. 24(9): p. 633-53.
[111] Jones, C., et al., Ciliary proteins link basal body polarization to planar cell polarity regulation. *Nat. Genet.*, 2008. 40(1): p. 69-77.
[112] Lin, F., et al., Kidney-specific inactivation of the KIF3A subunit of kinesin-II inhibits renal ciliogenesis and produces polycystic kidney disease. *Proc. Natl. Acad. Sci. USA*, 2003. 100(9): p. 5286-91.
[113] Ross, A.J., et al., Disruption of Bardet-Biedl syndrome ciliary proteins perturbs planar cell polarity in vertebrates. *Nat. Genet.*, 2005. 37(10): p. 1135-40.
[114] Montcouquiol, M. and M.W. Kelley, Planar and vertical signals control cellular differentiation and patterning in the mammalian cochlea. *J. Neurosci.*, 2003. 23: p. 9469-78.
[115] Montcouquiol, M., et al., Identification of Vangl2 and Scrb1 as planar polarity genes in mammals. *Nature*, 2003. 423: p. 173-7.
[116] Montcouquiol, M., et al., Asymmetric localization of Vangl2 and Fz3 indicate novel mechanisms for planar cell polarity in mammals. *J. Neurosci.*, 2006. 26: p. 5265-75.
[117] Curtin, J.A., et al., Mutation of Celsr1 disrupts planar polarity of inner ear hair cells and causes severe neural tube defects in the mouse. *Curr. Biol.*, 2003. 13(13): p. 1129-33.
[118] Lu, X., et al., PTK7/CCK-4 is a novel regulator of planar cell polarity in vertebrates. *Nature*, 2004. 430(6995): p. 93-8.
[119] Wang, Y., N. Guo, and J. Nathans, The role of Frizzled3 and Frizzled6 in neural tube closure and in the planar polarity of inner-ear sensory hair cells. *J. Neurosci.*, 2006. 26(8): p. 2147-56.
[120] Qian, D., et al., Wnt5a functions in planar cell polarity regulation in mice. *Dev. Biol.*, 2007. 306(1): p. 121-33.
[121] Etheridge, S.L., et al., Murine dishevelled 3 functions in redundant pathways with dishevelled 1 and 2 in normal cardiac outflow tract, cochlea, and neural tube development. *PLoS Genet*, 2008. 4(11): p. e1000259.
[122] Yamamoto, S., et al., Cthrc1 selectively activates the planar cell polarity pathway of Wnt signaling by stabilizing the Wnt-receptor complex. *Dev. Cell*, 2008. 15(1): p. 23-36.
[123] Tilney, M.S., et al., Preliminary biochemical characterization of the stereocilia and cuticular plate of hair cells of the chick cochlea. *J. Cell Biol.*, 1989. 109(4 Pt 1): p. 1711-23.
[124] Zine, A., A. Hafidi, and R. Romand, Fimbrin expression in the developing rat cochlea. *Hear Res.*, 1995. 87(1-2): p. 165-9.
[125] Zheng, L., et al., The deaf jerker mouse has a mutation in the gene encoding the espin actin-bundling proteins of hair cell stereocilia and lacks espins. *Cell*, 2000. 102(3): p. 377-85.
[126] Daudet, N. and M.C. Lebart, Transient expression of the t-isoform of plastins/fimbrin in the stereocilia of developing auditory hair cells. *Cell Motil Cytoskeleton*, 2002. 53(4): p. 326-36.

[127] Li, H., et al., Correlation of expression of the actin filament-bundling protein espin with stereociliary bundle formation in the developing inner ear. *J. Comp. Neurol.*, 2004. 468(1): p. 125-34.

[128] Zhu, M., et al., Mutations in the gamma-actin gene (ACTG1) are associated with dominant progressive deafness (DFNA20/26). *Am. J. Hum Genet*, 2003. 73(5): p. 1082-91.

[129] Procaccio, V., et al., A mutation of beta -actin that alters depolymerization dynamics is associated with autosomal dominant developmental malformations, deafness, and dystonia. *Am. J. Hum. Genet.*, 2006. 78(6): p. 947-60.

[130] Belyantseva, I.A., et al., Gamma-actin is required for cytoskeletal maintenance but not development. *Proc. Natl. Acad. Sci. USA*, 2009. 106(24): p. 9703-8.

[131] DeRosier, D.J., L.G. Tilney, and E. Egelman, Actin in the inner ear: the remarkable structure of the stereocilium. *Nature*, 1980. 287(5780): p. 291-6.

[132] Tilney, L.G., D.J. Derosier, and M.J. Mulroy, The organization of actin filaments in the stereocilia of cochlear hair cells. *J. Cell Biol.*, 1980. 86(1): p. 244-59.

[133] Kitajiri, S., et al., Actin-bundling protein TRIOBP forms resilient rootlets of hair cell stereocilia essential for hearing. *Cell*, 2010. 141(5): p. 786-98.

[134] Probst, F.J., et al., Correction of deafness in shaker-2 mice by an unconventional myosin in a BAC transgene. *Science*, 1998. 280(5368): p. 1444-7.

[135] Wang, A., et al., Association of unconventional myosin MYO15 mutations with human nonsyndromic deafness DFNB3. *Science,* 1998. 280(5368): p. 1447-51.

[136] Mburu, P., et al., Defects in whirlin, a PDZ domain molecule involved in stereocilia elongation, cause deafness in the whirler mouse and families with DFNB31. *Nat Genet*, 2003. 34(4): p. 421-8.

[137] Rzadzinska, A.K., et al., An actin molecular treadmill and myosins maintain stereocilia functional architecture and self-renewal. *J. Cell Biol.*, 2004. 164(6): p. 887-97.

[138] Belyantseva, I.A., et al., Myosin-XVa is required for tip localization of whirlin and differential elongation of hair-cell stereocilia. *Nat. Cell Biol.*, 2005. 7(2): p. 148-56.

[139] Delprat, B., et al., Myosin XVa and whirlin, two deafness gene products required for hair bundle growth, are located at the stereocilia tips and interact directly. *Hum. Mol. Genet*, 2005. 14(3): p. 401-10.

[140] Kikkawa, Y., et al., Mutant analysis reveals whirlin as a dynamic organizer in the growing hair cell stereocilium. *Hum. Mol. Genet*, 2005. 14(3): p. 391-400.

[141] Mburu, P., et al., Whirlin complexes with p55 at the stereocilia tip during hair cell development. *Proc. Natl. Acad. Sci. USA*, 2006. 103: p. 10973-8.

[142] Marfatia, S.M., et al., Identification of the protein 4.1 binding interface on glycophorin C and p55, a homologue of the Drosophila discs-large tumor suppressor protein. *J. Biol. Chem.*, 1995. 270(2): p. 715-9.

[143] Biederer, T. and T.C. Sudhof, CASK and protein 4.1 support F-actin nucleation on neurexins. *J. Biol. Chem.*, 2001. 276(51): p. 47869-76.

[144] Nayak, G.D., et al., Development of the hair bundle and mechanotransduction. *Int. J. Dev. Biol.*, 2007. 51(6-7): p. 597-608.

[145] Gillespie, P.G. and U. Muller, Mechanotransduction by hair cells: models, molecules, and mechanisms. *Cell,* 2009. 139(1): p. 33-44.

[146] Webb, S.W., et al., Regulation of PCDH15 function in mechanosensory hair cells by alternative splicing of the cytoplasmic domain. *Development,* 2011. 138(8): p. 1607-17.

In: Inner Ear Development and Hearing Loss
Editors: Saima Riazuddin and Zubair Ahmed
ISBN: 978-1-62417-011-9

Chapter 2

TIGHT JUNCTIONS - BARRIERS AGAINST HAIR CELL TOXICITY AND HEARING LOSS

G. D. Nayak, Z. M. Ahmed and S. Riazuddin*
Cincinnati Childrens's Hospital Medical Center,
Cincinnati, Ohio, US

ABSTRACT

In the cochlea, tight junctions are necessary to maintain the integrity of the hearing organ and defects in the proteins associated with these intercellular junctions can lead to hearing loss. The sensory epithelium in the cochlea is bathed in the K^+- rich endolymph, a pre-requisite for driving the mechanotransduction current. The tight junctions between the apical ends of the cells lining the scala media seal the sensory epithelium from the rest of the cochlear spaces.

Loss of this barrier leads to leakage of the endolymph through the reticular lamina into the intercellular spaces (space of Nuel) between the outer hair cells (OHCs). Exposure of the basolateral surfaces of OHCs to high levels of K^+ leads to toxicity and cell death. Several tight junction proteins are expressed in the inner ear and mutations in some of these are responsible for hereditary hearing loss. Transgenic mouse models for such mutations have not only helped characterize the proteins involved but also validated the importance of tight junctions in maintaining paracellularcation permeability barriers to prevent hair cell death.

This review focuses on the structure, function and localization of tight junctions in the sensory compartment of the cochlea. Emphasis will also be laid on the several inner ear tight junction proteins including the claudins, occludin, cingulin, ZO-1, ZO-2 and tricellulin. Interplay between these proteins is believed to be necessary for tight junction formation. Furthermore, we describe the clinical manifestations in humans due to loss of function of tight junction proteinsand discuss the phenotypes seen in mutant mouse models. Finally, we examine recent evidence that suggest a role for tight junction proteins in regulating gene expression.

* E-mail address: Saima.Riazuddin@cchmc.org

INTRODUCTION

Fluid Compartments in the Mammalian Cochlea and the Endolymph

The mammalian cochlea is composed of the bony labyrinth, which encloses the cellular structures that make up the membranous labyrinth. The bony labyrinthspirals around a central osseustube, the modiolus, and is partitioned into three spaces that house the fluid-filled compartments of the membranous labyrinth, the scalavestibuli, scala media and the scala tympani. The scalavestibuli and scala tympani are actually continuous, being connected at the apex of the cochlea via the helicotrema. Boththese compartments are filled with perilymph, a typical extracellular fluid with high levels of sodium and low amounts of potassium. The scala media on the other hand is filled with endolymph, a high-potassium solution (150mM) with low amounts of sodium (1.3 mM). This cochlear compartment houses the sensory epithelium and is isolated from the other two cochlear compartments (see Figure 1). The Reissner's membrane separates the scala mediafrom the scalavestibuli on the top, while parts of the osseus spiral lamina and the basilar membranedelimit it from the scala tympani below. The apical surfaces of the cells of the sensory epithelium are bathed in the endolymph of scala media and theirbasolateralsurfaces are exposed to cortilymph that is compositionally similar to and continuous with the perilymph ofscala tympani. Isolation of the scala media from the rest of the cochlea is brought about by tight junctions between all the epithelial cells lining the scala media (see Figure 1). Thus, the cells of the Reissner's membrane, the spiral ligament, sensory epithelium (sensory and non-sensory cells), inner sulcal cells and the cells lining the spiral limbus delimit the endolymphatic space within the cochlea and the tight junctions between these cells prevent any mixing of the endolymph and perilymph.

Another salient feature of the endolymph is its large positive potential known as the endocochlear potential, which in conjunction with the unique ionic composition of the endolymphis essential to cochlear function.

The cochlear sensory epithelium includes the sensory hair cells and the non-sensory supporting cells. When sound-induced mechanical stimuli displace the sensory structuresknown asstereocilia,that are present at the apical surface of hair cells, mechanically-gated cation channels open that lead to an influx of $K^+$and Ca^{2+}into hair cells. This leads to depolarization and release of neurotransmitters from the basolateral regions of hair cells. The neurotransmitters activate thenerve fibres that innervate the cochlear sensory epithelium and the acoustic stimuli are transmitted to the brain aselectrical signals. Thus, K^+ in the endolymph is the main charge carrier during sensory transduction and maintenance of the ionic composition of the endolymph and the endocochlear potential is crucial for sound signal transduction. The striavascularis in the lateral wall of the cochlea is responsible for the high-potassium content of the endolymph and generation of the endocochlear potential [1,2]. There is also evidence to suggest that K^+ is recycled between the cochlear compartments via the stria vascularis [1,2]. Briefly, the electrochemical potential for K^+ at the apical and basolateral pole of the hair cell allows for passive influx of K^+ at the apical pole and efflux from the basolateral pole. The K^+ that enters hair cells during acoustic stimulation is expelleddown its electrochemical gradient byvoltage-gated potassium channels like KCNQ4 that are located in the basolateral membrane of these cells [3].

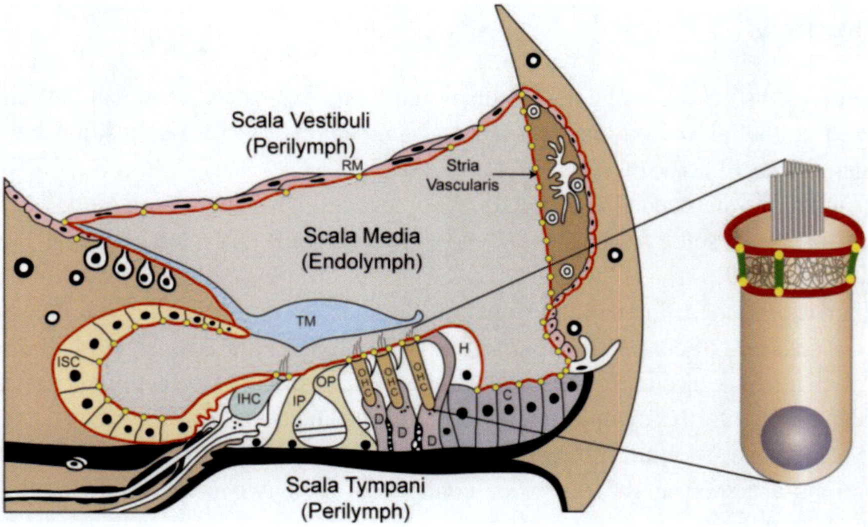

Figure 1. Illustration of the boundaries of the cochlear sensory compartment, the scala media. The filled red lines indicate the fluid-barrier formed by the tight junctions of the epithelia lining the scala media. Also shown are the striavascularis and the perilymphatic spaces, scalavestibuli and scala tympani. A single enlarged outer hair cell shows the localization of the bicellular tight junctions in red and the tricellular tight junctions in green.TM, tectorial membrane; IHC, inner hair cell; IPC, inner pillar cell; OPC, outer pillar cell; OHC, outer hair cell; D, Deiter's cell; H, Hensen's cell; C, Claudius' cell.

From here, the route of K^+ recycling has not been unequivocally proved but it is believed that the cation either diffuses into the perilymph or is quickly taken up by supporting cells and then delivered to the perilymph. The K^+ then reaches the spiral ligament and is taken up by the fibrocytes. An alternative route is via a gap-junction system connecting the supporting cells to the fibrocytes of the spiral ligament. The fibrocytes are in turn connected by gap junctions to the basal cells of the striavascularis, which are connected to the intermediate cells in the same way. Thus, the K^+ flowing into hair cells is recycled and returned to the endolymph via the stria vascularis [1,2].

The striavascularis is also responsible for generating the endocochlear potential [1,4,5]. The intrastrial compartment is enclosed by tight junctions between marginal cells on the scala media side and between basal cells on the spiral ligament side. The K^+ from the fibrocytes enters the intermediate cells via the basal cells. From here, the K^+ enters the intrastrial space via the KCNJ10 channels at the apical membrane of the intermediate cells. The K^+ in the intrastrial space is taken up against its electrochemical gradient by marginal cells via the Na^+–$2Cl^-$–K^+ co-transporter SLC12A2and theNa^+,K^+-ATPase ATP1A1/ATP1B2located in the basolateral membrane of these cells. Thus, the K^+ concentration of the intrastrial compartment is kept low compared to that of the cytosol of the intermediate cells resulting in the formation of a K^+ diffusion potential across the apical membrane of intermediate cells. Finally, the KCNQ1 channels on the endolymphatic side of the marginal cells extrude the K^+ into the endolymph. Thetwo K^+ diffusion potentials, one across the apical membrane of the intermediate cells and the otheracross the apical membrane of the marginal cells, together comprise the endocochlear potential [1,4,5].

Tight Junctions

Tight junctions belong to the apical junctional complexes that are seen at the luminal end of polarized epithelial and endothelialcells and are regions of close apposition between the plasma membranes of adjacent cells.

Tight junctions are needed to maintain the apical and basolateral membrane domains and prevent diffusion of solutes and solvent molecules through the intercellular spaces within epithelial sheets [6–9].

In other words, these intercellular junctions are necessary to maintain the polarized state of epithelial cells and to confer fluid-barrier properties to the epithelia. Tight junctions occupy a region that forms a circumferential belt around each epithelial cell, thus obliterating any intercellular space. On the cytoplasmic side, the tight junctions are associated with an actin cytoskeletal belt that provides anchorage and stability to the tight junctions [6]. Bicellular tight junctions are seen at the points of contact between two cells while tricellular tight junctions occur at the region where three cells meet (see figure 2).

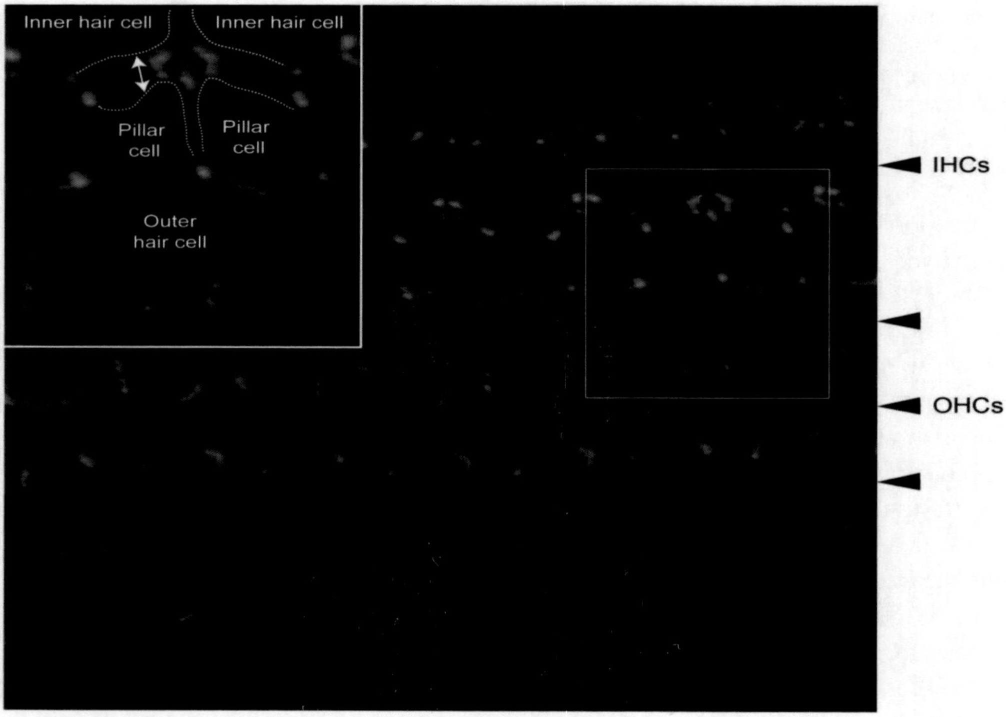

Figure 2. A confocal image of the mouse organ of Cortilabeled with ZO-1 (red) and tricellulin (green) antibodies. Shown in inset is a single outer hair cell (highlighted with double-dashed line marquee in main figure) and the four supporting cells (asterisks) surrounding it. ZO-1 is localized at bicellular junctions (dashed line tracing) that are seen between two supporting cells (homotypic junctions) and between a hair cell and the neighbouring supporting cell (heterotypic junctions). Tricellulin labels the tricellular tight junctions that are formed when the vertices of three adjacent cells converge. In the organ of Corti, the depth of the tricellular junctions is greater than that seen in other epithelia and tricellulinimmunoreactivity extends the full depth of these unique junctions (double headed arrow in inset). ZO-1 labeling intersects tricellulin at the apical and basal ends of the tricellular junctions.

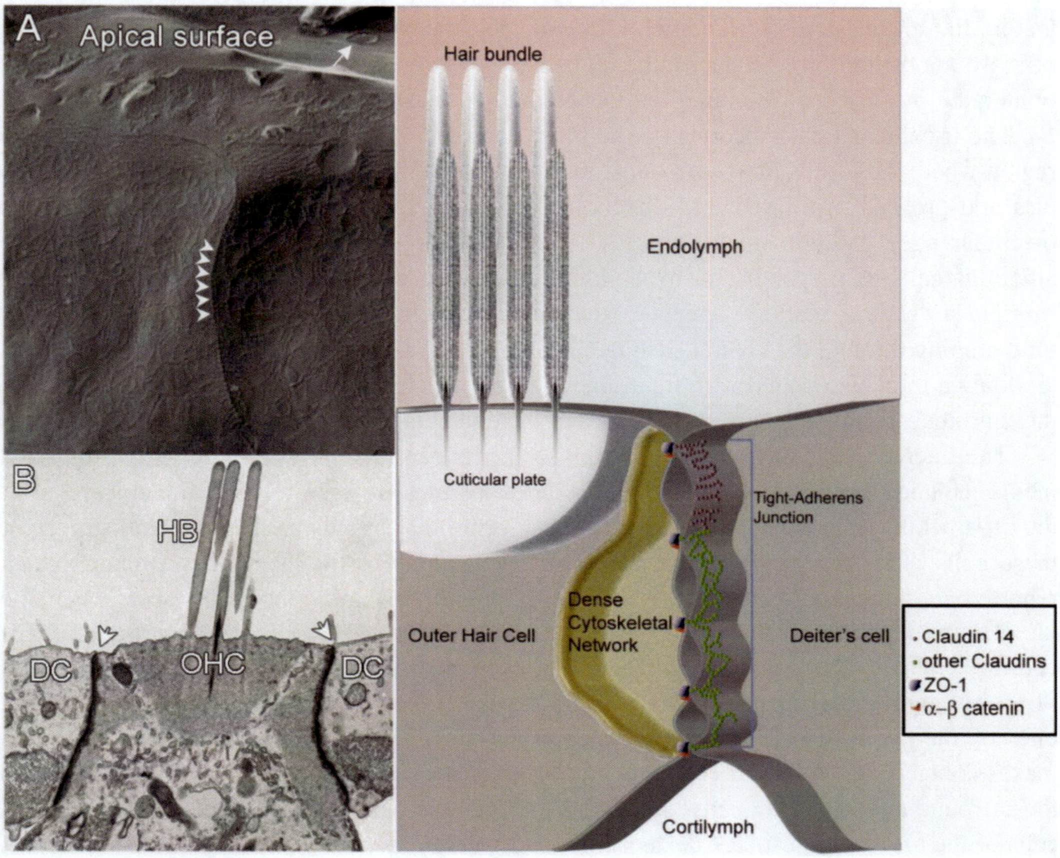

Figure 3. Electron microscopy images ofbicellular and tricellular tight junctions and illustration of a heterotypic tight junction in the organ of Corti. A)Freeze-fracture electron microscopy image of a tricellular tight junction between an OHC and two supporting cells in the organ of Corti. The arrow shows the site of cross-fracture of a stereocilium at the apical surface of the OHC. Arrowheads show the zipper-like tricellular junction running down the site of contact of the three cells. On either side of the tricellular tight junction, strands of bicellular junctions are apparent, where the apical strands are parallel to the apical surface and are followed by a web of interconnecting strands in the lower regions. B)Transmission electron microscopy image of two heterotypic junctions (arrows) between an OHC and the two Deiter's cells in the guinea pig organ of Corti[12]. Unlike the homotypic tight junctions between two supporting cells, the heterotypic junctions in the organ of Corti are associated with a dense cytoskeletal network that is a feature of adherens junctions. C)Illustration of a heterotypic tight junction between and an OHC and a Deiter'scell. These junctions isolate the endolymph of scala media from the cortilymph of space of Nuel.The dense cytoskeletal network observed in the OHC cytoplasm is shown. The claudins associated with these heterotypic junctions are also partitioned into subdomains. Claudin 14 is associated with the apical-most parallel strands, while the lower strands are made of claudins 9 and 6. Also, α and β catenin, two adherens junction proteins, co-localize with claudins 9 and 6.

Transmission electron microscopy and freeze-fracture scanning electron microscopy images have revealed the ultrastructure of tight junctions [6,8,9] (see figure 3, panels A and B). The latter technique shows bicellular tight junctions as a band of interconnected strands formed by chains of intramembranous particles (see figure 3, panel C). Depending on the site of fracture, the chains of intramembranous particles may be distributed predominantly to the protoplasmic or exoplasmic lipid leaflet of the plasma membrane. In either case, the particles appear as ridges on the lipid leaflet with corresponding vacant grooves on the opposing leaflet. In transmission electron microscopy images, the bicellular junctions appear as regions of close apposition of adjacent epithelial cells where the intercellular spaces are completely obliterated by fusion of the outer leaflets of the two plasma membranes (see figure 3, panel B). The tricellular tight junctions on the other hand are quite different in appearance. At the region where three cells meet, the apical-most strands of the bicellular tight junction appear to turn and proceed in a basalward direction, connecting the ends of the other strands of the bicellular tight junction in the process. The tricellular tight junction strands of the three adjoining cells lie perpendicular to the longitudinal axis of the cells and attach to each other forming a "central sealing element". Regulated paracellular diffusion occurs via a narrow tube running through the central sealing element. Thus far, several different types of proteins are known to be associated with tight junctions and the various combinations and amount of these proteins dictate the barrier properties of the epithelia [6,8,9].

The intercellular junctional complexes seen between the epithelial cells lining the scala media include tight junctions andadherens junctions that are seen towards the apical end of the cells, while desmosomes and gap junctions occur more basally along the lateral surface of these cells. The structure of most intercellular junctions in the cochlea is similar to that reported in other epithelia [10–12]. However, significant differences are seen when the intercellular junctions in the organ of Corti are observed [10–12]. The apical surfaces of hair cells are embedded in a rigid transcellular plate, the reticular lamina, formed by the processes of the supporting cells in the organ of Corti. Each hair cell is isolated from the surrounding ones by the processes of the adjacent supporting cells. Thus, while a single supporting cell makes contact with both hair cells and other supporting cells, a single hair cell only contacts the surrounding supporting cells (see figure 2). The apical junctional complexes between the cells of the organ of Corti lack desmosomes and gap junctions but display tight and adherens junctions. Adjacent supporting cells are connected by the characteristic apical tight junctions and adherens junctions [11,12]. The bicellular junctions between an outer hair cell and adjacent supporting cell, the Deiter's cell, however, are highly specialized [12] (see Figure 3, panels B and C). These junctions appear to have a combination of tight junction and adherens junction features, and extend down the depth of the reticular lamina, a region spanning 3-5 um. On the cytoplasmic side, except for the very apical region, these bicellular junctions are associated with an extensively developed cytoplasmic plaque similar to that seen in adherens junctions [12] (see figure 3, panels B and C). Tight junction proteins also appear to be differentially distributed between the very apical or lower regions of the junctions (see figure 3, panel C). It therefore appears that there may be subdomains within the bicellular junctions between OHCs and Deiter's cells and that the adherens junction-like features may provide the mechanical strength necessary to endure the shear and strain forces experienced by the reticular lamina [12].

TIGHT JUNCTION ASSOCIATED PROTEINS EXPRESSED IN THEMAMMALIAN COCHLEA

Over the last two decades a number of proteins that are associated with tight junctions have been discovered. These include integral membrane proteins and peripheral membrane proteins, as well as some nuclear and cytosolic proteins. Several of these have been shown to be expressed in the epithelia sheets lining the sensory compartment of the cochlea. The variability in the expression of these tight junction proteins between the different kinds of epithelia reflect the roles played by these cells in the hearing organ.

Zona Occludens

The zonaoccludens (ZO) proteins include ZO-1, 2 and 3 (also called TJP1, 2 and 3),where ZO-1 was the first tight junction protein to be cloned [13]. These proteins are essential for tight junction assembly and formation of adherens junctions [14,15]. The ZO proteins belong to the large family of membrane-associated guanylate kinase (MAGUK)-like proteins and behave as molecular scaffolds at sites of cell-cell contact. These proteins have the same general organization of their functional domains; three PDZ domains, one SH3 domain and a GUK domain [15]. ZO proteins interact with several of the tight junction proteins like the claudins, occludin, tricellulin, junctional adhesion molecules and coxsackie adenovirus receptor and anchor them to the actin cytoskeleton [15]. It is still unclear however, whether the ZO proteins are passively involved in stabilizing the tight junctions by anchoring them to the cytoskeleton or whether they play a more active role in the dynamic regulation of the cortical cytoskeleton [14]. While ZO-3 knock-out mice do not show a phenotype, which suggests that it is dispensable for tight junction function, ZO-1 and ZO-2 knock-out mice are embryonically lethal reflecting the non-redundant functions of these proteins [15–17]. Studies in epithelial cell lines have shown that loss of all the ZO proteins results in the absence of tight junctions and failure of other tight junction proteins to accumulate at regions of cell-cell contact [15]. Replacing ZO-1 or ZO-2 into these cells results in the formation of tight junction strands and incorporation of other tight junction proteins into them [15].

Quantitative RT-PCR of RNA from wild-type mice at different developmental time-points suggests that *Tjp2*transcriptlevels decrease steadily between embryonic day 16.5 and one week after birth [18]. In the adult mouse, the levels of *Tjp2* transcript are nearly half that seen at birth. Immunolocalization shows ZO-2 is found in the tight junctions of the cochlear and vestibular epithelia along the basolateral sides of hair cells [18].

There is also evidence that the ZO proteins act in signal transduction pathways and can regulate gene expression [19,20]. This is discussed in a later section.

Claudins

Claudins are a group of over 20 proteins and the first few of these were discovered in 1998 in the isolated junction fraction obtained from chicken liver [21].These 20-27 kDa proteins are the main constituents of the bicellular tight junction strands [22]. Although it is yet unclear how they form the ~10 nm particles seen in freeze-fracture images, the varying amounts and combinations of the different claudins govern several characteristics of the tight junction barriers, like its ionic charge and size selectivity [23–26]. Although there are differences between the different claudins, they have the same general structure with 4 transmembrane domains and short cytosolic amino and carboxy termini [21]. While the first and the fourth transmembrane regions as well as the extracellular loops are highly conserved among the different claudin species, the second and the third transmembrane regions are variable in their amino acid content [27]. The first extracellular loop of these proteins is longer and more hydrophobic than the second and is also the region that plays the most important role in homophilic interactions [28]. While most claudins are believed to readily interact with each other in the lateral plane (cis-interaction), and make homophilic interactions with their extracellular domain between adjacent cells (trans-interaction), not all claudins can make hetereophilic interactions intrans [29]. On the cytoplasmic side, the PDZ-binding motif has been shown to interact with the ZO proteins [30]. The intracellular regions of claudins also contain information necessary for the localization of these proteins at tight junctions and to maintain their stability at these sites [31,32]. In the cochlea, claudins 1, 2, 3, 8, 9, 10, 11, 12, 14 and 18 are expressed in the various epithelia that isolate the scala media from the rest of the cochlear spaces [33]. While some claudinsare expressed in multiple epithelia, and most epithelia express multiple claudins, at least one epithelia that is formed by the basal cells of the striavascularis express only claudin 11 [33]. Not surprisingly, claudin 11-deficient mice exhibit deafness due to defects in the striavascularis (discussed in detail later). The sensory epithelia was shown to express claudins 1, 2, 3, 9, 10, 12, 14 and 18, which in addition to claudin 8 are also expressed in the epithelial cells that form the Reissner's membrane, spiral limbus and the marginal cells of the stria vascularis [33]. Such an overlapping expression pattern suggests that functional redundancy may compensate for the loss of one of the claudins. On the contrary, mice with mutations in claudin 9 and 14 display hearing loss reflecting the indispensable functions played by some of the claudins [34,35].

Tight Junction-Associated MARVEL Protein Family

The tight junction-associated MARVEL protein (TAMP) family consists of occludin, MarvelD3 and tricellulin [36]. As the name suggests these proteins contain the MARVEL domain (for myelin and lymphocyte and related proteins for vesicle trafficking andmembrane link) and are associated with tight junctions [36].

Occludin

Occludin wasthe first integral tight junction protein to be identified and was considered to be the main constituent of tight junction strands until the discovery of claudins [37]. Like claudins, occludin is also a tetraspan membrane protein with two extracellular loops with the N- and C-termini localized in the cytoplasm [37]. The C-terminus contains the ELL domain and is required for protein interaction [38]. The extracellular domain of occludin isunusually rich in tyrosine and glycine residues and contains very few charged residues [37]. The C-terminus region of occludin has many serine, threonine and tyrosine residues, which are targets of several protein kinases. Phosphorylated occludin appears to preferentially localize to tight junctions [39].

Overexpression of occludin leads to an increase in the trans-epithelial resistance andan unexpected increase in paracellular flux [40]. Occludin also interacts with other tight junction proteins like ZO proteins and is incorporated into intramembranous strands formed by claudins [41–43]. Several studies have suggested that occludin plays an important role at tight junctions [40,44–46]. However, occludin-deficient epithelial cells display well-formed tight junction strands [47]. In addition, occludin-deficient mice display no abnormalities in the structure or function of tight junction barriers in the intestinal epithelia [48]. These mice however, display other significant gross phenotypes including post-natal growth retardation[48]. Occludin mutant male mice with normal spermatogenesis produce no litters when mated with wild-type females, while the occludin mutant females produce litters as normal but do not suckle them [48]. Histological irregularities that areevident in the occludinmutantmice include chronic inflammation and hyperplasiaof the gastric mucosa, brain calcification, thinning of the compact bone, testicular atrophy and loss ofcytoplasmic granules in the striated duct cells of thesalivary gland [48]. In the mammalian cochlea, occludin immunoreactivity is seen in the tight junctions between all the epithelial cells that line the scala media, including those of the sensory epithelium[33].However, the inner ear of occludin mutant mice has not been studied.

Tricellulin

The genes encoding tricellulinand occludin are located in tandem on mouse chromosome 13 and human chromosome 5 and it is thought that they arose by duplication events during phylogenic evolution [49]. Like occludin, tricellulin is also a tetraspan membrane protein, with cytoplasmic N and C-termini that confer differential targeting [49,50]. The C-terminus is required for basolateral targeting of the protein whereas the N-terminus probably directs it to tricellular contacts [50]. While the N-terminus of tricellulin is longer than that of occludin, the C-terminus of the former contains an ELL domain similar to occluding [49,51].

Tricellulin is found concentrated mostly at tricellular tight junctions although weak labeling at bicellular tight junctions is seen in some epithelia [49,51,52]. Occludin and lipolysis-stimulated lipoprotein receptor (LSR) have been reported to affect the localization of tricellulin [53,54]. Tricellulin exhibits cis- homomeric interactionsas well as heteromeric interactions with occluding [50]. Although the actual role of tricellulin in barrier function has not been unequivocally demonstrated, studies in epithelial cell lines suggest that tricellulin at tricellular tight junctions controls paracellular movement of macromolecules whereas its presence at bicellular tight junctions modulates ion permeation [49,53–55].

Recently, mutations in tricellulin were found to be the cause of autosomal recessive non-syndromic deafness at DFNB49 locus [51,56,57]. Tricellulinimmunoreactivity can be seen in the postnatal mouse inner in most of the epithelial cells of the cochlea and vestibule [51]. The protein appears to be concentrated at tricellular contacts with weaker labeling seen at bicellular tight junctions. At heterotypic junctions in the organ of Corti, where a single hair cell meets two supporting cells, tricellulinimmunoreactivity extends the full depth of the tricellular junction.

Thus, while ZO-1 outlines the top and bottom of the tricellular tight junctions in the organ of Corti, tricellulin perpendicularly intersects the two ZO-1 rings. The same pattern is also seen in the tricellular contacts in other non-sensory epithelia where the tricellular tight junctions are not as deep as in the organ of Corti [51].

Marvel Domain-Containing Protein 3 (MarvelD3)

MarvelD3 is the newest member of the TAMP family. Outside of the marvel domain marvelD3 has no similarities to occludin or tricellulin[58]. In many epithelial cell lines and mouse tissues tested, marvelD3 localizes to bicellular tight junctions [36]. Furthermore, RT-PCR analyses reveal the expression of marvelD3 in the rodent cochlea (Riazuddin et al., unpublished observation).

Co-immunoprecipitation studies show that marvelD3 interacts with tricellulin and occludin *in vitro*, while the latter two proteins do not interact with each other [36], which is in contrast to another study that suggest interaction between tricellulin and occluidin [50]. MarvelD3 may also modulate the ion permeability properties of an epithelia although it is not necessary for the development of the tight junctions itself [36,58].

Comparing the effects of each member of the TAMP family on the properties of the epithelial cells and the behavior of these proteins at the bi- and tricellular junctions reveal that these proteins may be able to partially compensate for the loss of one another but that there are unique functions that can be attributed to each of them [36].

OTHER TIGHT JUNCTION-ASSOCIATED PROTEINS IN THE COCHLEA

Cingulin

Cingulin is a 140-160 kDa protein seen in the cytoplasmic plaque associated with tight junctions [59]. This protein may bridge other tight junction proteins like ZO-1, ZO-2 and junctional adhesion molecule (JAM) to the acto-myosin cytoskeleton during tight junction assembly and regulation [60,61]. Knock-out of the cingulin gene in mouse embryonic stem cells does not disrupt tight junction formation but alters the expression of some tight junction proteins and transcription factors [62].

In the cochlea, cingulin localizes to both homotypic and heterotypic tight junctions in the organ of Corti [63,64].

Shroom2

The shroom family of proteins consists of shroom1 -4, which are PDZ-domain containing actin-binding proteins. The apical protein from Xenopus Iaevis1(APX1)/shroom domain2 is the most conserved domain among these proteins and has been shown to facilitate an acto-myosin based constriction event [65,66].

In the cochlea, shroom2 localizes to the tight junctions in the organ of Corti and interacts with F-actin, ZO-1 and myosin VIIa, an unconventional myosin that is necessary for auditory function [67].

TIGHT JUNCTION PROTEINS AS SIGNALLING MOLECULES AND MODULATORS OF GENE EXPRESSION

Over the last several years, there is increasing evidence that tight junction proteins participate in signal transduction pathways and can regulate gene expression [19,20,68,69]. One of the first indications that tight junction proteins may play a role in gene regulation came from observing dual localization of some nuclear and tight junction proteins. It was shown that ZO-1 and ZO-2 can transiently localize to the nucleus of proliferating epithelial cells and re-localize to newly forming tight junctions upon reaching confluency [70–72]. ZO-1 interacts with ZO-1 associated nucleic acid binding protein (ZONAB), a Y-box transcription factor, that in turn binds to the promoter regions of cyclin D1 and proliferating cell nuclear antigen (PCNA) and increases the expression of these proteins [73–75]. While cyclin D1 is involved in the regulation of G1/S transition of the cell cycle, PCNA is involved in DNA replication and repair [76–78]. ZONAB is known to localize to both the nucleus and tight junctions, depending on the proliferative state of the cell and the amount of ZO-1 present at the tight junctions [19,69]. Symplekin is another dual residency protein that is found both at tight junctions and in the nucleus [79]. Symplekin interacts with and regulates the transcriptional activity of ZONAB [80]. ZO-2 can interact with hnRNP protein scaffold attachment factor-B (SAF-B) has a role in modulating the chromatin structure and gene regulation [72]. Through interaction with the transcription factor MYC, ZO-2 binds the promoter region of cyclin D1 and regulates its expression [81]. ZO-2 also interacts with JUN, FOS and C/EBP (CCAAT/enhancer binding protein) both in the nucleus and at the plasma membrane [82]. Another way of tight junction protein-mediated regulation of gene expression and cell proliferation is via Rho GTPases. Specifically, cingulin has been shown to regulate the activity of RHOA, thereby controlling claudin 2 expression and cell proliferation in Madin-Darby Canine Kidney Cells (MDCK) cells [83,84]. In addition, protein kinase C signaling has long been known to modulate the epithelial barrier function of tight junctions [68]. Phosphatases like PP1, PP2A and PP2B also have modulatory effects on the permeability of tight junctions, either by direct phosphorylation of tight junction proteins or by inhibiting different PKC isoforms [68]. Thus, signaling to and from tight junctions can have profound effects on the barrier properties of an epithelium, its apico-basal polarity and the proliferative state of the cells involved.

CLINICAL PHENOTYPES IN HUMANS DUE TO MUTATIONS IN TIGHT JUNCTION PROTEINS

Owing to the importance of maintaining ion-homeostasis in the cochlea it is not surprising that mutations in tight junction proteins can cause hearing loss in humans. Interestingly, all of the known mutations in tight junction proteins lead to non-syndromic deafness despite widespread expression of the proteins. This suggests that although there may be functional redundancy in other tissues, these tight junction proteins have unique functions in the cochlea and are indispensable for hearing.

CLAUDIN 14 (DFNB29)

Mutations in claudin-14 are known to causeautosomal recessive non-syndromic deafness at*DFNB29* locus [85]. Using the parametric linkage analysis, mutations (p.Val85Asp and c.398delT) in *CLDN14* were identified as the cause of profound hearing loss in two large Pakistani families [85]. The deletion mutation, c.398delT, is located in the third transmembrane domain and is predicted to result in premature truncation of the encoded protein. The p.Val85Asp mutation is predicted to affect the secondary structure of claudin 14 but does not affect membrane targeting [85,86]. Besides profound hearing loss, the p.Val85Asp has been reported in a large family segregating severe hearing loss [87].

Variability seen in the severity of hearing loss due to the p.Val85Asp mutation of *CLDN14* may be caused by genetic modifiers and/or environmental factors.To date, several groups have reported six different pathogenic mutations in *CLDN14*as the cause for severe or severe to profound hearing loss in humans [86–89]. Recently, a genome-wide association study has shown association between the synonymous variants within the coding region of *CLDN14* gene and kidney stones and bone mineral density [90].

CLDN14 mRNA is detected in the human kidney and liver but small amounts of the transcript are also present in the brain. *In situ* hybridization and immunocytochemistry revealthat claudin14 is expressed postnatally in the mouse inner ear and the expression appears to be limited to the sensory epithelium of the inner ear organs [85].

TRICELLULIN (DFNB49)

Several groups have reported mutations in tricellulin, encoded by *TRIC*, as the underlying cause for autosomal recessive non-syndromic deafness, at *DFNB49* locus [51,56,57]. Audiograms of affected members of these families display moderate to profound hearing loss, with both interfamilial and intrafamilial variability seen in the degree of hearing loss [51].

Nearly all of the mutations reported so far are splice-site mutations [51,56,57]. However, one family segregates a transition mutation (c.1498C>T) that creates a nonsense codon, p.Arg500*, which is predicted to result in premature truncation of the protein in the occludin-ELL domain[51]. Intriguingly, all of the mutations reported so far are within or immediately flanking exons 4 and 5 of the TRIC [51,56,57]. It is estimated that mutations in *TRIC* underlie 1.30% (95% CI interval: 0.7-2.3) of autosomal non-syndromic hearing loss in the Pakistani population and are a significant cause of deafness in the Czech-Roma population [56,57].

Mice bearing a *Tric* knock-in mutation, p.Arg497*, which corresponds to the predicted nonsense mutation p.Arg500* in the DFNB49 family, display early onset, rapidly progressive hearing loss and the mice are profoundly deaf by P30 (Nayak et al., manuscript in preparation). Morphological examination of the organ of Corti at various time points during the first few weeks of life reveals severe outer hair cell loss in these mice by P16 and a near complete loss of all hair cells by P30. The hair cell phenotype is attributed to "leaky" tricellular tight junctions in the reticular lamina that allow diffusion of K^+ from the endolymph into the space of Nuel, thus creating a toxic environment for the OHCs (Nayak et al., manuscript in preparation).

TJP2 (DFNA51)

Genomic alterations in tight junction protein 2 (TJP2, also called ZO-2), cause autosomal dominant nonsyndromic deafness, DFNA51, due to defective signal transduction [18]. Audiological assessment of a family of Jewish ancestry revealshearing loss, with onset in the fourth decade. The auditory deficit that is initially progressive at high-frequencies ultimately encompasses all frequencies with severe to profound hearing loss with no vestibular defect.

The cause for hearing loss in this family is a tandem inverted duplication of ~270 kb containing the entire TJP2locus [18]. This genomic duplication causes a 2-fold increase in TJP2 level in the lymphoblastoid cell lines of affected individuals. Increase in the level of TJP2 leads to decrease in serine9 phosphorylation of GSK-3β and an increase inthe activity of the latter [18]. GSK-3β promotes the mitochondrial intrinsic apoptosis pathway, which suggests that the hearing loss observed in the DFNA51 family may be due to higher expression of apoptotic genes. Indeed, the lymphoblastoid cells from the affected individuals show an overall increase in the expression of *BCL2* family genes that favor apoptosis. This possibly heightens the susceptibility of cochlear hair cells to apoptosis resulting in hearing loss [18].

Evidence from Mouse Mutants

Much can be learned about the function of individual genes by studying the effects of their mutations in mice. Several tight junction mouse mutants have been studied so far. Among them, a few display non-syndromic deafness [34,35,91]. In addition, a double mutant obtained by breeding mice with mutations in two different claudins, was examined to determine the probable co-operation between the corresponding proteins [92].

Claudin 14

Cldn14$^{+/-}$mice were generated from recombinant embryonic stem cell clones where the three exons of *Cldn14* were replaced by a neomycin resistance cassette and the *lacZ* reporter gene by homologous recombination [34]. Intercrossing these mice produce *Cldn14*$^{+/-}$, *Cldn14*$^{+/+}$ and *Cldn14*$^{-/-}$ pups in the expected Mendelian ratio. The homozygous null mice are reportedly healthy and fertile and histopathological examination reveals no differences between the wild-type, heterozygous and homozygous null mice [34]. However, auditory brainstem responses at 5 week of age show that the *Cldn14*$^{-/-}$ mice are profoundly deaf with elevated thresholds of 50 dB-SPL or more over all frequencies tested. The *Cldn14*$^{+/-}$ mice meanwhile are indistinguishable from their wild-type litter mates in their hearing ability. The *Cldn14* null mice however, do not display any vestibular disorders although the protein is expressed in the vestibular sensory epithelium. The *Cldn14* null mice have normal endocochlear potential and hair cell development. However, widespread OHC loss is seenby postnatal day (P) 10, where the first observable phenotype before OHC death is disorganization and loss of stereocilia, followed by swelling of cell bodies and shortening of cell length.The cells finally appear to submerge under the reticular lamina and subsequently die. By P18, only a few OHCs bearing disorganized stereociliacan be seen. Loss of claudin 14 can affect the function of the tight junctions in the cochlear epithelium or may disregulate a signal transduction pathway leading to OHC death. However, the ultrastructure of tight junctions in the cochlear epithelium is unaffected in the *Cldn14*$^{-/-}$ mice and the cochlear epithelia from these mice survive intact *in vitro*, well past the equivalent postnatal time point when OHC death is observed. Claudin 14 may still affect tight junction permeability without affecting its ultrastructure. Electrophysiological studies in polarized epithelial cells lines overexpressing claudin 14 suggest that it strongly discriminates against the paracellular movement of cations. Thus, it is hypothesized that the OHC death observed in the *Cldn14* null mice is due to cationic barrier defects in the tight junctions of the cochlear epithelium [34]. Loss of claudin 14 may lead to leakage of the K^+-rich endolymph through the reticular lamina and into the extracellular spaces surrounding OHCs. Long-term exposure of OHC basolateral surfaces to high concentration of K^+ leads to prolonged depolarization of these cells and eventually cell death [1].

CLAUDIN 11

The first report on *Cldn11* null mice shows an absence of tight junctions in the central nervous system (CNS) myelin and between Sertoli cells [93]. The resulting effects were hindlimb weakness, slowed conduction velocities in the CNS and male sterility. Following the documentation of claudin 11expression in the basal cells of the striavascularis, the *Cldn11* null mice were examined for hearing deficits [33,91]. Interestingly, in the mouse cochlea, claudin11 is expressed only in the striavascularis, where no other claudins are detected [33].

Loss of claudin 11 leads to a complete absence of the intramembranous fibrils of tight junctions between adjacent basal cells[91]. It is thought that the extensive gap junction domains seen between closely apposed basal cells in *Cldn11* mutants is due to the loss of regulation of spatial organization of these junctions in the absence of tight junctions. Although the overall organization of the striavascularis is normal in these mice, the paracellular diffusion barrier of the basal cell layer is disrupted [91].

Auditory brainstem recordings of *Cldn11* null mice show that these animals have elevated hearing thresholds of ~50 dB SPL across all frequencies [91]. Distortion product otoacoustic emission measurements of adult *Cldn11*null mice reveal considerable deficiencies in OHC function compared to control mice. Also, the endocochlear potential is significantly reduced (29 mV) in the *Cldn11*null mice compared to control littermates (79 mV). Although a few OHCs show degenerative changes in the cochleae of adult *Cldn11*null mice, the loss is relatively low to account for the hearing deficits observed. There is no observable degeneration in any of the other cell types in the cochleae of the mutants, including spiral ganglion, strial marginal and endothelial cells.

Also, there are no changes in the expression of intercellular junction proteins, ion channels and pumps in the *Cldn11*null mice. Therefore, the hearing loss observed in

*Cldn11*null mice is attributed to dysfunctional striavascularis [91]. *Cldn11* and *Cldn14* double mutant mice display only the phenotypes seen in the single deletion mutants, which are deafness, neurological deficits and male sterility. There are no additional phenotypes despite the overlapping expression pattern in tissues like the kidney, which suggests an absence of functional co-operation between the two claudins [92].

CLAUDIN 9

The *Cldn9*deficient mouse strain, *nmf329*, was generated in the Jackson Laboratory by ENU-mutagenesis and the molecular and phenotypic characterization of these mice revealauditory deficits [35]. The *nmf329* mutation is a T to C point mutation 102 bases downstream of the start codon and results in a phenylalanine to leucine change in the predicted first extracellular loop of the protein. As the affected amino acid, p.Phe35, is conserved among all the claudin 9 orthologs identified thus far and is also highly conserved amongst many members of the claudin family, the mutation likely has functional consequences [35].

Auditory brainstem response analysis of *nmf329/nmf329* mutant mice reveal severe hearing loss by P16 and elevated thresholds of ~60 dB-SPL by P28 across all frequencies [35]. The hearing loss observed in these mice is recessive and non-syndromic and the homozygous mutant mice are viable. They do not exhibit any vestibular defects or any pathological changes in any of the tissues examined [35].

Temporal evaluation of the cochlear sensory epithelium of the *nmf329/nmf329* mutants shows normal hair cell development but preferential OHC loss at the onset of hearing and severe degeneration by P14 [35]. OHC death is severe in the basal turn of the cochlea, andis milder in the apical coil. Loss of the OHCs leads to "phalangeal scars", where the surrounding supporting cells replace the dying hair cells and re-seal the epithelium [35]. The initial rapid loss of OHCs appears to slow down during the first few weeks after birth such that at P80 some OHCs are still visible in the basal turn. Meanwhile, the inner hair cells are largely intact in the *Cldn9* mutants.

Electrophysiological studies on MDCK cells that express claudin 9 heterologously, show that the wild-type protein increases the transepithelial resistance of the MDCK layer by decreasing the paracellular permeability of Na^+.Thep.Phe35Leu mutation on the other hand, results in an increase in the paracellular permeability of cations through the MDCK layer and a subsequent decrease in transepithelial resistance [35].

Immunolocalization of claudin 9in the wild-type and homozygous *nmf329* mutants suggests that the point mutation does not affect the subcellular localization and organization of tight junctionstrands in the OHCs [35]. While the endocochlear potential is unperturbed in the mutants, the perilymphatic K^+ concentration is significantly higher than that observed in the wild-type littermates.

In contrast to the widespread OHC death observed *in vivo*, organotypic cultures of cochleae from the *nmf329* mutants do not display any hair cell loss. This suggests thatthe higher perilymphatic K^+ concentration *in vivo*may increase the levels of the cation around the basolateral spaces of OHCs and provide an unfavourable condition for their survival. To test this, the *nmf239* mutation was bred on to a mouse line that lacks POU3F4, a transcription factor that is necessary for K^+ recycling in the cochlea. In the absence of POU3F4, the mice have reduced endocochlear potential. The double mutant mice donot display OHC death, which suggests that reducing the driving force for K^+ rescues the OHCs from degeneration. Thus, the p.Phe35Leumutation in claudin 9 increases the permeability of the reticular lamina to K^+, which escapes into the extracellular spaces around the base of OHCs, similar to that suggested for *Cldn14* null mutants.

A high level of potassium in this region is known to prolong the depolarization of OHCs and is toxic to them[1]. Thus, in the *nmf329* mutant, loss of claudin 9-mediated barrier function leads to hair cell death due to K^+ toxicity.

Concluding Remarks

Tight junctions are key to maintaining fluid barriers in all epithelia that line a lumen or cavity and this compartmentalization is essential for homeostasis. In the inner ear, the scala media of the cochlea that houses the sensory cells is isolated from the rest of the organ by tight junctions between the epithelia lining this sensory compartment. These intercellular junctions are pre-requisites for cochlear function as they not only prevent intermixing of the compositionally distinct cochlear fluids, but are also an integral part of the machinery that generates the endocochlear potential. Several tight junction proteins are found in the mouse cochlea, including at least 15 different types of claudins, which suggests the complexity of the junctions involved. Moreover, functional redundancy may compensate for the loss of function or absence of one of the tight junction proteins due to mutations. However, some of these junctional proteins are indispensable for the hearing process as mutations in them cause hearing loss in humans and mice. While most of these mutations appear to affect the barrier function of the corresponding epithelia, at least one of them, the genomic duplication of *TJP2*, results in signal transduction defects. As more information about the cellular signaling roles of tight junction proteins becomes available, it is necessary to probe similar functions of these proteins in the cochlear epithelia. Pattern formation during development and its maintenance are processes that are likely to be dependent on signaling from tight junctions. Furthermore, the rigidity of the reticular lamina, a feature that is essential to cochlear sensitivity, may also be directly involved in signaling to and from the tight and adherence junctions. Thus, future efforts need to be directed towards elucidating the signal transduction roles played by tight junction proteins in the cochlea.

Acknowledgments

Research in the Riazuddin laboratory for human and mouse genomics is funded by the National Institutes of Health (NIDCD) R01DC011748; R01DC011803 and Action on Hearing Loss grants. Research in the Ahmed laboratory is funded by the National Institutes of Health (NIDCD) R00DC009287 andRPBCareer Development Award.

References

[1] Wangemann, P. Supporting sensory transduction: cochlear fluid homeostasis and the endocochlear potential. *The Journal of physiology* 576, 11-21 (2006).

[2] Zdebik, A. a, Wangemann, P. and Jentsch, T.J. Potassium ion movement in the inner ear: insights from genetic disease and mouse models. *Physiology (Bethesda, Md.)* 24, 307-16 (2009).

[3] Kros, C.J. *The Cochlea*. 8, (Springer New York: New York, NY, 1996).

[4] Nin, F. *et al.* The endocochlear potential depends on two K+ diffusion potentials and an electrical barrier in the stria vascularis of the inner ear. *Proceedings of the National Academy of Sciences of the United States of America* 105, 1751-6 (2008).

[5] Zdebik, A. a, Wangemann, P. and Jentsch, T.J. Potassium ion movement in the inner ear: insights from genetic disease and mouse models. *Physiology (Bethesda, Md.)* 24, 307-16 (2009).

[6] Tsukita, S., Yamazaki, Y., Katsuno, T. and Tamura, a Tight junction-based epithelial microenvironment and cell proliferation. *Oncogene* 27, 6930-8 (2008).

[7] Schulzke, J.-D. and Fromm, M. Tight junctions: molecular structure meets function. *Annals of the New York Academy of Sciences* 1165, 1-6 (2009).

[8] Anderson, J.M. and Van Itallie, C.M. Physiology and function of the tight junction. *Cold Spring Harbor perspectives in biology* 1, a002584 (2009).

[9] Steed, E., Balda, M.S. and Matter, K. Dynamics and functions of tight junctions. *Trends in cell biology* 20, 142-9 (2010).

[10] Jahnke, K. [Intercellular junctions in the guinea pig stria vascularis as shown by freeze-etching (author's transl)]. *Anatomy and embryology* 147, 189-201 (1975).

[11] Gulley, R.L. and Reese, T.S. Intercellular junctions in the reticular lamina of the organ of Corti. *Journal of Neurocytology* 5, 479-507 (1976).

[12] Nunes, F.D. *et al.* Distinct subdomain organization and molecular composition of a tight junction with adherens junction features. *Journal of cell science* 119, 4819-27 (2006).

[13] Stevenson, B.R., Siliciano, J.D., Mooseker, M.S. and Goodenough, D.A. Identification of ZO-1: a high molecular weight polypeptide associated with the tight junction (zonula occludens) in a variety of epithelia. *The Journal of cell biology* 103, 755-66 (1986).

[14] Fanning, A.S. and Anderson, J.M. Zonula occludens-1 and -2 are cytosolic scaffolds that regulate the assembly of cellular junctions. *Annals of the New York Academy of Sciences* 1165, 113-20 (2009).

[15] Tsukita, S. *et al.* Roles of ZO-1 and ZO-2 in establishment of the belt-like adherens and tight junctions with paracellular permselective barrier function. *Annals of the New York Academy of Sciences* 1165, 44-52 (2009).

[16] Katsuno, T. *et al.* Deficiency of Zonula Occludens-1 Causes Embryonic Lethal Phenotype Associated with Defected Yolk Sac Angiogenesis and Apoptosis of Embryonic Cells. *Molecular Biology of the Cell* 19, 2465-2475 (2008).

[17] Xu, J. *et al.* Early Embryonic Lethality of Mice Lacking ZO-2, but Not ZO-3, Reveals Critical and Nonredundant Roles for Individual Zonula Occludens Proteins in Mammalian Development. *Molecular and Cellular Biology* 28, 1669-1678 (2008).

[18] Walsh, T. *et al.* Genomic duplication and overexpression of TJP2/ZO-2 leads to altered expression of apoptosis genes in progressive nonsyndromic hearing loss DFNA51. *American journal of human genetics* 87, 101-9 (2010).

[19] Guillemot, L., Paschoud, S., Pulimeno, P., Foglia, A. and Citi, S. The cytoplasmic plaque of tight junctions: a scaffolding and signalling center. *Biochimica et biophysica acta* 1778, 601-13 (2008).

[20] Balda, M.S. and Matter, K. Tight junctions and the regulation of gene expression. *Biochimica et biophysica acta* 1788, 761-7 (2009).

[21] Furuse, M. Claudin-1 and -2: Novel Integral Membrane Proteins Localizing at Tight Junctions with No Sequence Similarity to Occludin. *The Journal of Cell Biology* 141, 1539-1550 (1998).

[22] Tsukita, S. and Furuse, M. The structure and function of claudins, cell adhesion molecules at tight junctions. *Annals of the New York Academy of Sciences* 915, 129-35 (2000).

[23] Yu, A.S.L., Enck, A.H., Lencer, W.I. and Schneeberger, E.E. Claudin-8 expression in Madin-Darby canine kidney cells augments the paracellular barrier to cation permeation. *The Journal of biological chemistry* 278, 17350-9 (2003).

[24] Colegio, O.R., Van Itallie, C.M., McCrea, H.J., Rahner, C. and Anderson, J.M. Claudins create charge-selective channels in the paracellular pathway between epithelial cells. *American journal of physiology. Cell physiology* 283, C142-7 (2002).

[25] Furuse, M., Furuse, K., Sasaki, H. and Tsukita, S. Conversion of zonulae occludentes from tight to leaky strand type by introducing claudin-2 into Madin-Darby canine kidney I cells. *The Journal of cell biology* 153, 263-72 (2001).

[26] Nitta, T. *et al.* Size-selective loosening of the blood-brain barrier in claudin-5-deficient mice. *The Journal of cell biology* 161, 653-60 (2003).

[27] Morita, K. Claudin multigene family encoding four-transmembrane domain protein components of tight junction strands. *Proceedings of the National Academy of Sciences* 96, 511-516 (1999).

[28] Lim, T.S., Vedula, S.R.K., Hunziker, W. and Lim, C.T. Kinetics of adhesion mediated by extracellular loops of claudin-2 as revealed by single-molecule force spectroscopy. *Journal of molecular biology* 381, 681-91 (2008).

[29] Furuse, M., Sasaki, H. and Tsukita, S. Manner of interaction of heterogeneous claudin species within and between tight junction strands. *The Journal of cell biology* 147, 891-903 (1999).

[30] Itoh, M. Direct Binding of Three Tight Junction-associated MAGUKs, ZO-1, ZO-2, and ZO-3, with the COOH Termini of Claudins. *The Journal of Cell Biology* 147, 1351-1363 (1999).

[31] Rüffer, C. and Gerke, V. The C-terminal cytoplasmic tail of claudins 1 and 5 but not its PDZ-binding motif is required for apical localization at epithelial and endothelial tight junctions. *European journal of cell biology* 83, 135-44 (2004).

[32] Van Itallie, C.M. and Anderson, J.M. The molecular physiology of tight junction pores. *Physiology (Bethesda, Md.)* 19, 331-8 (2004).

[33] Kitajiri, S.-iciro *et al.* Expression patterns of claudins, tight junction adhesion molecules, in the inner ear. *Hearing Research* 187, 25-34 (2004).

[34] Ben-Yosef, T. Claudin 14 knockout mice, a model for autosomal recessive deafness DFNB29, are deaf due to cochlear hair cell degeneration. *Human Molecular Genetics* 12, 2049-2061 (2003).

[35] Nakano, Y. *et al.* A claudin-9-based ion permeability barrier is essential for hearing. *PLoS genetics* 5, e1000610 (2009).

[36] Raleigh, D., Marchiando, A. and Zhang, Y. Tight Junction – associated MARVEL Proteins MarvelD3 , Tricellulin , and Occludin Have Distinct but Overlapping Functions. *Molecular Biology of the cell* 21, 1200-1213 (2010).

[37] Furuse, M. Occludin: a novel integral membrane protein localizing at tight junctions. *The Journal of Cell Biology* 123, 1777-1788 (1993).

[38] Li, Y., Fanning, A.S., Anderson, J.M. and Lavie, A. Structure of the conserved cytoplasmic C-terminal domain of occludin: identification of the ZO-1 binding surface. *Journal of molecular biology* 352, 151-64 (2005).

[39] Sakakibara, A. Possible Involvement of Phosphorylation of Occludin in Tight Junction Formation. *The Journal of Cell Biology* 137, 1393-1401 (1997).

[40] Balda, M.S. *et al.* Functional dissociation of paracellular permeability and transepithelial electrical resistance and disruption of the apical-basolateral intramembrane diffusion barrier by expression of a mutant tight junction membrane protein. *The Journal of cell biology* 134, 1031-49 (1996).

[41] Furuse, M. *et al.* Direct association of occludin with ZO-1 and its possible involvement in the localization of occludin at tight junctions. *The Journal of cell biology* 127, 1617-26 (1994).

[42] Furuse, M. A Single Gene Product, Claudin-1 or -2,Reconstitutes Tight Junction Strands and Recruits Occludin in Fibroblasts. *The Journal of Cell Biology* 143, 391-401 (1998).

[43] Itoh, M., Morita, K. and Tsukita, S. Characterization of ZO-2 as a MAGUK family member associated with tight as well as adherens junctions with a binding affinity to occludin and alpha catenin. *The Journal of biological chemistry* 274, 5981-6 (1999).

[44] McCarthy, K. *et al.* Occludin is a functional component of the tight junction. *Journal of Cell Science* 109, 2287-2298 (1996).

[45] Chen, Y., Merzdorf, C., Paul, D.L. and Goodenough, D.A. COOH terminus of occludin is required for tight junction barrier function in early Xenopus embryos. *The Journal of cell biology* 138, 891-9 (1997).

[46] Wong, V. and Gumbiner, B.M. A synthetic peptide corresponding to the extracellular domain of occludin perturbs the tight junction permeability barrier. *The Journal of cell biology* 136, 399-409 (1997).

[47] Saitou, M. *et al.* Occludin-deficient embryonic stem cells can differentiate into polarized epithelial cells bearing tight junctions. *The Journal of cell biology* 141, 397-408 (1998).

[48] Saitou, M. *et al.* Complex phenotype of mice lacking occludin, a component of tight junction strands. *Molecular biology of the cell* 11, 4131-42 (2000).

[49] Ikenouchi, J. *et al.* Tricellulin constitutes a novel barrier at tricellular contacts of epithelial cells. *The Journal of cell biology* 171, 939-45 (2005).

[50] K Westphal, J. *et al.* Tricellulin forms homomeric and heteromeric tight junctional complexes. *Cellular and molecular life sciences CMLS* 67, 2057-2068 (2010).

[51] Riazuddin, S. *et al.* Tricellulin is a tight-junction protein necessary for hearing. *American journal of human genetics* 79, 1040-51 (2006).

[52] Ohkuni, T. *et al.* Expression and localization of tricellulin in human nasal epithelial cells in vivo and in vitro. *Medical molecular morphology* 42, 204-11 (2009).

[53] Ikenouchi, J., Sasaki, H. and Tsukita, S. Loss of occludin affects tricellular localization of tricellulin. *Molecular biology of the cell* 19, 4687-4693 (2008).

[54] Masuda, S. *et al.* LSR defines cell corners for tricellular tight junction formation in epithelial cells. *Journal of cell science* 124, 548-55 (2011).

[55] Krug, S., Amasheh, S. and Richter, J. Tricellulin forms a barrier to macromolecules in tricellular tight junctions without affecting ion permeability. *Molecular biology of the cell* 20, 3713-3724 (2009).

[56] Chishti, M.S. *et al.* Splice-site mutations in the TRIC gene underlie autosomal recessive nonsyndromic hearing impairment in Pakistani families. *Journal of human genetics* 53, 101-5 (2008).

[57] Safka Brožková, D. *et al.* DFNB49 is an important cause of non-syndromic deafness in Czech Roma patients but not in the general Czech population. *Clinical genetics* (2011).doi:10.1111/j.1399-0004.2011. 01817.x.

[58] Steed, E., Rodrigues, N.T.L., Balda, M.S. and Matter, K. Identification of MarvelD3 as a tight junction-associated transmembrane protein of the occludin family. *BMC cell biology* 10, 95 (2009).

[59] Citi, S., Sabanay, H., Jakes, R., Geiger, B. and Kendrick-Jones, J. Cingulin, a new peripheral component of tight junctions. *Nature* 333, 272-6 (1988).

[60] Cordenonsi, M. Cingulin Contains Globular and Coiled-coil Domains and Interacts with ZO-1, ZO-2, ZO-3, and Myosin. *The Journal of Cell Biology* 147, 1569-1582 (1999).

[61] Bazzoni, G. *et al.* Interaction of junctional adhesion molecule with the tight junction components ZO-1, cingulin, and occludin. *The Journal of biological chemistry* 275, 20520-6 (2000).

[62] Guillemot, L. *et al.* Disruption of the cingulin gene does not prevent tight junction formation but alters gene expression. *Journal of cell science* 117, 5245-56 (2004).

[63] Raphael, Y. and Altschuler, R.A. Reorganization of cytoskeletal and junctional proteins during cochlear hair cell degeneration. *Cell motility and the cytoskeleton* 18, 215-27 (1991).

[64] Leonova, E.V. and Raphael, Y. Organization of cell junctions and cytoskeleton in the reticular lamina in normal and ototoxically damaged organ of Corti. *Hearing Research* 113, 14-28 (1997).

[65] Hildebrand, J.D. Shroom regulates epithelial cell shape via the apical positioning of an actomyosin network. *Journal of cell science* 118, 5191-203 (2005).

[66] Dietz, M.L., Bernaciak, T.M., Vendetti, F., Kielec, J.M. and Hildebrand, J.D. Differential actin-dependent localization modulates the evolutionarily conserved activity of Shroom family proteins. *The Journal of biological chemistry* 281, 20542-54 (2006).

[67] Etournay, R. *et al.* Shroom2, a myosin-VIIa- and actin-binding protein, directly interacts with ZO-1 at tight junctions. *Journal of cell science* 120, 2838-50 (2007).

[68] González-Mariscal, L., Tapia, R. and Chamorro, D. Crosstalk of tight junction components with signaling pathways. *Biochimica et biophysica acta* 1778, 729-56 (2008).

[69] Bauer, H., Zweimueller-Mayer, J., Steinbacher, P., Lametschwandtner, A. and Bauer, H.C. The dual role of zonula occludens (ZO) proteins. *Journal of biomedicine and biotechnology* 2010, 402593 (2010).

[70] Gottardi, C.J., Arpin, M., Fanning, A.S. and Louvard, D. The junction-associated protein, zonula occludens-1, localizes to the nucleus before the maturation and during the remodeling of cell-cell contacts. *Proceedings of the National Academy of Sciences of the United States of America* 93, 10779-84 (1996).

[71] Islas, S., Vega, J., Ponce, L. and González-Mariscal, L. Nuclear localization of the tight junction protein ZO-2 in epithelial cells. *Experimental cell research* 274, 138-48 (2002).

[72] Traweger, A. *et al.* The tight junction protein ZO-2 localizes to the nucleus and interacts with the heterogeneous nuclear ribonucleoprotein scaffold attachment factor-B. *The Journal of biological chemistry*278, 2692-700 (2003).

[73] Balda, M.S. and Matter, K. The tight junction protein ZO-1 and an interacting transcription factor regulate ErbB-2 expression. *The EMBO journal* 19, 2024-33 (2000).

[74] Balda, M.S., Garrett, M.D. and Matter, K. The ZO-1-associated Y-box factor ZONAB regulates epithelial cell proliferation and cell density. *The Journal of cell biology* 160, 423-32 (2003).

[75] Sourisseau, T. *et al.* Regulation of PCNA and cyclin D1 expression and epithelial morphogenesis by the ZO-1-regulated transcription factor ZONAB/DbpA. *Molecular and cellular biology* 26, 2387-98 (2006).

[76] Motokura, T. *et al.* A novel cyclin encoded by a bcl1-linked candidate oncogene. *Nature* 350, 512-5 (1991).

[77] Lehmann, A.R. and Fuchs, R.P. Gaps and forks in DNA replication: Rediscovering old models. *DNA repair* 5, 1495-8 (2006).

[78] Strzalka, W. and Ziemienowicz, A. Proliferating cell nuclear antigen (PCNA): a key factor in DNA replication and cell cycle regulation. *Annals of botany* 107, 1127-40 (2011).

[79] Keon, B.H., Schäfer, S., Kuhn, C., Grund, C. and Franke, W.W. Symplekin, a novel type of tight junction plaque protein. *The Journal of cell biology* 134, 1003-18 (1996).

[80] Kavanagh, E. *et al.* Functional interaction between the ZO-1-interacting transcription factor ZONAB/DbpA and the RNA processing factor symplekin. *Journal of cell science* 119, 5098-105 (2006).

[81] Huerta, M. *et al.* Cyclin D1 is transcriptionally down-regulated by ZO-2 via an E box and the transcription factor c-Myc. *Molecular biology of the cell* 18, 4826-36 (2007).

[82] Betanzos, A. *et al.* The tight junction protein ZO-2 associates with Jun, Fos and C/EBP transcription factors in epithelial cells. *Experimental cell research* 292, 51-66 (2004).

[83] Guillemot, L. and Citi, S. Cingulin regulates claudin-2 expression and cell proliferation through the small GTPase RhoA. *Molecular biology of the cell* 17, 3569-77 (2006).

[84] Citi, S. *et al.* The tight junction protein cingulin regulates gene expression and RhoA signaling. *Annals of the New York Academy of Sciences* 1165, 88-98 (2009).

[85] Wilcox, E.R. *et al.* Mutations in the gene encoding tight junction claudin-14 cause autosomal recessive deafness DFNB29. *Cell* 104, 165-72 (2001).

[86] Wattenhofer, M. *et al.* Different mechanisms preclude mutant CLDN14 proteins from forming tight junctions in vitro. *Human mutation* 25, 543-9 (2005).

[87] Bashir, R., Fatima, A. and Naz, S. Mutations in CLDN14 are associated with different hearing thresholds. *Journal of human genetics* 55, 767-70 (2010).

[88] Ahmed, Z.M. *et al.* Clinical manifestations of DFNB29 deafness. *Advances in oto-rhino-laryngology* 61, 156-60 (2002).

[89] Lee, K. *et al.* Novel CLDN14 mutations in Pakistani families with autosomal recessive non-syndromic hearing loss. *American journal of medical genetics. Part A* 158A, 315-21 (2012).

[90] Thorleifsson, G. *et al.* Sequence variants in the CLDN14 gene associate with kidney stones and bone mineral density. *Nature genetics* 41, 926-30 (2009).

[91] Gow, A. *et al.* Deafness in Claudin 11-null mice reveals the critical contribution of basal cell tight junctions to stria vascularis function. *The Journal of neuroscience* 24, 7051-62 (2004).

[92] Elkouby-Naor, L., Abassi, Z., Lagziel, A., Gow, A. and Ben-Yosef, T. Double gene deletion reveals lack of cooperation between claudin 11 and claudin 14 tight junction proteins. *Cell and tissue research* 333, 427-38 (2008).

[93] GOW, A. CNS Myelin and Sertoli Cell Tight Junction Strands Are Absent in Osp/Claudin-11 Null Mice. *Cell* 99, 649-659 (1999).

In: Inner Ear Development and Hearing Loss
Editors: Saima Riazuddin and Zubair Ahmed

ISBN: 978-1-62417-011-9

Chapter 3

USHER AND BARDET-BIEDL SYNDROME PROTEINS: NEW PIECES IN THE PLANAR CELL POLARITY PUZZLE

Arnaud P. J. Giese[1,2], Saima Riazuddin[1,2] and Zubair M. Ahmed[1,2*]

[1]Division of Pediatric Otolaryngology-Head and Neck Surgery, and
[2]Division of Pediatric Ophthalmology,
Cincinnati Children's Hospital Medical Center, Cincinnati, Ohio, US

ABSTRACT

The inner ear is one of the best systems in mammals to study planar cell polarity (PCP). During development of the inner ear, the PCP pathway controls the convergent extension and polarization of the stereociliary bundles of sensory hair cells of the organ of Corti. These two mechanisms are essential for the integrity of the sensory epithelium and for hearing. The discovery of several mutants, presenting a misorientation of the stereociliary bundles in the inner ear, permitted identification of the core genes that control PCP mechanisms. However, PCP proteins acting downstream in this pathway still remain unclear. Emerging evidences have shown that Usher proteins, which are essential for the establishment of various stereociliary links and mechanotransduction complex, and Bardet-Biedl Syndrome (BBS) proteins, which are involved in ciliogenesis, could be components of the PCP pathway. Regarding these new elements, it appears essential to put PCP proteins in a hearing context.

INTRODUCTION

The ear can be defined as the organ of hearing and balance. In mammals, the ear is composed of three components: the outer ear, the middle ear and inner ear (Figure 1). The outer ear collects sound by acting as a funnel. It is composed of the pinna and the auditory

[*] Email: Zubair.ahmed@cchmc.org

canal. The pinna, which is composed of an elastic cartilage, amplifies the sound and directs it to the auditory canal, a cartilaginous structure embedded in the temporal bone cavity. The middle ear transfers the sound from the outer to the inner ear. It is composed of the tympanic membrane and the ossicular chain that is composed of three small bones: the malleus, the incus, and the stapes. These three bones, also called ossicles, are articulated together and provide a link between the eardrum and the oval window of the inner ear. The vibrations of air in the auditory canal, caused by the emission of a sound, put the tympanic membrane in vibration. These vibrations are then transmitted through the ossicular chain to the inner ear. The inner ear is a complex structure and is composed of a rigid cavity called the bony labyrinth filled with perilymph and the membranous labyrinth that is floating in it. The membranous labyrinth is composed of the cochlear labyrinth, necessary for hearing and the vestibular labyrinth, which is essential for balancing. The organ of Corti is the sensory epithelium of the cochlea and is composed of neuro-sensory hair cells and non-sensory supporting cells. The organ of Corti receives vibration from the middle ear, and converts the mechanical movement into an electrical signal that is transmitted to the brain, through a mechanism known as mechano-electricaltransduction (MET). Deficits affecting MET lead to deafness.

In the US, deafness at birth affects one child in a thousand. 5% of the population aged under 45 and 30% of those over 70 years also suffer from hearing loss. Hearing loss can be classified into transmission deafness or perception deafness depending on which part of the ear is affected (Figure 1). Transmission deafness is hearing loss that can often be corrected with surgery or a hearing aid. Transmission deafness is due to a lesion in the outer or the middle ear. Impairment may result from a malfunction of the pinna, the external auditory canal, the eardrum or the ossicular chain. Perception deafness is a neuro-sensory hearing loss.

This is the most common type of hearing loss and is caused by lesions in the auditory system. This impairment is due to defects affecting the inner ear, the auditory nerve responsible for the electrical transmission of auditory information to the brain, or the auditory cortex that analyzes sound information.

Transmission and perception deafness are due to multiple factors such as environmental causes, diseases or neurological disorders. The most common environmental causes are elevated sound levels and trauma that can affect the middle and the inner ear. Ototoxicity due to antibiotics and other medication causes death of inner ear hair cells.

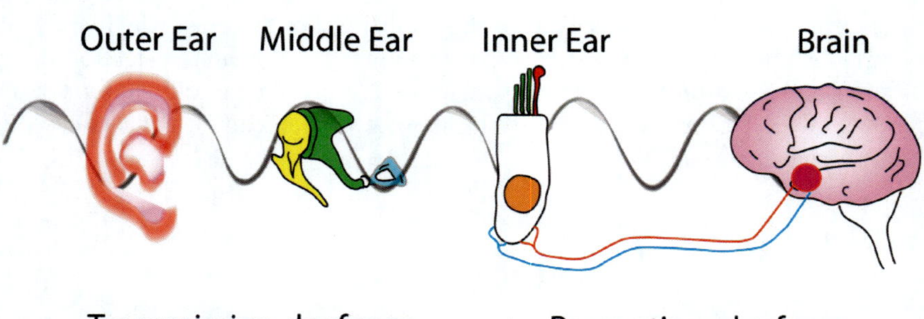

Figure 1. Schematic showing how the sound waves are transferred to the brain through the outer, middle and inner ear. The middle ear is composed of the malleus (yellow), the incus (green) and the stapes (blue).

Diseases such as Menière's, congenital rubella or meningitis can affect hearing. In adults, presbycusis is the most common cause with a hereditary predisposition and affects inner ear hair cells. In childhood, 30-45% of profound deafness is associated with a genetic disorder. 70% of these cases have been associated with non-syndromic diseases while 30% with syndromic diseases.

The most common human syndromes that include deafness are the Usher syndrome, the Pendred syndrome, Jervell and Lange-Nielsen syndrome, Waardenburg Type I and Type II syndromes and Alport syndrome. Usher syndrome (USH) is a group of autosomal recessively inherited disorders that leads to deaf-blindness. Usher syndrome is characterized by an impairment of the auditory system and a progressive retinal degeneration, which may be accompanied by vestibular areflexia. Inner ear impairment leads to hearing loss and balance-maintaining disorders, whereas retinitis pigmentosa (RP) leads to night blindness. Usher syndrome is classified into three clinical types: USH type I, USH type II and USH type III. Each clinical type is characterized by variability in the degree of hearing loss and the presence or absence of vestibular balance disorder. RP is common to all classes. For additional information, see (Yan and Liu, 2010).

Structure and Function of the Organ of Corti

In mammals, the organ of Corti is composed of multiple cell types: neuro-sensory hair cells and supporting cells. Hair cells are organized in three rows of outer hair cells (OHC), located on the distal side of the epithelium, and a single row of inner hair cells (IHC), located on the proximal side of the epithelium (Figure 2).

A supporting cell envelopes each hair cell. Hair cells possess characteristics of both epithelial cells, polarized along the apical basal axis, and neuronal cells, since they are responsible for converting the movement of the basilar membrane, generated by sound, into electrical signals understandable by the brain.

Hair cells of the organ of Corti contain, on their apical surface, an actin rich structure termed as stereociliary bundle. Stereocilia are embedded in and projected from the cuticular plate, an actin-rich firm laminar structure. Stereociliary bundles are composed of three rows of stereocilia with graduated heights and have a "W" or "V" shape. They are maintained together by various protein links including ankle links, lateral links, horizontal top connector, and tip-links. Planar Cell polarity pathway (PCP) controls the alignment of stereociliary bundles in the plane of the epithelium. In developing the mouse organ of Corti, a primary cilium or kinocilium is found at the vertex of the hair bundle, which regresses around P6-P7. The kinocilium, formed by acetylated tubulin, is supported by a basal body, and is the first polarized structure along the proximal distal axis followed by the stereociliary bundle polarization.

Hair cells depolarize in response to the deflection of their stereociliary bundle. Indeed, stereocilia are anchored into the tectoriale membrane and when the basilar membrane begins to move due to sounds vibration, they are able to detect. The rigidity of the stereocilia enables tension to develop in the tip links, which results in opening of the MET channels.

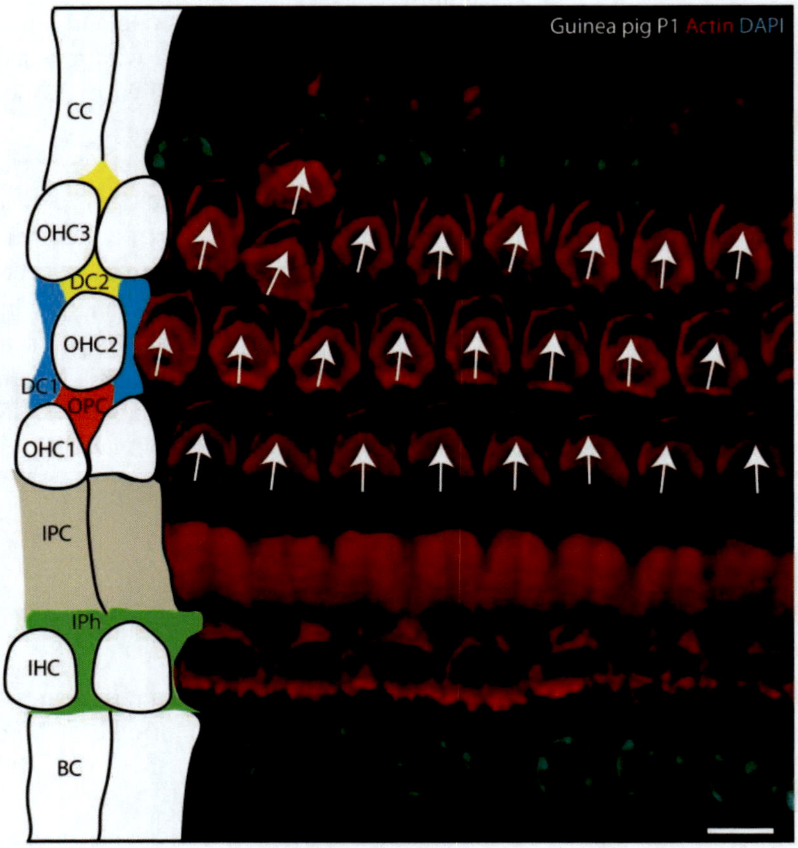

Figure 2. Top view of the organ of Corti: The organ of Corti is composed of three rows of outer hair cells (OHC1, 2, 3) and one row of inner hair cells (IHC). Outer hair cells have a cylindrical shape, while inner hair cells have a pear shape. Hair cells are enveloped by supporting cells such as Deiter's cells (DC1, 2), outer and inner pillar cells (OPC, IPC), and inner phalangeal cells (IPh). Hair bundles are stained with phalloidin (Red) and Nucleus with DAPI (Blue). The orientation of each outer hair bundle is represented by a white arrow. Scale bar: 10um.

Stereociliary Bundle: Sensor of the Hearing

Deflection of stereocilia converts sound signals into electrical signals (Figure 3). Thereby, the stereociliary bundle is the sensor of the hearing. To allow normal mechanotranscution multiple parameters are essential. Firstly, all the stereociliary bundles have to be oriented in the same direction along the medio-lateral axis of the cochlea. In 1999, Yoshida et al, showed that guinea pigs with congenital anomaly could show distinctly abnormal orientation of the W-shaped stereociliary bundle where some hair bundles are rotated up to 180 degrees from the normal orientation. Cochlear sensitivity was assayed via compound action potentials, and the thresholds in affected animals were elevated by 5 to 10 dB compared to normal controls (Yoshida and Liberman, 1999). Recent studies revealed that the orientation of stereociliary bundles is controlled by the PCP pathway, which is also linked to signaling from the primary cilia and basal bodies.

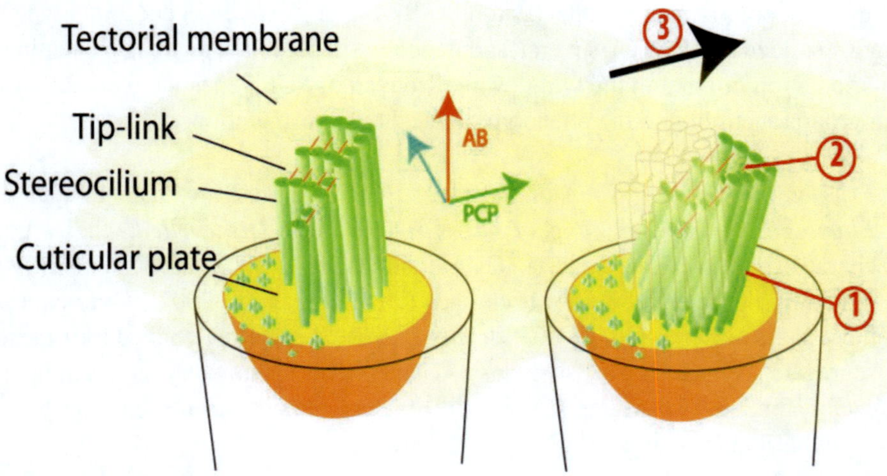

Figure 3. Schematic of stereociliary bundle structure: The stereociliary bundle is composed of stereocilia (green) and is anchored at its base into the cuticular plate (yellow) and in the tectorial membrane at its apex (light yellow). Tip links are represented in red. The sensory function of the stereociliary bundle is dependent on three parameters: (1) the stiffness of stereocilia due to actin polymerization. (2) the presence of tip-links that are stretched when the bundle is deflected. (3) the orientation of the bundle along the PCP axis, which allows an optimum tension of tip-links when the bundle is deflected.

Furthermore, kinocilium is indispensible for the establishment of PCP within the organ of Corti. Also, a few molecular components from the primary cilium and the basal body could act downstream of the PCP pathway. Secondly, the structure of the stereociliary bundle is essential to assure their deflection and the depolarization process. The height of the stereocilia and their rootlets, regulated by the polymerization of actin, are important for the anchorage of their tip into the tectorial membrane and in the cuticular plate, respectively.

Finally, stereocilia have to be held together by diverse extracellular links assured especially by the Usher protein. Usher proteins are also involved in the establishment of tip-links and absolutely necessary for hearing. Interestingly, recent publications have shown that the Usher protein could be directly linked to the PCP pathway, and act downstream.

In this chapter, we will further discuss how the PCP pathway, the cilia signaling pathway and the Usher protein pathway are connected together, and how this relationship is necessary for the hearing process.

Planar Cell Polarity in the Organ of Corti and Stereociliary Bundle Polarization

Generalities on PCP

PCP has been widely studied in *Drosophila melanogaster*, where it regulates several mechanisms including the uniform distal orientation of hairs localized on the epithelium of the wing and the rotation of ommatidia in the eye (Adler, 2002, Strutt, 2003, Klein and Mlodzik, 2005, Axelrod, 2009). In all these processes, PCP signaling results in cytoskeleton remodeling and polarization events (Eaton, 1997). The first few genes involved in PCP signaling were identified when several spontaneous drosophila mutants, presenting a non-uniform orientation of hairs in the wing, were discovered. *PCP* genes were classified into two signaling groups according to the phenotype caused by their mutations.

- *Frizzled / Flamingo* group or the Core *PCP* gene cassette that includes *Frizzled, Flamingo, Strabismus/Vang, Prickle, Diego* and *Dishevelled*: these genes are characterized by three criteria. (1) Mutations in these genes lead to PCP defects including the misdirection of trichomes (Lawrence et al., 2007). Over-expression of these genes also results in PCP defects. (2) PCP proteins, encoded by these genes, segregate asymmetrically in polarized cells. This asymmetry is essential for PCP establishment. (3) Mutants for any of these genes results in the loss of the asymmetric localization of all core PCP proteins.
- *Fat / Dachsous / Four-jointed* cassette: Mutations affecting *fat (ft), Dachsous (ds) or four-jointed (fj)* cause polarity defects but also growth defects of the wings and legs of Drosophila (Lawrence et al., 2007). To date, it is assumed that *Fat / Dachsous / Four-jointed* cassette acts parallel to the *Frizzled / Flamingo* cassette in order to establish PCP (Lawrence et al., 2007).

Planar Cell Polarity in Mammals

In mammals, *PCP* core genes were initially identified based on their homologs in drosophila. Several spontaneous mutant and knockout mice were used. Mutants for *PCP* genes show a PCP defect in the inner ear characterized by a misorientation of the stereociliary bundles of cochlear hair cells. Stereociliary bundles are not aligned along the proximal distal axis of the cochlea. The kinocilium, the first structure that is polarized along the PCP axis of the sensory epithelium, is also mispolarized. In mammals, *PCP* core genes include

- *Vangl1/2*, homolog of *Strabismus/Vang*. *Vangl2* was identified due to a spontaneous mutation in Loop-tail mutant mice (Montcouquiol et al., 2003).
- *Frizzled3/6* (Wang et al., 2006)
- *Dishevelled1/2/3*
- *Celsr1*, homolog of *Flamingo* (Curtin et al., 2003)
- *Prickle2 (Tao et al., 2011)*
- *Diversin,* homolog of *Diego*

In mammals, due to the complexity of the genome compared to drosophila, *PCP* genes are duplicated (or more) such that several genes belong to the same family and are redundant. It is sometimes necessary to have mutations in several *PCP* gene family members in order to establish a phenotype in the inner ear. For example, only double knock-outs of *Dishevelled 1 and 2, Dishevelled 2 and 3* (Etheridge et al., 2008), or *Frizzled 3 and 6* (Wang et al., 2006) develop a defective PCP phenotype in the inner ear. Besides the inner ear, most of the time homozygous core *PCP* gene mutants present additional phenotypes such as:

- Defect in the asymmetric morphogenesis of hair follicles (Guo et al., 2004, Devenport and Fuchs, 2008).
- Eye lid closure defect
- Gastrochisis
- Convergent extension defect
- Neural tube closure defect or "Neural Tube Defects" (NTDs), which in its most severe form, results in a Craniorachischisis.
- Pathologies associated with cilia syndromes such as Bardet Biedl syndrome and kidney (Polycystic Kidney Disease) (Ross et al., 2005)
- Asymmetric division defect due to misorientation of mitotic spindles
- Heart defects (Phillips et al., 2007, Phillips et al., 2008)
- Neuronal migration and axon guidance defects

Despite the diversity of mechanisms controlled by the *PCP* gene, remodeling and polarization of the cytoskeleton, similar to that observed in the drosophila, appear to be a common criterion.

New **PCP** *Gene in Mammals*

Several new *PCP* genes have appeared in mammals during evolution. These genes were found due to spontaneous mutation, or ENU mutagenesis screening. All of these genes were identified regardless to the PCP phenotype that was seen in the Organ of Corti or to the neural tube defect in corresponding mutant. *Ptk7*, a transmembrane Tyrosine-protein kinase-like receptor, was identified in 2004 (Lu et al., 2004). *Scribble1* was identified in 2003 in the spontaneous circle tail mutant (Montcouquiol et al., 2003). ENU mutatgenesis screenings permitted the identification of *Sec24b*, *chuzhoi*, and new mutant alleles for *Scribble1* as *PCP* genes (Wansleeben et al., 2010).

Core PCP Protein Asymmetry

As in the epithelium of the wing and the eye of drosophila, proteins encoded by core *PCP* genes are asymmetrically distributed along the PCP axis in several tissues. This asymmetrical distribution was shown in several PCP models such as the organ of Corti, the vestibular sensory epithelium, and hair follicles (Montcouquiol et al., 2006, Wang et al., 2006). In all these models, core PCP protein asymmetry is localized at the interface of two cell types. In the organ of Corti, asymmetrical distribution is localized at the junction between hair cells and supporting cells on both the proximal, and the distal side of cells. Due to this junction localization, it is still unclear in which cell type PCP proteins are localized. However, a recent study using a *Frizzled3* mosaic mouse model has shown that Frizzled3/6 were localized in the proximal side of hair cells (Wang et al., 2006). To date, proximal and distal asymmetrical localization was shown for the following PCP proteins:

Proximal Side of Hair Cells

- Vangl2 (Montcouquiol et al., 2006, Qian et al., 2007, Jones et al., 2008). Recently, it has been proposed that Vangl2 could be localized in both the proximal side of hair cells, and the distal side of supporting cells (Warchol and Montcouquiol, 2010, Giese Arnaud, 2012).
- Frizzled3/6 (Wang et al., 2006)

Distal Side of Hair Cells

- Dishevelled 1/2/3 (Etheridge et al., 2008).

These asymmetrical distributions are transitory and observable by embryonic day (E) 14.5 to postnatal day (P) 5 in the organ of Corti. Interestingly, mutation in a single *PCP* gene leads to the loss of all PCP protein asymmetry, reflecting the cooperation between these proteins.

Regulation of the Asymmetrical Distribution of Core PCP Proteins

Several mechanisms could explain how a protein can be asymmetrically distributed in a tissue during development.

- A protein can be targeted to one side of a cell. For example, SEC24B, a golgi budding protein, is necessary for Vangl2 membrane targeting and asymmetrical localization (Wansleeben et al., 2010).
- A transmembrane protein can be specifically endocytosed and recycled on one side of a cell (Giese Arnaud, 2012).
- A transmembrane protein can be degraded on one side of a cell. Recently, Smurfs proteins, involved in degradation of protein through an ubiquitination process, have been linked to PCP regulation (Narimatsu et al., 2009).
- A transmembrane protein can be specifically stabilized on one side. For example, Vangl2 has been shown to interact to the scaffolding protein Scribble1 (Montcouquiol et al., 2003).

Convergent Extension and PCP in the Organ of Corti Development

Convergent extension is the process by which a tissue of an embryo is restructured to converge along one axis and extend along a perpendicular axis by cellular movement. Convergent extension mechanisms are also involved in the cochlear development. Indeed, in the mouse, the cochlear duct gets thinner and stretches between E16 and E18. Convergent extension of the tissue is a post-mitotic process that occurs without cell division or apoptosis. Only cell movements, radial and planar intercalation, ensure that the sensory epithelium is organized into four rows of hair cells that are perfectly aligned. Convergent extension process is also known to regulate the neural tube closure. The primitive nervous system of chordates embryos, termed the neural tube, is formed from the ectoderm near the median line, which thickens to constitute the neural plate. The neural tube is developed during neurulation by invagination of the neural plate, which then forms a neural groove. This groove is closed by convergence and fusion of the neural crest. Then, the neural crest separates from the tube and the tube expands to form the cephalic vesicle, while the rest of the neural tube forms the spinal cord. All PCP mutants have two major defects: (1) a neural tube closure defect termed spina bifida. In the most severe form, the neural tube can be completely opened causing craniorachischisis (2) a shorter cochlear duct, where an accumulation of sensory hair cells at the apex of the organ of Corti and an unusual number of hair cell rows are seen. Recently, secreted Wnt factors have been implicated in the regulation of planar cell polarity in cochleae of vertebrates (Dabdoub and Kelley, 2005, Qian et al., 2007). This is a major difference between the PCP models of mammals and invertebrates. In drosophila, Wng/Wnt is not involved in the regulation of PCP, since the Wng mutant does not show any defect in the orientation of trichome in the wings. In xenopus and zebrafish, several *Wnt* mutants have been associated with convergent extension defects during gastrulation, notably "*Pipetail*" (*Wnt5*) mutant and the "*Silberblick*" (*Wnt11*) mutant in zebrafish. In mammals, the *Wnt5a* mouse mutant that also shows a convergent extension defect, results in shorter and thicker cochlea, and hair cell stereociliary bundles. Convergent extension defects are more severe in a *Wnt5a*$^{+/-}$ *Vangl2*$^{Lp/+}$ double mutant, showing a genetic interaction between *Vangl2* and *Wnt5a*. However, the hair bundle orientation defect was less severe showing that *Vangl2* and *Wnt5a* could act in two different signaling pathways (Qian et al., 2007).

Planar Cell Polarity and Deafness

Homozygous mutants for core *PCP* genes are embryonic lethal due to critical defects, such as craniorachisisis, hampering the use of these animals for hearing defects. To date, we only know that the misorientation of stereociliary bundles leads to a reduction in cochlear sensitivity (Yoshida and Liberman, 1999). Interestingly, a mutation in genes that belongs to the core PCP gene family leads to deafness. For example, a mutation in *Frizzled 4* leads to progressive auditory dysfunction (Wang et al., 2001).

Theoretically, mutation in non-core *PCP* genes, such as PCP regulators or effectors, could also cause hearing defects. To illustrate this idea, recently, Bonaglia et al have shown that four patients, presenting several defects, including deafness and mental retardation, had a deletion of a 359Kb region in the chromosome 19 (19p13.12). This locus contains six genes, including *GIPC1*, a gene that encodes a scaffolding protein that is implicated in many PCP processes in different species (Bonaglia et al., 2010). The authors have made the hypothesis that hearing loss in these patients was due to GIPC1 haplo-insufficiency and an alteration of GIPC1/Myosin VI complex in the organ of Corti. Indeed, in humans, mutations in myosin VI are associated with dominant (DFNA22) and recessively (DFNB37) inherited deafness (Ahmed et al., 2003, Sanggaard et al., 2008). Previously, *Kermit*, a homolog of *GIPC1* in *Xenopus*, was shown to bind to the C-terminal part of the core PCP protein Frizzled3. Frizzled receptors are known to regulate PCP mechanisms such as convergent extension during gastrulation (Djiane et al., 2000). In 2001, Tan et al have shown that Kermit is involved in neural tube development and that its over-expression inhibits the induction of the neural crest mediated by Frizzled 3 (Tan et al., 2001). Interestingly, *Myosin VIIa*, a gene involved in Usher syndrome type I and deafness in humans, leads to planar cell polarity defects in the Drosophila wing when it is mutated (Winter et al., 2001).

BARDET-BIEDL SYNDROME AND PCP

Generalities on Bardet-Biedl

Bardet-Biedl syndrome (BBS) is a ciliopathic autosomal recessive human genetic disorder. BBS occurs with a prevalence rate of 1:130,000 and results in a disorder of the cellular cilia and the ciliary anchoring structures. BBS is characterized by several phenotypes, such as obesity, retinitis pigmentosa, hexadactyly post-axial, hypogenitalism, kidney damage and mental retardation. Interestingly, in minor clinical features, BBS is associated with hearing loss. Mutations in twelve genes are casually linked to BBS. These genes encode BBS proteins, which are located in the basal body and involved in the assembly of cilia. So far, the following genes are implicated in Bardet Biedl syndrome: *BBS1, BBS2, BBS4, BBS5, BBS7, TTC8* (*BBS8*), *BBS9, BBS6, BBS10, BBS12, ARL6* (*BBS3*) and *TRIM32* (*BBS11*).

BBS proteins are assembled into a multiple protein complex, called "BBSome". BBSome is involved in a process termed intraflagellar transport (IFT). IFT is bi-directional within the cilia and BBS proteins are assumed to transport vesicles along the cilium, and so are essential in its maintenance and function.

BBS and PCP Gene Are Genetically Linked

In 2005, Ross et al have shown that the zebrafish *Tri* gene, the homolog of the mouse *Vangl2* gene, interacts genetically with *BBS4*. $BBS4^{MO}$ and $Tri^{-/-}$ double mutant has a specific defect in convergent extension mechanism, resulting in a shorter embryo, folded onto itself (Ross et al., 2005). Similarly, $BBS8^{MO}$ and $Tri^{-/-}$ double mutant revealed genetic interaction between *BBS8* and *Tri,* which regulate the left-right asymmetry determination (May-Simera et al., 2010a). These observations permitted linking the known regulator of convergent extension, *BBS* and *PCP*. In human epithelial cells, Vangl2 is located at the basal body of cilia and co-localized with other BBS proteins (BBS1, BBS2, BBS3, BBS4, BBS5, BBS6, BBS7, BBS8). The analysis of $Vangl2^{Lp/+}$ double mutant either with *BBS4* or $BBS1^{+/-}$ mice revealed defects in the orientation of stereociliary bundles in the inner ear along with an anencephaly and an eyelid closure defect. The data suggest a requirement for cilia-related pathway in convergent extension (May-Simera et al., 2010a). Taken together, these data suggest that cilia are involved in the establishment of planar cell polarity pathway (see table 1). In 2008, Dr. Ping Chen's team found that IFT88 and KIF3a, like the BBS proteins, are involved in the intraflagellar transport and maintenance of the cilium, by acting downstream of the PCP pathway. The analysis of $Ift88^{CKO/CKO}$ $Vangl2^{Lp/+}$ and $Kif3a^{CKO/CKO}$ mutant mice revealed that the primary cilium located at the vertex of the stereociliary bundle was absent, despite the fact that maintenance of the basal body and orientation of hair bundles was disrupted. These two mutants also revealed circularized hair bundles. Hair cells presenting such phenotype had a central basal body, further supporting the hypothesis that basal body and the kinocilium are necessary for the bundle structure and its polarization. Another interesting finding in these mutant mice was that the asymmetrical localization of PCP proteins was conserved in the organ of Corti, despite bundle misorientation.

Table 1. Major PCP, Usher, cilia and BBS genes

Gene	*Species*	*Mutant*	*Properties*	*Function*	*References*
Bbs8	*Zebrafish*	*Bbs8*^{MO} ; *Tri*$^{-/-}$	*Cilia*	Left-right asymmetry defect, ciliopathies	May-Simera et al, 2010
Ift88	*Mouse*	*Ift88*$^{CKO/CKO}$ *Vangl2*$^{Lp/+}$	*Cilia*	Craniorachisisis, Stereociliary bundle orientation, Basal Body/kinocilium localization, Photoreceptor assembly and maintenance	Jones et al, 2008 Pazour et al, 2002
Kif3a	*Mouse*	*Kif3a*$^{CKO/CKO}$	*Cilia*	Stereociliary bundle orientation, Basal Body/kinocilium localization	Jones et al, 2008 Sipe et al, 2011
Bbs1	*Mouse*	*BBS1*$^{+/-}$; *Vangl2*$^{Lp/+}$	*Cilia*	Stereociliary bundle orientation, Craniorachisisis	May-Simera et al, 2010
Bbs4	*Zebrafish*	*Bbs4*^{MO} ; *Tri*$^{-/-}$	*Cilia*	Convergent extension	Ross et al, 2005
Bbs4	*Human*		*Cilia*	Deafness	Ahmad, J., et al. 2005
Fat4	*mouse*	*Fat4*$^{-/-}$; *Vangl2*$^{LP/+}$	*PCP*	Polycystic kidney syndrome	Saburi et al, 2008
GIPC1	*Human*	*Deletion*	*PCP*	Deafness	Bonaglia et al, 2010
GIPC1	*Mouse*	*shRNA*	*PCP*	PCP regulator, Vangl2 interactor	Giese et al. 2012
xGIPC1	*Xenopus*	-	*PCP*	Convergent extension, Regulator of Frizzled pathway	Tan et al, 2001
Frizzled3/6	*Mouse*	-	*PCP*	Stereociliary bundle orientation, Craniorachischisis	Wang et al, 2006
Dishevelled1 /2/3	*Mouse*	-	*PCP*	Stereociliary bundle orientation, Craniorachischisis	Etheridge et al, 2008
Vangl2	*Mouse*	*Loop tail*	*PCP*	Stereociliary bundle orientation, Craniorachischisis	Montcouquiol et al, 2003
Celsr1	*Mouse*	*Spin Cycle*	*PCP*	Stereociliary bundle orientation, Craniorachischisis	Curtin et al, 2003
Prickle	*Mouse*	-	*PCP*	Stereociliary bundle orientation, Craniorachischisis	Ueno et al, 2009
MyoVIIa	*Mouse*	*Myo7a*$^{4626SB/4626SB}$	*Usher*	PCP inner ear, Kinocilium polarization, Deafness	Lefevre et al, 2008
MyoVIIa	*Human*	*DFNB2*	*Usher*	Deafness	Weil et al, 1995
Cdh23	*Mouse*	*Cdh23*$^{v2J/v2J}$	*Usher*	Stereociliary bundle orientation	Lefevre et al, 2008
Pcdh15	*Mouse*	*Pcdh15*$^{av3J/av3J}$	*Usher*	Stereociliary bundle orientation, tip links structure	Lefevre et al, 2008
Pcdh15-CD2	*Mouse*	*Pcdh15*$^{\Delta CD2}$	*Usher*	Stereociliary bundle orientation, tip links structure	Webb et al, 2011
Sans	*Mouse*		*Usher*	Scaffolding protein	

In regular development, when PCP begins to establish within the cochlea, the transient asymmetrical localization of PCP proteins is the first event that occurs. This major work was the first evidence that ciliary proteins are acting downstream of PCP proteins (Jones et al., 2008). These results were further validated in 2011 but the authors specified that Kif3a regulates planar polarization of auditory hair cells through both ciliary and non-ciliary mechanisms (Sipe and Lu, 2011).

Interestingly, Bardet Biedl syndrome is characterized by RP and hearing loss, two criteria found in Usher syndrome. Several contributions have shown that Usher proteins are localized to the centrosome and basal body, and that they could act downstream the PCP pathway.

Recently, it has been shown that mutations of the centrosomal protein CEP290 lead to Leber congenital amaurosis (LCA), a hereditary cause of blindness like the Usher syndrome. CEP290 interacts with MKKS, another BBS protein.

MKKS mutations, implicated in the BBS syndrome, disrupted the interaction with CEP290. Interestingly, the combination of mutations in both CEP290 and MKKS improved ciliogenesis, probably by affecting the integrity of multi-protein complexes at the cilia transition zone and basal body (Rachel et al., 2012).

Usher Syndrome and Planar Cell Polarity

Usher syndrome (USH) is classified into three subtypes: USH1, USH2 and USH3, USH1 being the most severe. To date, 11 distinct loci have been correlated to Usher syndrome (see table 1). Proteins involved in each Usher syndrome subtypes are the following:

- USH 1: Myosin 7A (*USH1B*), an unconventional myosin, Harmonin (*USH1C*) and Sans (*USH1G*), two scaffold proteins, Cadherin 23 (*USH1D*), and Protocadherin 15 (*USH1F*), two cadherin domains containing proteins.
- USH 2: Usherin (*USH2A*), VLGR1 (*USH2C*), Whirlin (*USH2D*)
- USH 3: Clarin-1 (*USH3*)

The discovery of spontaneous mouse mutants for *USH1* genes has shown that the proteins encoded by these genes maintain the organization of the inner ear hair bundles.

Thereby, *deaf circler*, *shaker 1*, *Ames waltzer*, *waltzer* and *Jackson shaker* mutant mice, for harmonin, myosin 7a, protocadherin 15, sans and cadherin 23, respectively, have a bundle defect and a hearing loss (Gibson et al., 1995, Alagramam et al., 2001, Di Palma et al., 2001, Johnson et al., 2003, Kikkawa et al., 2003).

Usher proteins are the main components of Ankle links and Tip-links. Ankle links connect stereocilia of hair cells at their base. Tip-links connect the tip of each stereocilium, termed lower tip link density (LTLD) to the side of the adjacent taller stereocilium, termed upper tip-link density (UTLD). Tip-links are believed to interact with the transduction channel, and stereocilia movements change the tension in the tip-link. Upper and lower parts of tip-links are composed of cadherin 23 and protocadherin 15, respectively (Siemens et al., 2004, Ahmed et al., 2006, Kazmierczak et al., 2007). The increase of the tension results in the opening of transduction channels. Cadherin 23 and protocadherin 15 also participate in the establishment of transient lateral links that connect the kinocilium to the nearest stereocilia (Michel et al., 2005, Ahmed et al., 2006, Webb et al., 2011).

Usher Proteins Form a Variety of Complexes

Usher proteins form a multi-assembly complex and several interactions between USH1 proteins have been shown. Thereby, Harmonin and Whirlin, owing to their PDZ domains, are able to interact with the four other USH1 proteins and allow the formation of large molecular complexes (Boeda et al., 2002, Siemens et al., 2002, Adato et al., 2005, Reiners et al., 2005). Myosin 7a, an actin filament plus-end-directed myosin, can interact with protocadherin 15 and sans (Adato et al., 2005, Grati and Kachar, 2011) and is believed to bring these proteins from the base to the apex of stereocilia.

PCP Defects in the Inner Ear of Usher Mice Mutants

Several Usher mouse mutants present a PCP phenotype in the inner ear. Recently, analysis of many Ush1 mutant mice, including *MyoVIIa, Cdh23, Pcdh15, Sans* and *Harmonin* revealed defects in the proper positioning of kinocilium in the developing hair bundles of the inner ear. In *Cdh23* and *Pcdh15* mutants, most of the time the kinocilium was dissociated with the stereociliary bundle (Lefevre et al., 2008). More recently, it has been reported that *PCDH15-CD2* deficient mice have an abnormal polarization of hair bundles, an absence of kinociliary links and hearing impairment. Interestingly, these mice present circular hair bundles with a centered kinocilium, a phenotype similar to that seen in *Ift88* KO mutant. Like the *Ift88* KO mutant, *PCDH15-CD2* deficient mice present a normal distribution of PCP proteins in the sensory epithelia, suggesting that PCDH15-CD2 acts downstream of the PCP signaling pathway (Webb et al., 2011).

Based on these results, it is believed that the Usher proteins, like the BBS proteins may act downstream of PCP components to control polarity in the cochlea.

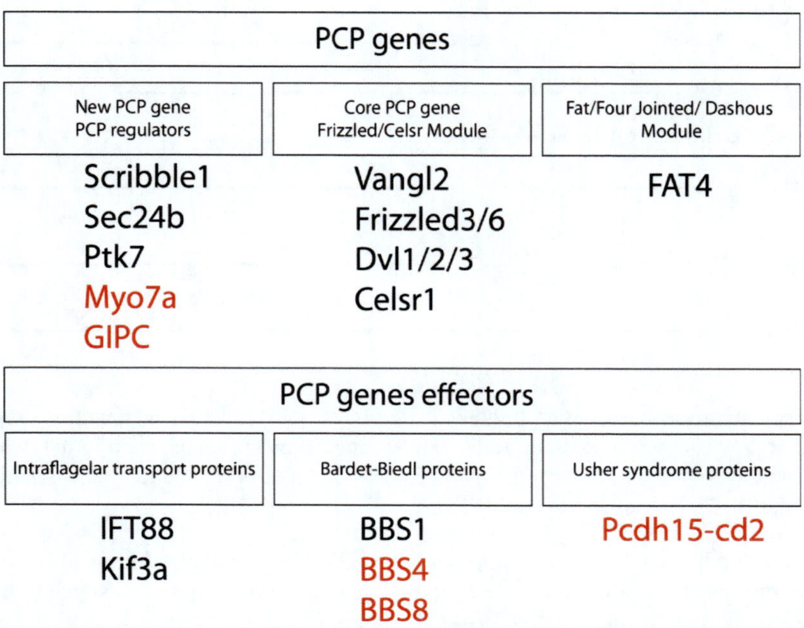

Figure 4. Molecular components acting downstream the Planar cell polarity pathway. Genes highlighted in red are involved in deafness.

Usher and BBS Proteins, New Pieces in the PCP Puzzle

Pathways downstream of PCP, involved in inner ear development, are mainly unknown. In this chapter, we have seen that Usher proteins and BBS proteins could act downstream of the PCP signaling pathway in the inner ear but it is still unclear how BBS, Usher and PCP proteins are interconnected. In the mouse organ of Corti, asymmetry of PCP proteins is detected around E14.5. At this point, due to basal body, BBS and cilia proteins, the kinocilium is already built and positioned at the center of the apical surface of hair cells (Figure 5).

From E15.5, when the asymmetry of PCP proteins is more prominent, the kinocilium migrates from the center to the periphery of the cell apical surface. It is believed that PCP proteins send an intracellular signal into the cell in order to initiate the migration of the kinocilium. Around E16.5, stereocilia from the basal coil of the cochlea are differentiated and are assembled into a bundle. At this stage, a reorientation of the hair bundle occurs, (Figure 5).

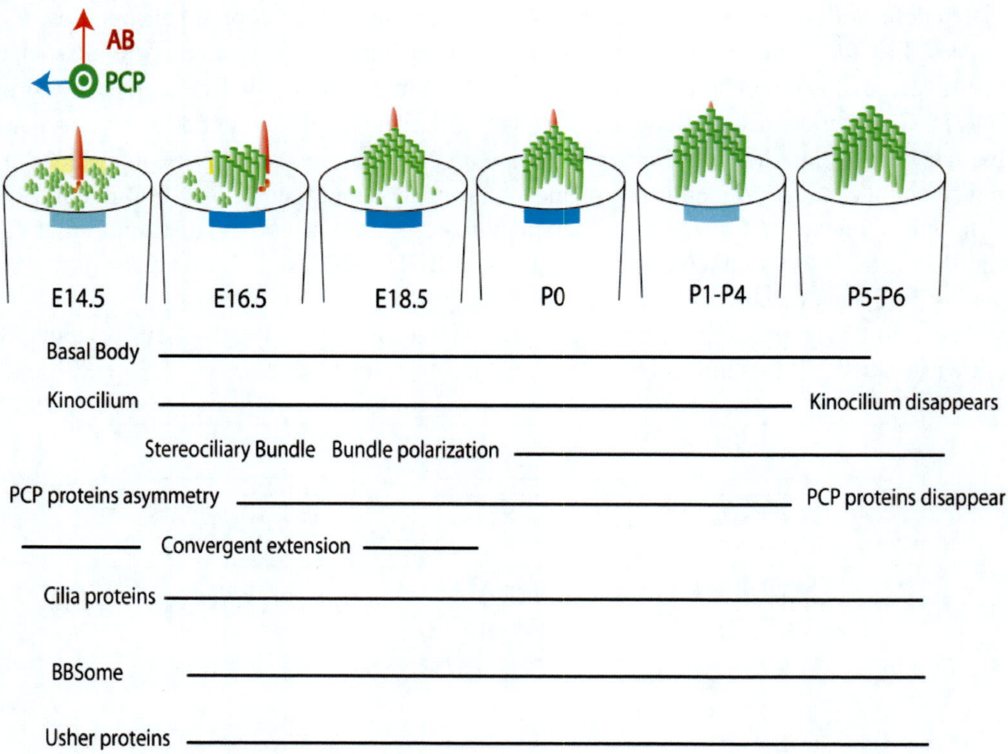

Figure 5. Schematic of the stereociliary bundle development. PCP proteins asymmetry is represented with blue and yellow squares. The Basal body and the kinocilium are represented in red, whereas the stereociliary bundle is in green. Embryonic days (E), Post natal days (P), Apico-basal polarity (AB), Planar Cell Polarity (PCP).

The stereociliary bundle and the kinocilium progressively reach their final location and are polarized along the proximo-distal axis around E18.5. Thereby, the kinocilium may send a signal to the hair bundle in order to align them along the PCP axis (Figure 5, 6).

This could explain why a mispolarization of the stereocilia bundles occurs when the kinocilium is missing in ciliary mutants. Interestingly, Usher proteins are localized to the centrosome and basal body in several systems, and participate in the establishment of transient links between the kinocilium and the hair bundle. Usher proteins may transmit the PCP signal from the kinocilium to the hair bundle (Figure 6). This hypothesis could explain why some Usher mice mutants present a defect in the stereociliary bundle orientation in the absence of these transient links, while PCP protein asymmetry is still present. We can also imagine that BBS and cilia proteins may also participate in the targeting of Usher protein to the kinocilium. From P1 to P6, PCP proteins asymmetry decreases and disappears after P5. At this point, the kinocilium disappears too, suggesting that PCP components may be essential for maintaining the kinocilium.

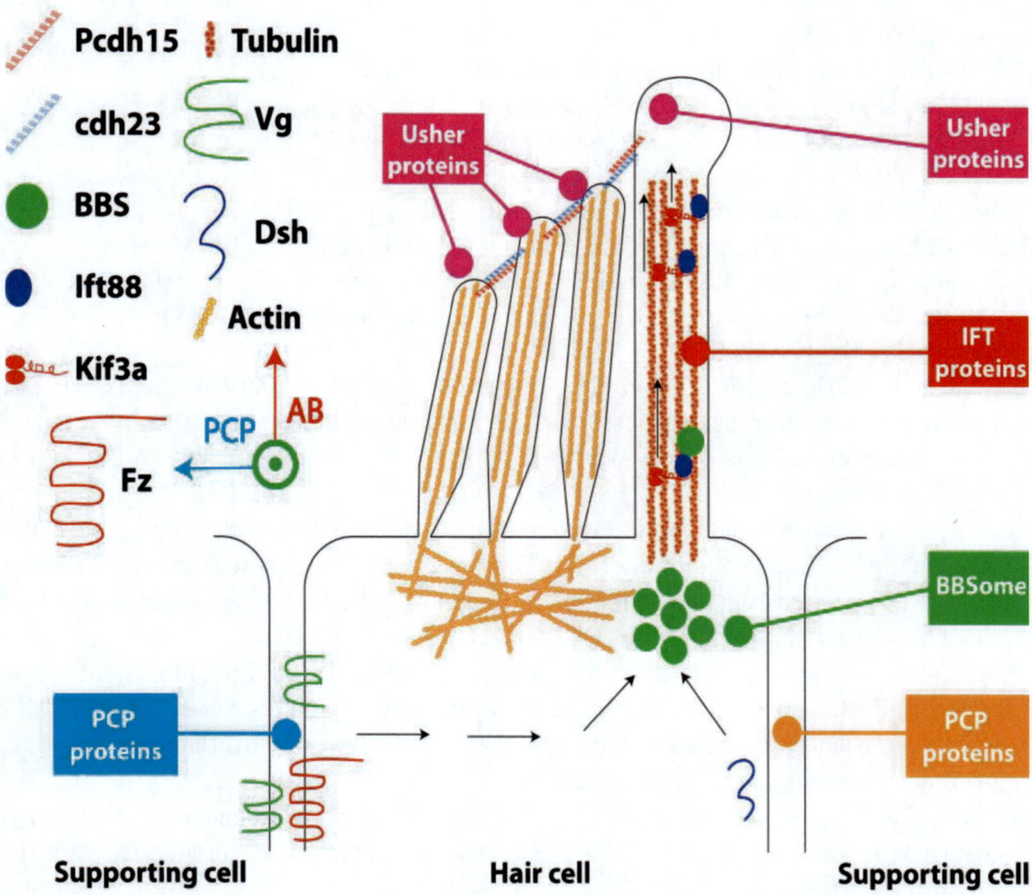

Figure 6. Schematic diagram of PCP signaling in a single hair cell. PCP proteins asymmetry is represented with blue and yellow squares. BBSome, IFT and Usher proteins are represented in green, red and pink respectively. PCP signal is represented with black arrows.

Acknowledgments

Research in the Ahmed laboratory for human and mouse genetics is funded by the National Institutes of Health (NIDCD) R00DC009287 and RPB Career Development Award. Research in the Riazuddin laboratory is funded by the National Institutes of Health (NIDCD) R01DC011748; R01DC011803 and Action on Hearing Loss grants.

References

Adato A, Lefevre G, Delprat B, Michel V, Michalski N, Chardenoux S, Weil D, El-Amraoui A, Petit C (Usherin, the defective protein in Usher syndrome type IIA, is likely to be a component of interstereocilia ankle links in the inner ear sensory cells. *Hum. Mol. Genet.* 14:3921-3932.2005).

Adler PN (Planar signaling and morphogenesis in Drosophila. *Dev. Cell* 2:525-535.2002).

Ahmed ZM, Goodyear R, Riazuddin S, Lagziel A, Legan PK, Behra M, Burgess SM, Lilley KS, Wilcox ER, Griffith AJ, Frolenkov GI, Belyantseva IA, Richardson GP, Friedman TB (The tip-link antigen, a protein associated with the transduction complex of sensory hair cells, is protocadherin-15. *J. Neurosci.* 26:7022-7034.2006).

Ahmed ZM, Morell RJ, Riazuddin S, Gropman A, Shaukat S, Ahmad MM, Mohiddin SA, Fananapazir L, Caruso RC, Husnain T, Khan SN, Griffith AJ, Friedman TB, Wilcox ER (Mutations of MYO6 are associated with recessive deafness, DFNB37. *Am. J. Hum. Genet.* 72:1315-1322.2003).

Alagramam KN, Murcia CL, Kwon HY, Pawlowski KS, Wright CG, Woychik RP (The mouse Ames waltzer hearing-loss mutant is caused by mutation of Pcdh15, a novel protocadherin gene. *Nat. Genet.* 27:99-102.2001).

Axelrod JD (Studies of epithelial PCP. *Semin. Cell Dev. Biol.* 20:956.2009).

Boeda B, El-Amraoui A, Bahloul A, Goodyear R, Daviet L, Blanchard S, Perfettini I, Fath KR, Shorte S, Reiners J, Houdusse A, Legrain P, Wolfrum U, Richardson G, Petit C (Myosin VIIa, harmonin and cadherin 23, three Usher I gene products that cooperate to shape the sensory hair cell bundle. *EMBO J.* 21:6689-6699.2002).

Bonaglia MC, Marelli S, Novara F, Commodaro S, Borgatti R, Minardo G, Memo L, Mangold E, Beri S, Zucca C, Brambilla D, Molteni M, Giorda R, Weber RG, Zuffardi O (Genotype-phenotype relationship in three cases with overlapping 19p13.12 microdeletions. *Eur. J. Hum. Genet.* 2010).

Curtin JA, Quint E, Tsipouri V, Arkell RM, Cattanach B, Copp AJ, Henderson DJ, Spurr N, Stanier P, Fisher EM, Nolan PM, Steel KP, Brown SD, Gray IC, Murdoch JN (Mutation of Celsr1 disrupts planar polarity of inner ear hair cells and causes severe neural tube defects in the mouse. *Curr. Biol.* 13:1129-1133.2003).

Dabdoub A, Kelley MW (Planar cell polarity and a potential role for a Wnt morphogen gradient in stereociliary bundle orientation in the mammalian inner ear. *J. Neurobiol.* 64:446-457.2005).

Devenport D, Fuchs E (Planar polarization in embryonic epidermis orchestrates global asymmetric morphogenesis of hair follicles. *Nat. Cell Biol.* 10:1257-1268.2008).

Di Palma F, Holme RH, Bryda EC, Belyantseva IA, Pellegrino R, Kachar B, Steel KP, Noben-Trauth K (Mutations in Cdh23, encoding a new type of cadherin, cause stereocilia disorganization in waltzer, the mouse model for Usher syndrome type 1D. *Nat. Genet.* 27:103-107.2001).

Djiane A, Riou J, Umbhauer M, Boucaut J, Shi D (Role of frizzled 7 in the regulation of convergent extension movements during gastrulation in Xenopus laevis. *Development* 127:3091-3100.2000).

Eaton S (Planar polarization of Drosophila and vertebrate epithelia. *Curr. Opin. Cell Biol.* 9:860-866.1997).

Etheridge SL, Ray S, Li S, Hamblet NS, Lijam N, Tsang M, Greer J, Kardos N, Wang J, Sussman DJ, Chen P, Wynshaw-Boris A (Murine dishevelled 3 functions in redundant pathways with dishevelled 1 and 2 in normal cardiac outflow tract, cochlea, and neural tube development. *PLoS Genet.* 4:e1000259.2008).

Gibson F, Walsh J, Mburu P, Varela A, Brown KA, Antonio M, Beisel KW, Steel KP, Brown SD (A type VII myosin encoded by the mouse deafness gene shaker-1. *Nature* 374:62-64.1995).

Giese AP, Ezan J, Wang L, Lasvaux L, Lembo F, Mazzocco C, Richard EM, Reboul J, Borg JP, Kelley MW, Sans N, Brigande J, and Montcouquiol M (Gipc1 has a dual role in Vangl2 trafficking and hair bundle integrity in the inner ear. Accepted in *Development* 2012).

Grati M, Kachar B (Myosin VIIa and sans localization at stereocilia upper tip-link density implicates these Usher syndrome proteins in mechanotransduction. Proc. Natl. Acad. Sci. USA 108:11476-11481.2011).

Guo N, Hawkins C, Nathans J (Frizzled6 controls hair patterning in mice. *Proc. Natl. Acad. Sci. USA* 101:9277-9281.2004).

Johnson KR, Gagnon LH, Webb LS, Peters LL, Hawes NL, Chang B, Zheng QY (Mouse models of USH1C and DFNB18: phenotypic and molecular analyses of two new spontaneous mutations of the Ush1c gene. *Hum. Mol. Genet.* 12:3075-3086.2003).

Jones C, Roper VC, Foucher I, Qian D, Banizs B, Petit C, Yoder BK, Chen P (Ciliary proteins link basal body polarization to planar cell polarity regulation. *Nat. Genet.* 40:69-77.2008).

Kazmierczak P, Sakaguchi H, Tokita J, Wilson-Kubalek EM, Milligan RA, Muller U, Kachar B (Cadherin 23 and protocadherin 15 interact to form tip-link filaments in sensory hair cells. *Nature* 449:87-91.2007).

Kikkawa Y, Shitara H, Wakana S, Kohara Y, Takada T, Okamoto M, Taya C, Kamiya K, Yoshikawa Y, Tokano H, Kitamura K, Shimizu K, Wakabayashi Y, Shiroishi T, Kominami R, Yonekawa H (Mutations in a new scaffold protein Sans cause deafness in Jackson shaker mice. *Hum. Mol. Genet.* 12:453-461.2003).

Klein TJ, Mlodzik M (Planar cell polarization: an emerging model points in the right direction. *Annu. Rev. Cell Dev. Biol.* 21:155-176.2005).

Lawrence PA, Struhl G, Casal J (Planar cell polarity: one or two pathways? *Nat. Rev. Genet.* 8:555-563.2007).

Lefevre G, Michel V, Weil D, Lepelletier L, Bizard E, Wolfrum U, Hardelin JP, Petit C (A core cochlear phenotype in USH1 mouse mutants implicates fibrous links of the hair bundle in its cohesion, orientation and differential growth. *Development* 135:1427-1437.2008).

Lu X, Borchers AG, Jolicoeur C, Rayburn H, Baker JC, Tessier-Lavigne M (PTK7/CCK-4 is a novel regulator of planar cell polarity in vertebrates. *Nature* 430:93-98.2004).

May-Simera HL, Kai M, Hernandez V, Osborn DP, Tada M, Beales PL (Bbs8, together with the planar cell polarity protein Vangl2, is required to establish left-right asymmetry in zebrafish. *Dev. Biol.* 2010a).

May-Simera HL, Kai M, Hernandez V, Osborn DP, Tada M, Beales PL (Bbs8, together with the planar cell polarity protein Vangl2, is required to establish left-right asymmetry in zebrafish. *Dev. Biol.* 345:215-225.2010b).

Michel V, Goodyear RJ, Weil D, Marcotti W, Perfettini I, Wolfrum U, Kros CJ, Richardson GP, Petit C (Cadherin 23 is a component of the transient lateral links in the developing hair bundles of cochlear sensory cells. *Dev. Biol.* 280:281-294.2005).

Montcouquiol M, Rachel RA, Lanford PJ, Copeland NG, Jenkins NA, Kelley MW (Identification of Vangl2 and Scrb1 as planar polarity genes in mammals. *Nature* 423:173-177.2003).

Montcouquiol M, Sans N, Huss D, Kach J, Dickman JD, Forge A, Rachel RA, Copeland NG, Jenkins NA, Bogani D, Murdoch J, Warchol ME, Wenthold RJ, Kelley MW (Asymmetric localization of Vangl2 and Fz3 indicate novel mechanisms for planar cell polarity in mammals. *J. Neurosci.* 26:5265-5275.2006).

Narimatsu M, Bose R, Pye M, Zhang L, Miller B, Ching P, Sakuma R, Luga V, Roncari L, Attisano L, Wrana JL (Regulation of planar cell polarity by Smurf ubiquitin ligases. *Cell* 137:295-307.2009).

Phillips HM, Hildreth V, Peat JD, Murdoch JN, Kobayashi K, Chaudhry B, Henderson DJ (Non-cell-autonomous roles for the planar cell polarity gene Vangl2 in development of the coronary circulation. *Circ. Res.* 102:615-623.2008).

Phillips HM, Rhee HJ, Murdoch JN, Hildreth V, Peat JD, Anderson RH, Copp AJ, Chaudhry B, Henderson DJ (Disruption of planar cell polarity signaling results in congenital heart defects and cardiomyopathy attributable to early cardiomyocyte disorganization. *Circ. Res.* 101:137-145.2007).

Qian D, Jones C, Rzadzinska A, Mark S, Zhang X, Steel KP, Dai X, Chen P (Wnt5a functions in planar cell polarity regulation in mice. *Dev. Biol.* 306:121-133.2007).

Rachel RA, May-Simera HL, Veleri S, Gotoh N, Choi BY, Murga-Zamalloa C, McIntyre JC, Marek J, Lopez I, Hackett AN, Brooks M, den Hollander AI, Beales PL, Li T, Jacobson SG, Sood R, Martens JR, Liu P, Friedman TB, Khanna H, Koenekoop RK, Kelley MW, Swaroop A (Combining Cep290 and Mkks ciliopathy alleles in mice rescues sensory defects and restores ciliogenesis. *J. Clin. Invest.* 122:1233-1245.2012).

Reiners J, van Wijk E, Marker T, Zimmermann U, Jurgens K, te Brinke H, Overlack N, Roepman R, Knipper M, Kremer H, Wolfrum U (Scaffold protein harmonin (USH1C) provides molecular links between Usher syndrome type 1 and type 2. *Hum. Mol. Genet.* 14:3933-3943.2005).

Ross AJ, May-Simera H, Eichers ER, Kai M, Hill J, Jagger DJ, Leitch CC, Chapple JP, Munro PM, Fisher S, Tan PL, Phillips HM, Leroux MR, Henderson DJ, Murdoch JN, Copp AJ, Eliot MM, Lupski JR, Kemp DT, Dollfus H, Tada M, Katsanis N, Forge A, Beales PL (Disruption of Bardet-Biedl syndrome ciliary proteins perturbs planar cell polarity in vertebrates. *Nat. Genet.* 37:1135-1140.2005).

Sanggaard KM, Kjaer KW, Eiberg H, Nurnberg G, Nurnberg P, Hoffman K, Jensen H, Sorum C, Rendtorff ND, Tranebjaerg L (A novel nonsense mutation in MYO6 is associated with progressive nonsyndromic hearing loss in a Danish DFNA22 family. *Am. J. Med. Genet. A.* 146A:1017-1025.2008).

Siemens J, Kazmierczak P, Reynolds A, Sticker M, Littlewood-Evans A, Muller U (The Usher syndrome proteins cadherin 23 and harmonin form a complex by means of PDZ-domain interactions. *Proc. Natl. Acad. Sci. USA* 99:14946-14951.2002).

Siemens J, Lillo C, Dumont RA, Reynolds A, Williams DS, Gillespie PG, Muller U (Cadherin 23 is a component of the tip link in hair-cell stereocilia. *Nature* 428:950-955.2004).

Sipe CW, Lu X (Kif3a regulates planar polarization of auditory hair cells through both ciliary and non-ciliary mechanisms. *Development* 138:3441-3449.2011).

Strutt D (Frizzled signalling and cell polarisation in Drosophila and vertebrates. *Development* 130:4501-4513.2003).

Tan C, Deardorff MA, Saint-Jeannet JP, Yang J, Arzoumanian A, Klein PS (Kermit, a frizzled interacting protein, regulates frizzled 3 signaling in neural crest development. *Development* 128:3665-3674.2001).

Tao H, Manak JR, Sowers L, Mei X, Kiyonari H, Abe T, Dahdaleh NS, Yang T, Wu S, Chen S, Fox MH, Gurnett C, Montine T, Bird T, Shaffer LG, Rosenfeld JA, McConnell J, Madan-Khetarpal S, Berry-Kravis E, Griesbach H, Saneto RP, Scott MP, Antic D, Reed J, Boland R, Ehaideb SN, El-Shanti H, Mahajan VB, Ferguson PJ, Axelrod JD, Lehesjoki AE, Fritzsch B, Slusarski DC, Wemmie J, Ueno N, Bassuk AG (Mutations in prickle orthologs cause seizures in flies, mice, and humans. *Am. J. Hum. Genet.* 88:138-149.2011).

Wang Y, Guo N, Nathans J (The role of Frizzled3 and Frizzled6 in neural tube closure and in the planar polarity of inner-ear sensory hair cells. *J. Neurosci.* 26:2147-2156.2006).

Wang Y, Huso D, Cahill H, Ryugo D, Nathans J (Progressive cerebellar, auditory, and esophageal dysfunction caused by targeted disruption of the frizzled-4 gene. *J. Neurosci.* 21:4761-4771.2001).

Wansleeben C, Feitsma H, Montcouquiol M, Kroon C, Cuppen E, Meijlink F (Planar cell polarity defects and defective Vangl2 trafficking in mutants for the COPII gene Sec24b. *Development* 137:1067-1073.2010).

Warchol ME, Montcouquiol M (Maintained expression of the planar cell polarity molecule Vangl2 and reformation of hair cell orientation in the regenerating inner ear. *J. Assoc. Res. Otolaryngol.* 11:395-406.2010).

Webb SW, Grillet N, Andrade LR, Xiong W, Swarthout L, Della Santina CC, Kachar B, Muller U (Regulation of PCDH15 function in mechanosensory hair cells by alternative splicing of the cytoplasmic domain. *Development* 138:1607-1617.2011).

Winter CG, Wang B, Ballew A, Royou A, Karess R, Axelrod JD, Luo L (Drosophila Rho-associated kinase (Drok) links Frizzled-mediated planar cell polarity signaling to the actin cytoskeleton. *Cell* 105:81-91.2001).

Yan D, Liu XZ (Genetics and pathological mechanisms of Usher syndrome. *J. Hum. Genet.* 55:327-335.2010).

Yoshida N, Liberman MC (Stereociliary anomaly in the guinea pig: effects of hair bundle rotation on cochlear sensitivity. *Hear Res.* 131:29-38.1999).

In: Inner Ear Development and Hearing Loss
Editors: Saima Riazuddin and Zubair Ahmed
ISBN: 978-1-62417-011-9

Chapter 4

AUTOIMMUNE INNER EAR DISEASE (AIED)

Roberto Bovo and Chiara Faccioli
ENT Department,
University Hospital of Padua, Italy

ABSTRACT

Autoimmune inner ear disease (AIED) is probably a rare disease accounting for less than 1% all cases of hearing impairment or dizziness, but its incidence might be overlooked because of the lack of specific diagnostic test. Many cases are analogous to rapidly progressive glomerulonephritis in that inner ear inflammation progresses to severe, irreversible damage within 3 months of onset (and often much more quickly). On the other hand, steroid responsiveness is high and with prompt treatment, the hearing loss may be reversible. Nowadays experimental models of autoimmune hearing loss have been developed in a variety of animals. The correlation between experimental models in animals and serological findings in human might be significant. Several studies seem to demonstrate that genetically controlled aspects of the immune system may increase or otherwise be associated with increased susceptibility to different inner ear diseases.

This chapter offers a practical tool for the diagnosis and treatment of AIED.

INTRODUCTION

AIED is probably a rare disease accounting for less than 1% all cases of hearing impairment or dizziness, but its incidence might be overlooked because of the lack of specific diagnostic test.

The concept that the immune system may have a role in some idiopathic hearing loss has been introduced during the early decades of the past century by Joannovic and Masugi [1,2]. In 1958 Lehnard [3] suspected that some cases of sudden bilateral hearing loss could be related to the production of anticochlear antibodies. In 1961 Beickert [4], and three years later Terayama [5] presented data supporting autoimmunity in experimental guinea pig cochleae. In 1979 McCabe [6] first described a cohort of 18 patients with bilateral asymmetric hearing loss progressing over weeks to months which responded to steroid therapy. He proposed the definition of autoimmune hearing loss and asserted the importance of a high index of suspicion in these patients since, if diagnosed early, they could be treated and their hearing preserved. His work stimulated research into this topic.

Nowadays experimental models of autoimmune hearing loss have been developed in a variety of animals and the correlation between these models and serological findings in human might be significant [7,8,9]. Several studies seem to demonstrate that genetically controlled aspects of the immune system may increase or otherwise be associated with increased susceptibility to different inner ear diseases [10].

Clinical Features

The disease seems more common in female between 20 and 50 years of age and manifests with the occurrence of a rapidly progressive, often fluctuating, bilateral sensory-neural hearing loss (SNHL) over a period of weeks to months [11]. The progression of hearing loss is too rapid to be diagnostic for presbycusis and too slow to conclude a diagnosis of sudden SNHL. Generalized imbalance, ataxia, motion intolerance, positional vertigo and episodic vertigo may be present in almost 50% of patients [12]. Bilateral hearing loss occurs in 80% of patients [13], with symmetric or asymmetric audiometric thresholds, although only one ear may be affected at an early stage. Almost 25-50% of patients have also tinnitus and aural fullness, which can fluctuate.

Systemic autoimmune diseases coexist in 15-30% of patients (systemic lupus erythematosus, rheumatoid arthritis, disseminated vasculitis, Sjögren's syndrome, myasthenia gravis, Hashimoto's thyroiditis, Cogan's syndrome, Behçet's disease, sarcoidosis, Wegener's granulomatosis, colitis ulcerosa, relapsing polychondritis).

A detailed history may rarely disclose endocrine diseases and/or recurrent fever. Otoscopy is usually normal, nevertheless external ear skin and/or cartilage inflammation and/or facial palsy may rarely occur (e.g. relapsing polychondritis), as well as tissue destruction of the tympanic membrane, middle ear and mastoid (e.g. Wegener's granulomatosis). Differential diagnosis comprehend : both sides Menière's disease, luetic inner ear disease, Lyme disease, toxoplasmosis, treatment with ototoxic drugs (gentamicin, cisplatin), Charcot-Marie-Tooth disease (hereditary neuropathy), enlarged vestibular aqueduct syndrome, endocranic hypertension.

Laboratory Studies

While specific tests for autoimmunity to the inner ear would be desirable, at this writing there are none that are both commercially available and proven to be useful. Antigen specific tests include: migration inhibition test (MIT), lymphocyte transformation test (LTT) and Western blot analysis for antibodies to inner ear antigen. MIT use is limited because of inherent technical difficulties. Results obtained by LTT are still greatly controversial [14,15]. Western blot analysis has been extensively used in the clinical practice. In fact, a commercially available test, called "anti-68 kD (hsp-70) Western blot" (*OTOblotTM*) was reported to detect a local autoimmune inner ear process in the absence of any systemic autoimmune process and to be correlated with steroid responsiveness [16]. The test uses purified hsp-70 kDa antigen from a bovine kidney cell line and is based on the assumption that the 68 kDa protein is the heat shock protein 70 (hsp—70) [17]. Unfortunately, this assumption has now been refuted: in fact, there is mounting evidence that the target antigen of the 68 kDa antibody is not the HSP 70 (as was believed over the last 15 years), but the human "choline transporter—like protein 2" (CTL2) [18]. Furthermore, the sensibility reported in different studies is low [19,20] and antibodies to HSP-70 can also be found in Lyme disease, ulcerative colitis, cancers, and in about 5% of healthy individuals. In Meniere's disease, Hornibrook et al. found no significant difference between 80 subjects with definite Meniere's disease and controls [21].

On the other hand, there is seldom convincing evidence also from broader laboratory tests indicating autoimmunity. A non specific antigen screening test is useful for evidence of systemic immunologic dysfunction; yet do not strictly correlate with a diagnosis of immune-mediated inner ear disease. In the clinical practice the antigen-non-specific test usually recommended are:

I. blood tests for autoimmune disorders: levels of circulating immune complexes, Sed Rate, antinuclear antibodies (ANA), Raji-Cell, Rheumatoid Factor, Complement C1Q, Smooth Muscle Antibody, TSH and anti-microsomal antibodies, anti-gliadin antibodies (for Celiac disease), HLA testing
II. blood tests for conditions that resemble autoimmune disorders: FTA (for Syphilis), Lyme titre, HBA1C (for diabetes, which is often autoimmune mediated also), HIV (HIV is associated with auditory neuropathy)

Nevertheless, Garcia-Berrocal et al. [22] confronted the efficiency of two immunologic work-up study in patients with a high clinical suspicion of autoimmune inner ear disease (AIED). The restricted examination consisting of ANA and immunophenotype of peripheral blood lymphocytes (PBL), demonstrated similar efficiency when compared with a classical work-up study, whose cost is about 5 times higher. Therefore, an exhaustive immunologic work-up study is not recommended if financial resources are limited.

Medical Therapy for AIED

Treatment for AIED seems to be rapidly changing and new protocols are constantly being attempted. As the natural history of untreated immune-mediated inner ear disease is unknown the efficacy of these protocols is evaluated on empirical clinical data gathered during the last two decades. The mainstay of this treatment is the positive response to anti-inflammatory drugs, particularly corticosteroids, in term of improved hearing. In McCabe's clinical study [6] and in several subsequent ones [23,24], the efficacy of immunosuppressive therapy is well demonstrated in a vast subset of patient. In cases with a classic rapidly progressive bilateral hearing impairment, an initial treatment with high-dose steroids is generally tried, assuming that there are no contraindications as peptic ulcer disease, diabetes, glaucoma, hypertension and history of tuberculosis. Since inner ear inflammation in AIED can rapidly progress to a severe and irreversible damage, these patients are treated with a sense of urgency. A standardised regimen for steroid therapy doesn't exist, yet many recommend prednisone 1 mg/Kg/day for four weeks, followed by a slow taper over several weeks to a maintenance dose of 10-20 mg/die or every other day. Shorter-term or lower dose long-term therapy has either been ineffective or appears to increase the risk of relapse. Patients often learn what maintenance dose is necessary to preserve hearing as disease activity often waxes and wanes. If hearing suddenly worsens or tinnitus reappears in one or both ears during the taper it is indicate to repeat the initial high dose treatment. Nevertheless, not all patients respond to corticosteroid therapy in the same manner: some demonstrate improvement in threshold, discrimination scores or both, while others have fluctuation without a definite improvement and still others progress to profound hearing loss despite aggressive immunosuppressive treatment. Steroid treatment is inexpensive, but in some patients it is difficult to maintain because of side effects or because hearing loss becomes refractory to them. In most cases of patients with no response to steroids within 6-8 weeks, a cytotoxic chemotherapy type of medication such as methotrexate (MTX) and cyclophsphamide has been used over the long term [25,26]. These agents are associated with considerable toxicity and adverse effects: myelosuppression, haemorrhagic cystitis, infertility and increased risk of malignancy. When dealing with cytotoxic drugs the following consultations are recommended: rheumatologic, immunologic and haematological. Furthermore, these consultations in addition with ophthalmologic and neurological ones are useful in ruling out systemic diseases. As suggested by Ryan et al. [28] it is questionable whether every suspicious case should be treated with these powerful drugs: the decision regarding when and how to treat should always be multidisciplinary. It is to be considered that the real benefit of these treatment is still not well established. In fact, in a multicentric study methotrexate was no more effective than placebo in maintaining the hearing improvement achieved with prednisone treatment [27]. The normal oral dose of MTX is 7.5-20 mg weekly with folic acid, and with this dosage MTX seems to be less toxic and to be associated with a lower risk of neoplasia in respect to cyclophosphamide. However the patient needs to be regularly monitored by means of complete blood count, platelet count, determination of urea nitrogen and creatinine levels, liver function tests and urinalysis. Cyclophosphamide in addition to steroids has been recommended by McCabe [6] as a first-line treatment with the following regimen: intravenous cyclophosphamide 5mg/Kg per day for 2 weeks, followed by a rest period of 2 weeks, and then a final 2 weeks of infusions. Liberal amounts of fluids intake is recommended and again peripheral blood counts at regular intervals. Administration in children and young people must be avoided for the risk of permanent sterility. If symptoms recur cyclophosphamide and steroids are restarted. Three month cycles are continued until patients can be weaned. No patient required more than 24 months of treatment in McCabe's study.

In 1989 Luetje [29] introduced the use of plasmapheresis in patients with AIED. Improvement of auditory function occurred in 6 of 8 patients, 3 of whom were able to discontinue immunosuppressive medication. Plasmapheresis is only suitable to disorders mediated by antibodies or immune complexes, is expensive and its application remains to be further investigated.

Antagonist against proinflammatory cytokines, such as IL-1 and tumour necrosis factor (TNF) have been tested. Among them, Etanercept (Enbrel), a TNF receptor blocker drug, seemed initially to demonstrate good efficacy [30,31], but in following trials the results were no better than placebo [32,33]. Enbrel is given as a subcutaneous injection once/week, usually between 25 and 50 units and at this dosage it is generally well tolerated. Nevertheless, according to the manufacturer's information there is a low risk of serious infections (2%), nervous system disorders, and depression / personality disorders (1%).

Van Wijk et al [34], found that transtympanic delivery of another TNF-alpha blocker, Infliximab, once weekly for 4 weeks allowed steroids to be tapered off, resulted in hearing improvement and reduced disease relapses, but this study was based on only 9 cases. Among the other anti-TNF drugs, Humira (Adalimumab) was approved by the FDA (2002), but it is not known so far whether it is useful in AIED. In controlled studies of all TNF-alpha blocking drugs, more cases of lymphoma have been noted in treated patients than controls. It is also generally felt that when these drugs are in use there should be increased vigilance for reactivation of tuberculosis.

In animals, attempts have been made to induce tolerance by administration of antigens that cause autoimmunity or peptide competition: variants of AIED have been treated with oral collagen [35]. Oral tolerization to antigen has been applied to autoimmune disease patients, although the exact mechanisms involved are still not clear. Most probably active suppression and clonal anergy or clonal deletion are the main mechanisms of oral tolerance. For these reasons, the identification of auto-antigens in AIED would be of paramount importance for better management of these patients. Monoclonal antibodies against surface antigens (e.g.CD3) or the T-cell receptor might be used to block lymphocytes.

Local application of steroids in animal middle ear led to higher and more sustained perilymph levels than systemic treatment [36]. For this reason, several clinical trials have been carried out on transtympanic administration of steroids. In a small study, Garcia-Berrocal et al. showed the improvement of hearing and balance symptoms in AIED [37]. On the other hand, round window application of different immune-suppressive drugs via an osmotic mini-pump was ineffective in reducing immune-mediated hearing loss [38]. Larger trials are needed to determine the true effectiveness of this type of treatment [39, 40].

Several laboratories have researched the possibility of cell or gene therapy to replace damaged ear cells in AIED. Laboratory tests with animal models are promising, but much more research is needed to determine the effectiveness and safety of these therapies [41, 42].

Interstitial cell adhesion molecule-1 (ICAM-1) is a molecule present on activated endothelial cells that recruits lymphocytes into the inner ear [43]. Intravenous anti-ICAM-1 has proven to reduce the recruitment of leucocytes into the scala tympani, the 8th nerve and the perivascular spaces around the vessels of the SMV and modiolar veins [44].

Cochlear Implant and AIED

Reportedly, 6% of the AIED patients progress to the point of profound loss. Most do extremely well with a cochlear implant (CI). With regard to Cogan syndrome the percentage of profound loss raise up to 60% and CI remains the only treatment option. Because of the fact that cochlear ossification may progress very rapidly, in most cases implantation should not be delayed. Literature data agree that once the electrode array is properly inserted, functional outcomes are good [45,46].

Conclusion

Based on clinical and experimental data there is today strong evidence that immune mechanisms are involved in the aetiopathogenesis of inner ear damage, together with viral infection, trauma, vascular damage and genetic factors.

While specific tests for autoimmunity to the inner ear would be desirable, at this writing there are none that are both commercially available and proven to be useful. Till now most of the identified antigens lack a clear association with localized inner-ear pathology and the diagnosis of AIED is based either on clinical criteria and/or on a positive response to steroids. In the clinical practice we recommend an antigen-non-specific test battery including blood test for autoimmune disorders and for conditions that resemble autoimmune disorders [46, 47, 48]. Nevertheless, if financial resources are limited a very restricted work-up study may have a similar efficiency.

The severity of autoimmune inner ear disease is analogous to the one found in rapidly progressive glomerulonephritis. If not treated, the inner ear inflammation progresses quickly to a severe irreversible damage within 3 months of onset, or even in a shorter period. Fortunately, the steroid responsiveness is high and with a prompt treatment, the hearing can be rescued. Nevertheless, 6% of the AIED patients progress to the point of profound loss and CI can be the only treatment option.

References

[1] Joannovic D. Zur Wirkung fermentativ gewonner spaltungsprodukte aus Geweben und Bakterien. *Wein Klin Wschr* 1920;70:1410-11.

[2] Masugi M, Tomizuka Y. Über die spezifisch zytotoxischen Veränderungen der Niere und sehr Leber durch das spezifische Antiserum (Nephrotoxin und Hepatoxin). *Trans. Jap. Pathol.* oc 1931;21:329-41.

[3] Lehnhardt E. Plotzliche horstorungen auf beiden seiten gleichzeitig oder nacheinander aufgetreten. *Z. Laryngol. Rhinol. Otol.* 1958;37:1.

[4] Beickert V. Zur Frage der empfindungs Schwerhörigkeit under Autoallergie. *Z. Laryngol. Rhinol. Otol.* 1961;40:837-42.

[5] Terayama Y, Sasaki U. Studies on experimental allergic (isoimmune) labyrinthitis in guinea pigs. *Acta Oto-Laryngol.* 1964;58:49-64.

[6] McCabe, B. Autoimmune Sensorineural Hearing Loss. *Ann. Otol.* 1979;88:585-589.

[7] Gloddek B, Arnold W. Clinical and Experimental Studies of Autoimmune Inner Ear Disease. *Acta Otolaryngol.* 2002; Suppl 548:10-14.

[8] Yoo TJ, Yazawa Y. Immunology of cochlear and vestibular disorders. In: Luxon L, editor. Audiological Medicine -- Clinical aspects of hearing and balance. London: Taylor and Francis; 2003 p. 61-87.

[9] Hefeneider SH, McCoy SL, Hausman FA, Trune DR. Autoimmune mouse antibodies recognize multiple antigens proposed in human immune-mediated hearing loss. *Otol. Neurotol.* 2004;25:250-6.

[10] Bernstein JM, Shanahan TC, Schaffer FM. Further observations on the role of the MHC genes and certain hearing disorders. *Acta Otolaryngol.* 1996;116:666-71.
[11] Bovo R, Aimoni C, Martini A. Immune-mediated inner ear disease. *Acta Otolaryngol.* 2006;126:1012–1021.
[12] Bovo R, Berto A, Ciorba A, Martini A. Vertigo and Autoimmunity. In: Dizziness: Vertigo, Disequilibrium and Lightheadedness . Eds: A. Lindqvist and G. Nyman. 2009 Nova Science Publishers, Inc.NewYork. pp.119-137.
[13] Hughes G, Kinney S, Barna B, Calabrese L, Hamid M. Autoimmune reactivity in Menière's disease: preliminary report. *Laryngoscope* 1983;43:410-17.
[14] Berger P, Hillman M, Tabak M, Vollrath M. The lymphocyte transformation test with type II collagen as a diagnostic tool of autoimmune sensorineural hearing loss. *Laryngoscope* 1991;101:895-9.
[15] Harris J, Sharp P. Inner ear autoantibodies in patients with rapidly progressive sensorineural hearing loss. *Laryngoscope* 1990;100: 526-24.
[16] Bloch DB, San Martin JE, Rauch SD, Moscicki RA, Bloch KJ. Serum antibodies to heat shock protein 70 in sensorineural hearing loss. *Arch. Otolaryngol. Head Neck Surg.* 1995;121:1167-1171.
[17] Billings P, Keithley E, Harris J. Evidence linking the 68 kilo Dalton antigen identified in progressive sensorineural hearing loss patient sera with heat shock protein 70. *Ann. Otol. Rhinol. Laryngol.* 1995;104:181-188.
[18] Nair TS, Kozma KE, Hoefling NL et al. Identification and characterization of choline transporter-like protein **2,** an inner ear glycoprotein of 68 and 72 kDa that is the target of antibody-induced hearing loss. *J. Neurosc.* 2004; 24:1772-1779.
[19] Gottschlich S, Billings PB, Keithley EM, Weisman MH, Harris JP. Assessment of serum antibodies in patients with rapidly progressive sensorineural hearing loss and Meniere's disease. *Laryngoscope* 1995;105:1347-1352.
[20] Yeom K, Gray J, Nair TS, Arts HA, Telian SA, Disher MJ, El-Kashlan H, Sataloff RT, Fisher SG, Carey TE (2003) Antibodies to HSP-70 in normal donors and autoimmune hearing loss patients. *Laryngoscope* 113: 1770-1776.
[21] Hornibrook J, George P, Spellerberg M, Gourley J. HSP70 antibodies in 80 patients with "clinically certain" Meniere's disease. Ann. Otol. Rhinol. Laryngol. 2011;120:651-5.
[22] García Berrocal JR,. Ramírez-Camacho R, Vargas J A, Millan. I. Does the Serological Testing Really Play a Role in the Diagnosis Immune-mediated Inner Ear Disease? *Oto-Laryngologica* 2002;122:243-248.
[23] Helfgot S, Mosciscki R, San Martin J et al. Correlation between antibodies to type II collagen and treatment outcome in bilateral progressive sensorineural hearing loss. *Lancet* 1991;337:387-9.
[24] Tomoda K, Suzuka Y, Iwai H, Yamashita T, Kumazawa T. Menière's disease and autoimmunity: clinical study and survey. *Acta Otolaryngol* Suppl 1993;500:31-4.
[25] Sismanis A, Thompson T, Willis HE. Methotrexate therapy for autoimmune hearing loss: a preliminary report. *Laryngoscope* 1994;104:932-934.

[26] Sismanis A, Wise CM, Johnson GD. Methotrexate management of immune-mediated cochleovestibular disorders. *Otolaryngol. HNS* 1997;116:146-52.

[27] Harris JP, Weisman MH, Derebery JM, Espeland MA, Gantz BJ, Gulya AJ, et al. Treatment of corticosteroid-responsive autoimmune inner ear disease with methotrexate: a randomized controlled trial. *JAMA* 2003;290:1875-83.

[28] Ryan A, Harris J, Keithley E. Immune-mediated Hearing Loss: Basic Mechanisms and Options for Therapy. *Acta Otolaryngol.* 2002; Suppl 548:38- 43.

[29] Luetje CM, Berliner KI. Plasmapheresis in autoimmune inner ear disease: long-term follow-up. *Am. J. Otol.* 1997;18:572-576.

[30] Rahman MU, Poe DS, Choi HK. Etanercept therapy for immune-mediated cochleovestibular disorders: preliminary results in a pilot study. *Otol. Neurotol.* 2001;22:619-624.

[31] Wang X, Truong T, Billings PB, Harris JP, Keithley EM. Blockage of immune-mediated inner ear damage by etanercept. *Otol. Neurotol.* 2003;24:52-7.

[32] Cohen S, Shoup A, Weisman MH, Harris J. Etanercept treatment for autoimmune inner ear disease: results of a pilot placebo-controlled study. *Otol. Neurotol.* 2005;26:903-7.

[33] Matteson EL, Choi HK, Poe DS, Wise C, Lowe VJ, McDonald TJ, Rahman MU. Etanercept therapy for immune-mediated cochleovestibular disorders: a multi-center, open-label, pilot study. *Arthritis Rheum.* 2005; 53:337-42.

[34] Van Wijk F, Staecker H, Keithley E, Lefebvre PP. Local perfusion of the tumor necrosis factor alpha blocker infliximab to the inner ear improves autoimmune neurosensory hearing loss. *Audiol. Neurootol.* 2006;11(6):357-65.

[35] Kim N, Cheng KC, Kwon SS, Mora R, Barbieri M, Yoo TJ. Oral administration of collagen conjugated with cholera toxin induces tolerance to type II collagen and suppresses chondritis in an animal model of autoimmune ear disease. *Ann. Otol. Rhinol. Laryngol.* 2001;110:646-54.

[36] Parnes L, Sun A, Freeman D. Corticosteroid pharmacokinetics in the inner ear fluids: an animal study followed by clinical application. *Laryngoscope* 1999;109:1-17.

[37] Berrocal JR, Ramírez-Camacho R. Sudden sensorineural hearing loss: supporting the immunologic theory. *Ann. Otol. Rhinol. Laryngol*. 2002;111:989-97.

[38] Yang G, Song H, Keithley E, Harris J. Intratympanic immunosuppressive for prevention of immune-mediated sensorineural hearing loss. *Am. J. Otol.* 2000; 21:499-504.

[39] Alles MJ, der Gaag MA, Stokroos RJ. Intratympanic steroid therapy for inner ear diseases, a review of the literature. Eur. Arch. Otorhinolaryngol. 2006;263:791-7.

[40] Rauch SD. Intratympanic steroids for sensorineural hearing loss. Otolaryngol. Clin. North Am. 2004; 37:1061-74. .

[41] Nakagawa T. Ito J. Application of cell therapy to inner ear diseases. *Acta Oto-Laryngol. Supplement*. 2004; 551:6-9.

[42] Pau H. Clarke RW. Advances in genetic manipulations in the treatment of hearing disorders. *Clin. Otolaryngol. and Al Sci*. 2004; 29:574-6.

[43] Suzuki M, Harris J. Expression of intercellular adhesion molecule-1 during inner ear inflammation. *Ann. Otol. Rhinol. Laryngol.* 1995;104:69-75.

[44] Takasu T, Harris J. Reduction of inner ear inflammation by treatment with anti-ICAM-1 antibody. *Ann. Otol. Rhinol. Laryngol.* 1997; 106:1070-5.

[45] Bovo R, Ciorba A, Trevisi P, Aimoni C, Cappiello L, Castiglione A, Govoni M, Martini A. Cochlear implant in Cogan syndrome. *Acta Otolaryngol.* 2011; 131:494-7.

[46] Wang JR, Yuen HW, Shipp DB, Stewart S, Lin VY, Chen JM, Nedzelski JM. Cochlear implantation in patients with autoimmune inner ear disease including Cogan syndrome: a comparison with age- and sex-matched controls. *Laryngoscope.* 2010;120:2478.

[47] Agrup C, Luxon LM. Immune-mediated inner ear disorders in neuro-otology. *Curr. Opin. Neurol.* 2006;19:26-32.

[48] Bovo R, Ciorba A, Martini A. The diagnosis of autoimmune inner ear disease: evidence and clinical pittfalls. *Eur. Arch. Otorhinolaryngol.* 2009; 266:37-40.

In: Inner Ear Development and Hearing Loss
Editors: Saima Riazuddin and Zubair Ahmed
ISBN: 978-1-62417-011-9

Chapter 5

LABYRINTHINE APLASIA, MICROTIA, AND MICRODONTIA (LAMM) SYNDROME AND *FGF3* MUTATIONS

Kumarie Latchman and Mustafa Tekin*
Dr.John T.Macdonald Foundation Department of Human Genetics and
John P.Hussman Institute for Human Genomics,
University of Miami Miller School of Medicine, Miami, Florida, US

ABSTRACT

Hearing loss presents as a clinical finding in more than 400 genetic syndromes, some of which are associated with inner ear anomalies. Congenital deafness with labyrinthine aplasia (also known as Michel aplasia), microtia, and microdontia (LAMM syndrome; MIM 610706) was described in 2007 as an autosomal recessive syndrome. Mutations in *FGF3* were demonstrated in affected subjects. Since the initial description, 56 individuals with LAMM syndrome from 13 unrelated families have been reported. Microdontia was the most constant finding that was present in all affected individuals. Michel aplasia was present in most cases although other severe inner ear anomalies were detected in some individuals, especially with the p.R95W mutation. Microtia typically affected the upper pinna and was associated with anteverted ears, large skin tags or lobulation. Microtia was not observed in a few cases with the p.R95W mutation. Clinical findings do not appear to involve the other systems and in particular cognitive development is not affected. Reported mutations include missense, nonsense, and small deletions leading to a frameshift suggesting that the LAMM syndrome is caused by the loss of FGF3 function. The presence of severe inner ear anomalies, complete labyrinthine aplasia in most cases, limits the usage of cochlear implants. Auditory brain stem implantation may be considered as in other cases with severe inner ear anomalies. Recognition of LAMM syndrome and detection of *FGF3* mutations in a deaf individual is important because it leads to better genetic counseling and empower families to have informed reproductive decisions.

* E-mail address: mtekin@med.miami.edu

Introduction

It is the intent of this paper to summarize what is known about the recently recognized genetic syndrome characterized by complete labyrinthine aplasia, microtia, and microdontia. Approximately one-third of individuals with hereditary deafness have additional finding leading to the diagnosis of a genetic syndrome. Overall, there are greater than 400 syndromes in which deafness is a significant clinical finding [1]. In 2007, a new autosomal recessive deafness syndrome was described that involved the occurrence of an external ear anomaly (microtia), inner ear anomaly (labyrinthine aplasia) associated with congenital profound deafness, and microdontia [2]. This condition was named as Labyrinthine Aplasia, Microtia, and Microdontia (LAMM) syndrome (MIM 610706) [3] and was found to be caused by mutations in the *FGF3* gene (MIM 164950), coding for fibroblast growth factor 3. Thus far 56 affected subjects from 13 unrelated families have been reported [2-8]. LAMM syndrome affects males and females equally and it is inherited in an autosomal recessive manner in which both parents carry a single copy of an *FGF3* mutation. Reported families thus far originated from Turkey, Pakistan, Saudi Arabia, Somalia, Albania, and Italy. Parental consanguinity was present in most of the reported families reflecting its facilitative effect for the phenotypic expression of rare autosomal recessive mutations.

Clinical Phenotype

The primary phenotypic effects resulting from mutations in *FGF3* are profound congenital sensorineural deafness, microtia with shortening of the auricles above the crura of the antihelix, and microdontia with widely spaced teeth.

Congenital deafness associated with severe inner ear anomalies: All 56 reported individuals with bilateral *FGF3* mutations had bilateral congenital-onset profound deafness. CT scan and/or MRI images of the temporal bone were reported in 33 individuals. Twenty-five cases did not have any inner ear structure present and were diagnosed with bilateral complete labyrinthine aplasia (Table 1 and Figure 1). Complete labyrinthine aplasia, also known as Michel aplasia as it was first described by Michel in 1863 [9], refers to a rare form of inner ear anomaly in which there is a complete absence of the inner ear bony and membranous structures. Five individuals had complete labyrinthine aplasia in one ear and some structures visible in the other ear. These were, in most cases, small vestibule-like structures with no differentiation into the cochlear or vestibular systems. Remaining three individuals had some inner ear structure demonstrated bilaterally. In one case it was bilateral tiny vestibule-like formation [2]. In another individual, it was bilateral common cavity [5]. And finally in one individual, the bony internal acoustic canals were present bilaterally with some cochlear and vestibular structures [6].

Microtia: According to the clinical classification suggested by Weerda [10], type 1 microtia refers to the presence of a small auricle with mostly normal auricular structure and an intact external auditory meatus. In LAMM syndrome, the typical external ear anomaly is type 1 microtia with shortening of the auricle above the crura of the antihelix (Figure 2). This anomaly was present in both ears in 27 of 37 individuals clinically evaluated (Table 1).

Table 1. Characteristics of reported individuals with LAMM syndrome

Family	# of Affected Individuals in Each Family	Right Inner Ear[a]	Left Inner Ear[a]	Right Auricle[a]	Left Auricle[a]	Teeth[a]	*FGF3* Mutations	Ref.
1	5	-Michel aplasia 5/5	-Michel aplasia 5/5	-Microtia 5/5	-Microtia 5/5	-Microdontia 5/5	p.S156P	2
2	3	-Michel aplasia 3/3	-Michel aplasia 3/3	-Microtia 3/3	-Microtia 3/3	-Microdontia 5/5	p.R104X	2
3	1	-Michel aplasia 1/1	-Michel aplasia 1/1	-Microtia 1/1	-Microtia 1/1	-Microdontia 1/1	p.V206SfsX 117	2
4	1	-Michel aplasia 1/1	-Michel aplasia 1/1	-Microtia with a tag on the upper helix 1/1	-Microtia with a tag on the upper helix 1/1	NA	p.I85Mfs15	3
5	3	-Small vestibule-like structure 1/3 -Michel aplasia 2/3	-Small cystic structure 1/3 -Michel aplasia 2/3	-Microtia 3/3 A tag on the upper helix 1/3	-Microtia 3/3 A tag on the upper helix 1/3	-Microdontia 3/3	p.L6P	3
6	21	-Michel aplasia 2/2	-Small cystic structure 2/2	-Microtia with tag 2/2	-Microtia 2/2	-Microdontia 2/2	p.G66C	4
7	4	-Michel aplasia 3/4 -Common cavity 1/4	-Michel aplasia 1/4 -Common cavity 2/4 -1 ½ turn cochlea; absence of LSC 1/4	-Microtia 1/4 -Normal 3/4	-Microtia 3/4 -Normal 1/4	-Microdontia 3/4	p.R95W	5
8	7	-Michel aplasia 4/6 - Bony IAC(+), dysplastic SCC, single cochleovestibular nerve 1/6 -Reminiscent of cochlear basal turn 1/6	-Michel aplasia 5/6 -1 ½ turn cochlea, short broad cystic LSC confluent with the vestibule, bony IAC(+) 1/6	-Normal 7/7	-Normal 7/7	-Microdontia 5/7 -Possible microdontia 2/7	p.R95W	6
9	4	-Michel aplasia 2/2	-Michel aplasia 2/2	-Microtia 4/4	-Microtia 4/4	-Microdontia 4/4	p.R104X	6
10	3	-Michel aplasia 2/2	-Michel aplasia 2/2	-Microtia 3/3	-Microtia 3/3	-Microdontia 3/3	p.R132GfsX 26	6
11	2	-Michel aplasia 2/2	-Michel aplasia 2/2	-Microtia 2/2 -Lobulation of upper helix 1/2	-Microtia 2/2	-Microdontia 2/2	p.Y106C; p.W153Vfs X51	7
12	1	-Michel aplasia 1/1	-Michel aplasia 1/1	-Microtia 1/1	-Microtia 1/1	-Microdontia 1/1	p.Y49C; p.R104X	7
13	1	-Michel aplasia 1/1	-Michel aplasia 1/1	-Microtia 1/1	-Microtia 1/1	-Microdontia 1/1	p.C50X	8

IAC: internal acoustic canal; SCC: superior semicircular canal; LCC: lateral semicircular canal

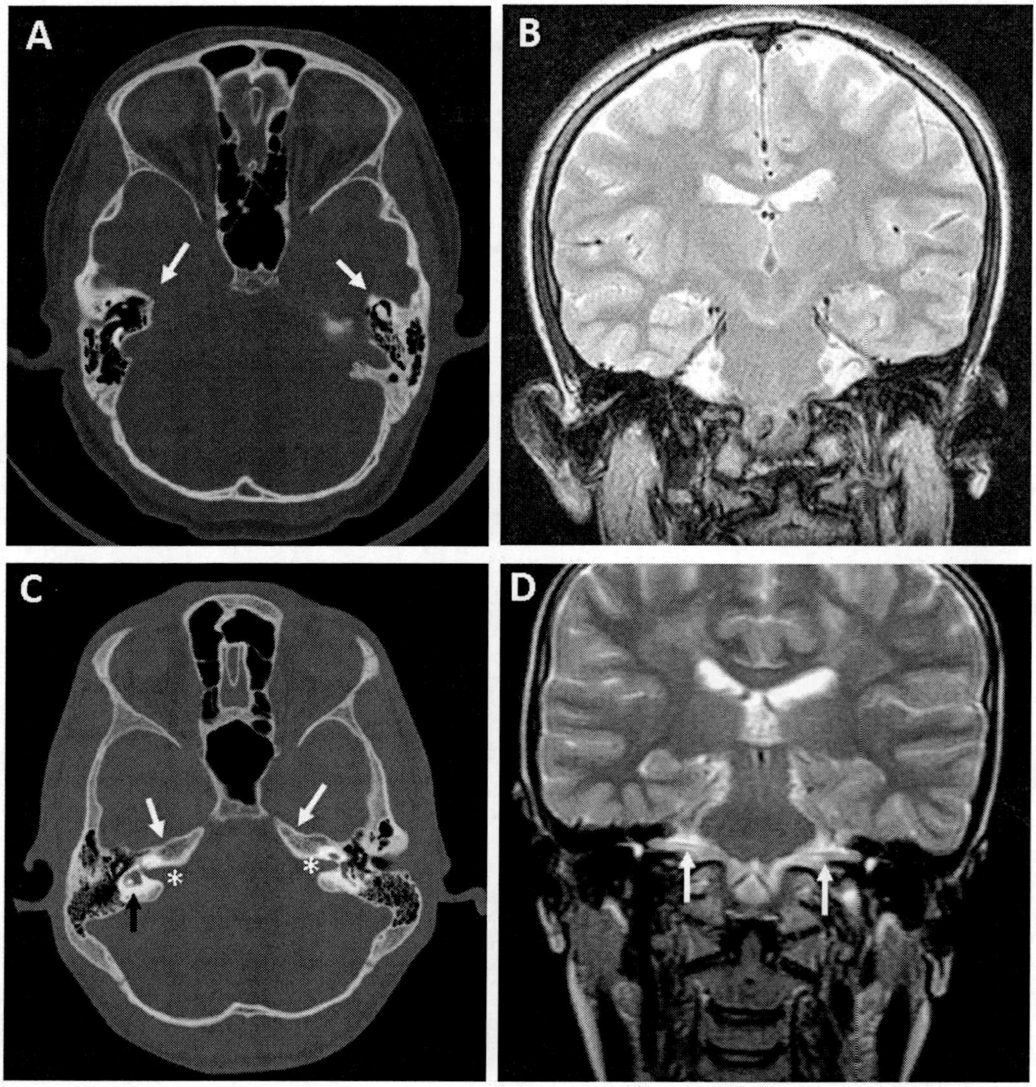

Figure 1. A) Bilateral absence of inner ear structures in an individual with LAMM syndrome. Note normal development of middle ear cavity with flattened medial walls and malleus and incus on the left (arrows). **B)** In an individual with LAMM syndrome coronal MR image clearly shows the absence of cochleovestibular nerve in cerebellopontine angle. **C)** Normal temporal bone CT image. At a level of ossicles, internal acustic canals (asterisks), vestibule (black arrow) and petrous apex of temporal bones (white arrows) are well seen. **D)** Normal MR findings. Cochlear and vestibuler nerves (white arrows) in the acustic canal along with the cohlear and vestibular structures are easily seen on a coronal image.

Microtia was unilateral in two cases and was not observed in the remaining eight people (Table 1). Individuals who had unilateral microtia or no microtia at all had the same homozygous p.R95W mutation. Other external ear anomalies included anteverted ears and large skin tags or lobulation of the upper side of auricle (Figure 2).

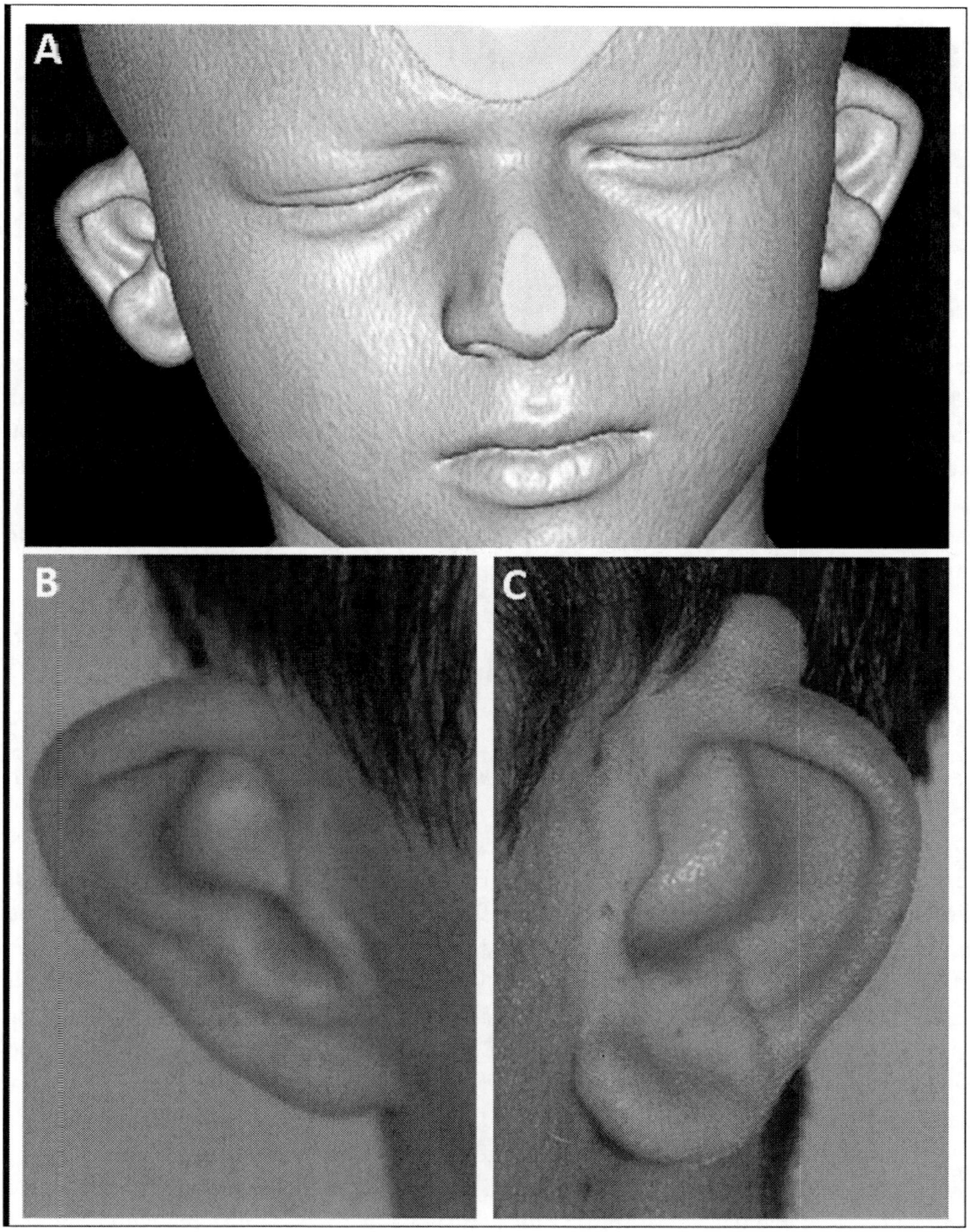

Figure 2. A) 3D rendering of MR images shows bilateral type I microtia with anteverted ears in an individual with LAMM syndrome. B,C) Typical microtia in two different individuals. Note the lobulation on the upper helix (C).

Microdontia: Small-sized teeth were observed in all reported individuals with LAMM syndrome. Other dental anomalies observed are conical tooth and decreased diameter of a tooth resulting in widely-spaced teeth (Figure 3). Hypodontia or any dental anomalies in the tooth roots were not observed in this syndrome.

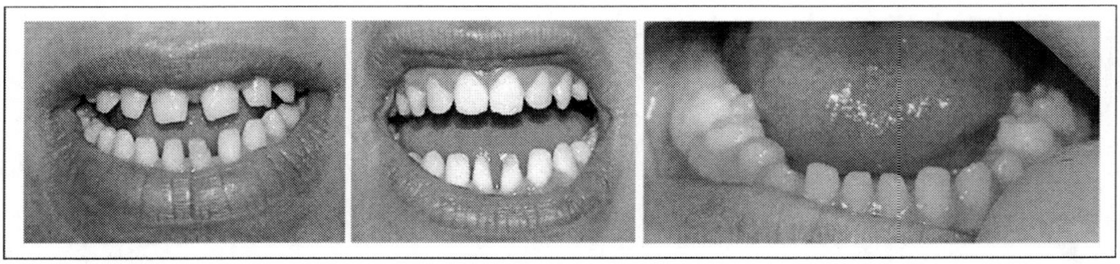

Figure 3. A-C) Microtia with widely spaced teeth in three different individuals. Note the involvement of all teeth.

Other observed findings in some of the reported individuals are distinctive facial findings including a long face, downslanting palpebral fissures, deep set eyes, high nasal bridge with hypoplastic alae nasi, mild micrognathia, hypoplasia/dysplasia of middle ear anatomical structures, stenosis of the jugular foramen with enlarged emissary vein formation, and gross motor developmental delay during infancy. Many of these findings are not likely to be a part of the clinical spectrum of *FGF3* mutations or specific to LAMM syndrome. There are multiple adults with normal cognitive function reported with LAMM syndrome.

THE *FGF3* GENE AND REPORTED MUTATIONS

The *FGF3* gene is located on chromosome 11q13.3 and contains 3 exons (DNA size is 9.45 kilobases and the mRNA transcript size is 1,548 base pairs). It codes for the fibroblast growth factor 3 protein.

There are 22 known fibroblast growth factor (FGF) genes in humans. Fibroblast growth factor proteins are known to function in embryonic development, cell growth, morphogenesis, tissue repair, tumor growth and invasion [11]. They mainly function through three pathways including the RAS/MAP kinase pathway (the main pathway), phosphoinositides 3 kinase/AKT pathway, and the phospholipase C gamma pathway. Physiologically, FGF3 binds to the FGFR (fibroblast growth factor receptor) 1b and 2b to activate its signaling cascade whereby it regulates cellular proliferation, survival, migration, and differentiation [12]. A unique feature of FGFs is that they act in concert with heparin or heparin sulfate proteoglycans at the level of the FGFR to activate the signaling cascade and induce a variety of cellular processes. Along with Fgf8 and Fgf10, Fgf3 plays a crucial role in the embryonic development of the otic placode (forms the inner ear) and its eventual differentiation into the vestibular and cochlear structures [13-18]. Studies of the Fgf3 gene in various species also show that it plays a primary role in the development of the teeth [19,20].

A total of 12 *FGF3* mutations have been reported in 13 unrelated families (Table 2). Six mutations were missense and six were nonsense or small deletions leading to truncated proteins or possibly nonsense mediated mRNA decay. Each mutation was reported in only one family except for p.R104X which was observed in Turkish, Pakistani, and Italian families [1,6,7].

Table 2. *FGF3* Mutations in LAMM syndrome

Nucleotide Change	Amino Acid Change	Location in the Gene	Ref.
c.17T>C	p.L6P	Exon1	3
c.146A>G	p.Y49C	Exon 1	7
c.150C>A	p.C50X	Exon 1	8
c.196G>T	p.G66C	Exon 1	4
c.255delT	p.I85MfsX15	Exon 2	3
c.283C>T	p.R95W	Exon 2	5, 6
c.310C>T	p.R104X	Exon 2	2, 6, 7
c.317A>G	p.Y106C	Exon 2	7
c.394delC	p.R132GfsX26	Exon 3	6
c.466T>C	p.S156P	Exon 3	2
c.616delG	p.V206SfsX117	Exon 3	2
c.457-458delTG	p.W153VfsX51	Exon 3	7

Genotype-Phenotype Correlation

In general, genotype-phenotype correlations can be made when a specific gene mutation consistently results in a predictable phenotypic effect. In LAMM syndrome, intra and interfamilial variability of the clinical phenotype is minimal except for the p.R95W mutation. Here affected individuals have less severe phenotypic effects compared to the other *FGF3* gene mutations [5,6]. Eight out of 11 reported individuals with the homozygous p.R95W mutation did not have microtia. None of the reported individuals with other mutations had normal appearing external ears. Moreover, in seven out of 20 inner ears of individuals with homozygous p.R95W mutation there was discernible inner ear formation present. None of the individuals with other mutations had inner ear components except for primitive vesicle-like structures in the inner ear.

Conclusion

LAMM syndrome is an autosomal recessive condition that presents with profound sensorineural deafness. It is caused by homozygous and compound heterozygous mutations of the *FGF3* gene. There appears to be a genotype-phenotype correlation especially with the p.R95W mutation leading to a milder phenotype, thus providing important clinical assessment tools for clinicians. It is important to recognize that *FGF3* mutations cause radiologically detectable inner ear anomalies even without microtia and difficult-to-distinguish microdontia. Mutation analysis of the *FGF3* gene is clinically available (www.genetests.org). Because of severe inner ear anomalies, the usage of cochlear implantation is limited in most individuals. However, providing the clinical and molecular diagnosis to affected families leads to better genetic counseling and empower families to have informed reproductive decisions.

REFERENCES

[1] H.V. Toriello, W. Reardon, R.J. Gorlin, *Hereditary Hearing Loss and Its Syndromes*, 2nd Ed., Oxford University Press (2004).

[2] M. Tekin, B.O. Hişmi, S. Fitoz, H. Ozdağ, F.B. Cengiz, A. Sirmaci, I. Aslan, B. Inceoğlu, E.B. Yüksel-Konuk, S.T. Yilmaz, O. Yasun, N. Akar. Homozygous mutations in fibroblast growth factor 3 are associated with a new form of syndromic deafness characterized by inner ear agenesis, microtia, and microdontia. *Am. J. Hum. Genet.* 80, 338-44 (2007).

[3] M. Tekin, H. Oztürkmen Akay, S. Fitoz, S. Birnbaum, F.B. Cengiz, L. Sennaroğlu, A. Incesulu, E.B. Yüksel Konuk, A. Hasanefendioğlu Bayrak, S. Sentürk, I. Cebeci, G.E. Utine, E. Tunçbilek, W.E. Nance, D. Duman. Homozygous FGF3 mutations result in congenital deafness with inner ear agenesis, microtia, and microdontia. *Clin. Genet.* 73, 554-65 (2008).

[4] O. Alsmadi, B.F. Meyer, F. Alkuraya, S. Wakil, F. Alkayal, H. Al-Saud, K. Ramzan, M. Al-Sayed.Syndromic congenital sensorineural deafness, microtia and microdontia resulting from a novel homoallelic mutation in fibroblast growth factor 3 (FGF3). *Eur. J. Hum. Genet.* 17, 14-21 (2009).

[5] R. Ramsebner, M. Ludwig, T. Parzefall, T. Lucas, W.D. Baumgartner, O. Bodamer, F.B. Cengiz, C. Schoefer, M. Tekin, K. Frei. A FGF3 mutation associated with differential inner ear malformation, microtia, and microdontia. *Laryngoscope.* 120, 359-64 (2010).

[6] S. Riazuddin, Z.M. Ahmed, R.S. Hegde, S.N. Khan, I. Nasir, U. Shaukat, S. Riazuddin, J.A. Butman, A.J. Griffith, T.B. Friedman, B.Y. Choi. Variable expressivity of FGF3 mutations associated with deafness and LAMM syndrome. *BMC Med. Genet.* 12,21 (2011).

[7] A. Sensi, S. Ceruti, P. Trevisi, F. Gualandi, M. Busi, I. Donati, M. Neri, A. Ferlini, A. Martini. LAMM syndrome with middle ear dysplasia associated with compound heterozygosity for FGF3 mutations. *Am. J. Med. Genet. A.* 155A, 1096-101 (2011).

[8] P. Dill, J. Schneider, P. Weber, D. Trachsel, M. Tekin, C. Jakobs, B. Thöny, N. Blau.Pyridoxal phosphate-responsive seizures in a individual with cerebral folate deficiency (CFD) and congenital deafness with labyrinthine aplasia, microtia and microdontia (LAMM). *Mol. Genet. Metab.* 104, 362-8 (2011).

[9] P. Michel. Memoire sur les anomalies congenitales de poreille intern. *Gazette Med de Strasburg* 23, 55–58 (1863).

[10] H. Weerda. Classification of congenital deformities of the auricle. *Facial Plast. Surg.* 5, 385-388 (1988).

[11] P. Krejci, J. Prochazkova, V. Bryja, A. Kozubik, W.R. Wilcox. Molecular pathology of the fibroblast growth factor family. *Hum. Mutat.* 30, 1245-55 (2009).

[12] M.E. Pownall, H.V. Isaacs. FGF *Signalling in Vertebrate Development*. San Rafael (CA): Morgan (2010).

[13] S.L. Mansour, J.M. Goddard, M.R. Capecchi. Mice homozygous for a targeted disruption of the proto-oncogene int-2 have developmental defects in the tail and inner ear. *Development.* 117,13–28 (1993).

[14] L.C. Zelarayan, V. Vendrell, Y. Alvarez, E. Domínguez-Frutos, T. Theil, M.T. Alonso, M. Maconochie, T. Schimmang. Differential requirements for FGF3, FGF8 and FGF10 during inner ear development. *Dev. Biol.* 308,379-91 (2007).

[15] J. Represa, Y. Leon, C. Miner, F. Giraldez. The int-2 protooncogene is responsible for induction of the inner ear. Nature. 353:561–563 (1991).

[16] V. Vendrell, E. Carnicero, F. Giraldez, M.T. Alonso, T. Schimmang. Induction of inner ear fate by FGF3. *Development.* 127,2011–2019 (2000).

[17] T.J. Wright, S.L. Mansour. Fgf3 and Fgf10 are required for mouse otic placode induction. *Development.* 130,3379–3390 (2003).

[18] R.K. Ladher, T.J. Wright, A.M. Moon, S.L. Mansour, G.C. Schoenwolf. FGF8 initiates inner ear induction in chick and mouse. *Genes Dev.* 19, 603–613 (2005).

[19] P. Kettunen, J. Laurikkala, P. Itäranta, S. Vainio, N. Itoh, I. Thesleff. Associations of FGF-3 and FGF-10 with signaling networks regulating tooth morphogenesis. *Dev. Dyn.* 219,322-32(2000).

[20] W. Jackman, B. Draper, D. Stock. Fgf signaling is required for zebrafish tooth development. *Dev. Biol.* 274, 139–157 (2004).

In: Inner Ear Development and Hearing Loss
Editors: Saima Riazuddin and Zubair Ahmed
ISBN: 978-1-62417-011-9

Chapter 6

Social Implications of Cochlear Implantation in Children

Matthew Provenzano and Daniel I. Choo*

Division of Pediatric Otolaryngology Head & Neck Surgery,
Cincinnati Children's Hospital Research Foundation, Cincinnati, Ohio, US

Abstract

Cochlear implantation has a profound impact on deaf individuals. Patients undergoing implantation demonstrate significant changes in their methods of communication and interaction with society. Many implanted children have speech and reading skills that track with their hearing counterparts and successfully use the telephone. Equally important are the social consequences of this technology. Long established institutions such as schools for deaf individuals find the number of students dwindling. Deaf society must determine the proper place of cochlear implantation within Deaf culture and education. At the same time, society grapples with the financial consequences of implanting thousands of these devises into children and the elderly. The merits of unilateral versus bilateral implantation, and the associated costs, are often debated by medical providers and healthcare policy experts. As healthcare resources become increasingly limited, medical necessity versus quality of life arguments become increasingly important for technology such as cochlear implantation. In this chapter we will explore some of the social consequences of cochlear implantation. Special attention will be made to the financial consequences of these programs and changes to the deaf culture.

Introduction

Numerous book chapters have described varying aspects of cochlear implantation. The surgical technique and outcomes have been well documented. A body of evidence points to the benefits these devices provide to elderly patients who have lost hearing and children who

* Correspondence to: Daniel.choo@cchmc.org

have never experienced it. The lay press has also provided myriad stories of patients' experiences after undergoing cochlear implantation. Researchers continue to search for technologic enhancements of current implant devices such that those individuals opting to receive a cochlear implant can benefit from improved access to sound and speech.

Apart from these potential benefits to the patient, cochlear implantation also presents significant social ramifications for society. This chapter will explore two aspects of societal changes cause by cochlear implantation: the response from the Deaf community and the financial costs of widespread cochlear implantation.

Use of these devices was initially unfavorably viewed by the Deaf community. This perspective continues to evolve as Deaf culture incorporates people who have received an implant and those who have chosen not to. In contrast to the Deaf community's response to implantation, a substantial portion of the hearing society has enthusiastically embraced this technology and now works to reconcile the tensions between technological capabilities and social/ethical norms, limited financial healthcare resources and the large costs associated with these devices.

Cochlear Implantation and the Deaf Community

In 1991, the National Association of the Deaf's (NAD) task force presented a position statement that "deplores the decision of the Food and Drug Administration [to approve cochlear implantation in children aged 2-17 years old] which was unsound scientifically, procedurally, and ethically." "The parents who make the decision for the child are often poorly informed about the Deaf community, its rich heritage and promising future."[1] This was the position statement from the NAD in response to the decision to allow cochlear implantation in children. The group describes itself as "the nation's premier civil rights organization of, by and for deaf and hard-of-hearing individuals in the United States of America."

The NAD statement, while seemingly inflammatory and controversial, appears almost timid compared to some of the additional publications on this subject. The literature is replete with comparisions of cochlear implantation to atrocities in human history that invoke extremes of emotions [2]. Such strong sentiments and opinions on this topic reflect the core beliefs and values upon which hearing, deafness and communication are founded for people.

Opposition to implantation has not only been based upon the surgical risks of the procedure but several other very relevant ramifications of cochlear implantation. Some opponents of implantation have focused on the ethics of performing an elective procedures on children who are deaf or hard of hearing, prior to an age or stage at which they could competently decide for themselves as to whether or not this was appropriate for them. This poses a potentially challenging scenario for some families who desire to take their child's wishes into consideration but are pressed by a substantial body of clinical and development evidence that shows early (developmental) windows of opportunity for children to learn an auditory-oral mode of communication and the potential consequences of missing that temporal window. For other opponents of implantation, the ethical implications of trying to "correct" or "treat" an intrinsic trait (such as being deaf or hard of hearing), presents the greatest individual dilemma. One analogous perspective is that it would be ethically wrong to surgically alter someone's skin color (or any other given ethnic trait) even if the capability was readily available and effective. For the Deaf community as a whole, there is also an understandable perspective that widespread cochlear implant practices could potentially have a negative impact (at a populational level) for the deaf and hard of hearing community. [3] Such considerations underscore that cochlear implantation is less about a novel surgical technique for individuals who are deaf, but is instead, more about preventing the eradication of a vibrant culture and community.

Its very apropos to review some of these viewpoints by the NAD and the larger Deaf community in the larger historical and cultural context of deafness in America. Over the centuries, deafness has clearly been regarded (particularly by physicians) as an ailment to be "cured" by the medical community. In contradistinction, deafness has been long viewed as a civil rights issue in the Deaf community. This core difference in this worldview is essential to understanding the initial resistance to cochlear implantation to children. Viewed through the lens of civil rights, "curing" these children of deafness through implantation is tantamount to the abhorrent historical practices involving reeducation and "civilization" of other racial or ethnic groups. As is the case with all issues of civil rights advances, the historical record demonstrates that the Deaf community's progress has been made in the face of significant challenges.

America's Deaf community began to flourish in the early nineteen century as centers of education developed throughout the country. Pioneering educators developed American Sign Language (ASL). This development created a linguistic minority within the larger English speaking society. The development of this distinct language helped set apart the deaf individuals as a distinct ethnic community.[4, 5]

Deaf education was well grounded in the Deaf community. It grew from within, largely free of externally imposed notions of deaf education and training. This system of education produced impressive results. Many deaf people achieved significant educational and professional gains.[5]

These achievements were challenged by a movement in the later part of the nineteenth century to promote Oralism in deaf education. Oralism employs lip reading and mouth movements so that the deaf student can communicate orally. Oralism posed a potential threat to those who saw ASL as a critical component of Deaf culture. Removing ASL from the Deaf community, in an effort to assimilate them into the hearing community, was akin to sacrificing a portion of their cultural heritage in order to conform to the societal norms. The parallels between these attitudes and those similarly employed with other historical instances of cultural and ethnic "reeducation" are clearly seen.[6]

The external application of Oralism further infuriated the Deaf community. Championed by hearing individuals such as Alexander Graham Bell, Oralism appeared to be imposed on the Deaf community by people who poorly understood Deaf culture or education. The autonomy previously experienced by Deaf educators and students was replaced by solutions from hearing people.[5]

It was within the context of these developments that control and preservation of Deaf culture, education, and communication fully evolved to become a matter of civil rights. The middle portion of the twentieth century witnessed the reestablishment of American Sign Language's prominence in Deaf society. This was obviously within the larger social context of a renewed focus on civil rights. Deaf culture and ASL were components of a group that fought successfully to protect and preserve a distinct culture. Deaf society argued that its culture and language were distinct entities and not simply adaptations of hearing culture and spoken English. The externally imposed changes to education and language were not simply matters of pedagogical technique but were instead seen as blatant efforts to change Deaf culture and erode civil rights; these were attempts to force Deaf society to conform to hearing culture.[7]

It was within the context of this struggle to reclaim previously eroded civil rights that cochlear implantation was introduced. Here again was a new method of communication that rid deaf individuals of their "disability" and allowed them to achieve spoken English. Deaf culture and American Sign Language were no longer needed now that this medical condition could be "cured" or at least managed. Deafness again became an abnormal deviation from the normal "healthy" individual. From one perspective, this was oralism reborn; this time supplemented with cochlear implant assisted hearing in order to improve the results.

The consequences of implantation expand beyond the preservation of hard fought gains; the very existence of ASL and Deaf culture have been suggested to be in jeopardy. Some have estimated that Sign Language could become a dead language. One such study, conducted in Australia, estimated that the number of people using Sign Language has significantly decreased. In that work, up to 84% of children who were deaf or hard of hearing were being implanted. Those who were not implanted usually had significant other medical problems that precluded them from meaningful communication of any means.[8] As the number of people using Sign Language approaches the minimal requirement for a "critical language mass" the future of the language itself becomes more precarious.[8]

The controversy surrounding implantation is complicated by the heterogeneity of the Deaf community. Many individuals who received implants, notably previously hearing individuals, do not see themselves as part of the Deaf community. These individuals regarded themselves as hearing people who now suffered from a medical ailment that robbed them of their previous life. For this group, cochlear implantation appeared to be a medical solution to a medical problem. Issues of culture or civil rights never entered the equation. Likewise, hearing parents of deaf children sought out implantation in order for their children to have more typical lives in a largely hearing world.

Implantation of these children brought the two cultures, Hearing and Deaf, into conflict. Hearing parents wanted their offspring firmly within the hearing culture. As deafness became "curable" its position as a "disease", and not a cultural attribute, solidified. Hearing parents wanted their children "cured." Deaf culture wanted the child to be recognized as a normal individual who communicated by a different means comparable to a foreign language. "Curing" a deaf child via implantation made no more sense than "curing" a non-English speaking immigrant by teaching them English.

While the majority of hearing parents would elect for implantation of a deaf child, this choice is clearly not universal. Byrd and colleagues report a case out of Michigan involving hearing parents fluent in ASL that elected not to have their twin deaf boys implanted.[9] The authors note that this appears to be one of the rare cases in the literature documenting the refusal of hearing parents to proceed with implantation. At one extreme, such a decision by the parents raises the question as to whether this decision constitutes legal medical neglect. The authors' site Michigan case law that has severed parental rights based upon neglect for non-critical care of the child. The authors conclude that preventing implantation in these boys will "indelibly impact their lives and limit their potential" despite the fact that the parents "may believe that that they are acting in the best interest of their children."[9]

Other works offer a response to the Bryd article. Robert Crouch's article entitled "Let the deaf be Deaf" offers a scathing criticism of medical deconstruction of the individual; he refutes the dissection of the patient into functional and diseased components, the later to the corrected through medical intervention.[10] He employs, with withering effect, quotes from prominent American neurotologists that appear to demonstrate an almost complete lack of understanding of deaf individuals and Deaf culture. The effect is a picture of medical paternalism at its worst. Crouch offers a contrasting view of the parents' choice from that posited by Bryd et al. Byrd describes the parents' choice as one that will "limit their [sons'] potential." Crouch describes the choice as one that has saved the sons from implantation and the "arduous" task of acquiring spoken language which is "beset with many pitfalls, where there seems to be no guarantee that the destination will be reached."[9] He explains that these parents have chosen a "different, but no less human, expressive potential." They have opted to forgo a still "unproven" medical treatment for their prelingual children and have, instead, chosen a path previously tread and clearly defined; one that leads to a rich and fulfilling life within the Deaf culture and American Sign Language.

Deaf parents of deaf children face an even greater challenge in that they recognize the rich cultural heritage of the Deaf culture, yet are cognizant that they are a minority residing within a hearing majority. Their struggle is no different from those who endeavor to preserve a distinct and different cultural heritage while integrating into the majority society. Superimposed upon this struggle is the recent memory of civil rights discrimination again the Deaf culture.

The 1991 NAD statement also highlights the potential benefits the Deaf community can offer to deaf patients and their families.[1] Deaf community resources and counseling are often not incorporated into the perioperative education and consent process. Patients and families rarely hear the benefits of deaf education, the support offered by deaf individuals and the impressive professional and academic achievements of deaf individuals.

Failure to provide complete information to a patient undergoing cochlear implantation strikes at the heart of the informed consent process. Patients and their families need to know all the alternatives to a proposed surgical procedure. Survey data from parents of children who received implants report that only 50% had even met a deaf adult.[11] These parents especially would likely have little information about the benefits of American Sign Language and the resources offered by the Deaf community. Those familiar with Deaf culture may have a bias against implantation and harbor misinformation that needs to be addressed by the physician.[12] Hearing parents often have no desire to discuss alternatives that would allow for the child to remain deaf. Likewise, adults who have lost their hearing want to reenter the hearing culture and have no desire to learn a second language or integrate into a new community

It is within the complexity of these decisions and the benefits of implantation that the NAD issued a revised statement on implantation in 2000. In part, this statement reads "The NAD recognizes the rights of parents to make informed choices [and] respects their choice to use cochlear implants and all other assistive devices, and strongly supports the development of the whole child and of language and literacy. While there are some successes with implants, success stories should not be over-generalized to every individual."[13] As the statement clearly indicates, the opinion about cochlear implant in the Deaf community is evolving.

The evolving views on cochlear implantation expressed in the revised statement are manifest in other actions in the Deaf community as it works to incorporate those individuals who have chosen implantation. By demonstrating a more receptive attitude towards implantation, the Deaf community, it's history, educational opportunities and support are no longer cut off from implanted deaf individuals. National centers of deaf education such as Gallaudet University are tailoring new educational methods for cochlear implant recipients. The University's Cochlear Implant Center works to create auditory and visual educational programs for people who have a cochlear implant.[11] Combining American Sign Language and voicing, in order to help accommodate the CI recipient, remains an area of continued controversy. Deaf and hearing individuals disagree about the merits of this pursuit.[11] There is also disagreement over which method of communication should be emphasized, which taught first and the overall benefits of a blended linguistic education for implant recipients. These debates will continue within the context of widespread cochlear implantation and have ramifications for the Deaf community and the recipients of these devices.

The revised NAD statement, in conjunction with the changing pedagogical practices, demonstrates a significant shift in the opinion of cochlear implants in Deaf culture. While this transition certainly cannot negate the important historical challenges faced by the Deaf community, it demonstrates that some of the more controversial positions have been modified. These changes appear to mirror an evolving sentiment held by the larger Deaf community with research demonstrating some agreement on the use of bilingual education (Gale E). The relationship between ASL and speech through cochlear implantation has move from one of hostility to one of mutually complimentary linguistic cohabitation.

It remains to be seen how growing implantation will ultimately affect the Deaf community. What is clear is that the rich history, educational achievements and culture within the Deaf community are invaluable resources for society. Cochlear implantation and the Deaf community will continue to work in concert to improve the lives of those with hearing impairment.

Cost Analysis of Cochlear Implantation

Cochlear implantation cost also creates significant challenges for societies attempting to allocate limited healthcare resources in a logical and equitable manner. Any benefit of implantation provided to the individual patient must be balanced against the larger, societal cost of that implantation. In a healthcare system with limited resources, any costly medical intervention must be weighed against competing use of resources. The problem of financial allocation has become more acute over the last decade as health care costs escalate. These challenges transcend boarders; many countries struggle to contain spending while providing the most cost efficient interventions.

Methods of Analyzing the Efficacy of Intervention

Cost analysis of any medical intervention must begin with a logical analysis of the intervention's benefit to the individual patient. A number of different methods exist to make this determination. All of these various methods attempt to assess the intervention's impact across various aspects of the patient's life. Comparison of pre and post intervention scores determines the intervention's impact on the patient. The EuroQol is one such assessment tool. It examines various aspects of the patient's health such as mood, pain, social relationships and mobility.[14] The study asks patients to read various descriptions of their lifestyle and then draw a line from those descriptions to a scaled bar (0-100) indicating the best and worst possible health state.[14] Examples of such description include "being dead" or "confined to bed and unable to feed self". Although examination of mood and social relationship can indirectly measure the effects of cochlear implantation, the EuroQol did not directly assess the patient's hearing or communication ability.

Wyatt and Niparko utilized another quality of life instrument, the Ontario Health Utilities Index, to measure the effect of cochlear implantation.[15, 16] The Ontario index, developed to assess treatment for childhood cancer, examines seven attributes of quality of life: sensation, mobility, emotion, cognition, self-care, pain and fertility. Of these seven catagories, only one, "sensation", deals specifically with hearing. The "sensation" category asks patients to rank their health status from one to four; deaf being ranked as a four and normal hearing as a one. However, this category also encompasses vision and speech, thereby introducing possible confounders into the assessment.

Unlike many of its counterparts, the Sintonen health related quality of life instrument does specifically address hearing as well as related topics such as speech and distress.[17] Like its counterparts, this grading system does assess qualities of life likely unaffected by implantation such as vision and sexual function. Patients are asked to grade their hearing on a 1 to 5 scale with 1 being completely normal hearing and 5 being completely deaf. A 3 on this scale indicates that the patient can hear normal speech with considerable difficulty, requiring conversations to be louder than normal. A 2 indicates hearing normal speech with little difficulty. Using the Sintonen system, patient surveys have demonstrated that patients can move from a pre-operative score of 5 to a post-operative score of 2 or 3.[18]

The pre-operative condition and post-operative results greatly effect these surveys. Profoundly deaf patients who experienced great success with cochlear implantation have a larger improvement in quality of life compared to someone with partial deafness and minimal post-operative improvement. Carter's work examined outcomes based upon three tiers of results: high value, middle value and low value. Those patients with a low value improvement saw an increase of 13% in their quality of life while those with high improvement saw a 32% improvement.[18] As will be discussed later, these varying results significance effect the cost efficiency of cochlear implantation.

Data from these various quality of life measurements are then converted to a Quality Adjusted Life Year (QALY). Although detail discussion of the assumptions and mathematics used to model the QALY are beyond the scope of this manuscript, a simple explanation demonstrates its importance in determining the cost utility of cochlear implantation. Quality adjusted life years are measured on a scale from 1 (perfect health) to 0 (death). An intervention that saved a child's life, had no associated morbidity and was shown to allow for a normal life span would have a very high QALY score. Alternatively, an intervention that provided minimal, short term improvement for an elderly patient would have a low QALY score The QALY score can then be adjusted for the intervention's cost.

Comparison of Cost Efficiency for Various Medical Interventions

Cost analysis allows for various procedures and treatments to be compared in order to determine the most efficient use of healthcare resources. Unfortunately, comparison of cost calculations are inherently flawed for multiple reasons. Any calculation is linked to currency valuations. The value of a currency changes both relative to other currencies in the form of exchange rate fluctuations and also to itself across time as inflation erodes its value. Exchange rates present a particularly difficult aspect of cost comparison. Cost analysis performed in another country must be converted to the currency of another country for accurate comparisons. These rates can also effect the cost of medical equipment manufactured in another country, a problem of particular importance as many cochlear implants are manufactured outside the country of implantation. It is possible that a cost efficient medical procedure could become cost prohibitive due to fluctuations in exchange rates. While long term contracts and price negotiation can help mitigate this fluctuation, monetary changes remain a challenge when estimating cost. In addition to these confounders, the cost of the intervention itself may change over time. Given these variables, it is possible that an intervention that was cost efficient at one time may cease being cost appropriate at a future date. Despite these limitations, calculated cost efficiency remains an important tool in helping to determine the economic appropriateness of a medical intervention.

Once calculated, an intervention's cost efficiency can be viewed in both absolute and relative terms. Society may deem expenditures of a certain amount to be too costly, regardless of outcome. For example, although every society has chosen to invest ample resources into the care of sick children, no society allows for billions of dollars[1] to be spent on each individual child. The World Health Organization (WHO) has recognized a bench march of three times the annual earnings as a reasonable level of spending to attain an additional year of life.[19] In 2010, the real median household income in the United States of America was $49,445.[20]

Any formula used to determine the financial appropriateness of medical care, such as that posited by the WHO, carries significant moral, economic and health policy implications. It is also clear that healthcare decisions, using this definition, would be vastly different depending upon the country of practice. Those countries with high annual earnings would tolerate significantly higher levels of spending compared to those with lower earnings. Pegging the worthiness of a specific intervention to a function of gross national product and income creates a situation whereby the appropriateness of a medical intervention has a distinctly nationalistic flavor. In effect, poorer countries place a lower monetary value on a year of human life compared to their rich counterparts. This also creates difficulty when comparing the worthiness of certain interventions between countries; what may be an acceptable expenditure in one nation may be unacceptable in another.

Cost comparison between specific interventions is another way to determine the cost efficacy. By examining the expenditure of cochlear implants, relative to other interventions, one can get a better sense for the fiscal appropriateness of this procedure. The resources allocated for implantation, while large in absolute cost, may be quite low relative to other procedures when adjusted for QALY.

---

[1] Of note: throughout this manuscript, dollars ($) will refer to United States of America dollars unless otherwise noted.

Cost comparisons are contained in Table 1. Cochlear implantation fairs well compared to a variety of other interventions. Some interventions, such as positron emission tomography (PET) imaging for Alzheimer's disease, carry costs ranging from $74,000 to $1.9 million dollars for each QALY.[21] The average cost for this intervention exceeded $598,000. In 2010 US dollars, this represents approximately 12 times the annual household income. Other interventions have greater cost efficiency. Research has demonstrated that intensive care unit care of even extremely low birth weight babies is relatively inexpensive ($3130 – Australian Dollars) when adjusted for the total life years gained.[22] This equates to 0.06 times the 2010 annual household income in the United States even without accounting for the exchange rate between US and Australian dollars and inflation changes. Most other medical interventions fall within these extreme ranges. As will be demonstrated later in this text, the cost of cochlear implantation per QALY compares favorably to many of these other interventions.[23].

Table 1. Cost comparison of various medical interventions

Intervention	Cost/QALY*	Source
Laser therapy for retinopathy of prematurity	$737	[33]
Initial cataract surgery	$2020	[34]
NICU care low birth weight babies	$3130/yr gained**	[22]
Cochlear implantation in children	$9741	[29]
Radiation therapy following conservative surgery for early stage breast cancer	$30,800	[35]
MRI for equivocal neurologic symptoms	$114,755	[36]
Kidney/Pancreas transplant	$167,224	[37]
PET imaging for Alzheimer	$598,000	[21]
Treatment for central retinal artery occlusion	$3.9 million	[38]

* All currencies in US dollars unless otherwise specified
** Australian dollars

Detailed Analysis of the Cost Efficiency of Cochlear Implantation

A number of variables effect the cost efficiency calculation of cochlear implants. In one examination of cochlear implant cost analysis, Wyatt et al identified fourteen different factors and assumptions that effected their calculations: 1) Average age at implantation and life expectancy 2) Type of device used 3) Lack of an alternative treatment 4) The percentage of patients able to be implanted 5) Device failure did not occur twice in the same patient 6) Maintenance fees and warranty terms 7) Failure rate and reliability of the hardware 8) Patients not implanted had no change in overall health utilization 9) Amount of time lost due to implantation 10) Patients were selected correctly on the basis that there was a viable nerve present 11) Amount of rehabilitation time required to implant use 12) Outpatient versus inpatient implantation 13) Percentage of patients who fully utilize the device once implanted 14) Discounting of future cash flow and quality of life resulting from implantation.[16] Each of these fourteen categories contain a number of different components that could effect the outcome. In their study, Wyatt and colleagues calculated the probability of certain estimates (such as percentage of device failures) being true. They then used these probabilities to determine the cost of implantation as well as the cost efficiency of implantation. However, cost estimates could be significantly effected if these estimates provided to be inaccurate. Cost estimation of minor complications is one such example of the difficulties in estimating the total cost of cochlear implantation. The authors estimated the average cost of a minor complication at $814. However, the maximum cost of a minor complication could reach $20,000. Likewise, while the base estimate for surgical cost was approximately $12,000, the estimated range was as high as $30,000. Despite these acknowledged limitations, Wyatt and colleagues estimated the cost of implantation at $15,593/QALY with a range of $12,000 to $30,000.[16] Analysis was performed using cost in US dollars with prices from the early 1990s.

Similar research by Summerfield and colleagues was published out of Great Britain the same year that Wyatt et al published their results. Summerfield calculated that the cost of gaining 1 QALY for an adult using a multichannel device was between £8,624 and £25,871.[24] Assuming an exchange rate of 1.56 US dollars per British Pound, the cost of implantation would range from $13,453 to $40,358. Summerfield estimated that the difference between the British estimates and his American counterparts could be explained mostly by the estimated costs of device maintenance and processor upgrades. Such variations further demonstrate how the overall cost estimates can be greatly effected by estimations of various aspects of implantation and device management. Despite these variations in cost, both studies demonstrated that cochlear implantation was, relative to other medical interventions, a sound investment of healthcare resources. These studies also demonstrate the importance of controlling costs associated with implantation.

Work later that decade examined, on a prospective basis, the cost of multichannel implantation in an adult population. A study conducted in the United States by Palmer and colleagues examined the cost of 62 individuals with an average age of 54 years old.[25] In this study, charges were determined by examining patient's medical bills, thus allowing the authors to calculate the exact expense of implantation and avoided estimating the entire cost. For those patients with a 22-year life expectancy, the cost of implantation was $14,670 per QALY. As their analysis shows, projection of the cost over the extended period of time is essential to lowering the cost/QALY to an acceptable level. For example, the cost in post implant year one exceeds $180,000/QALY but drops precipitously thereafter as the cost is spread over a number of years. Despite the prospective nature of the study, there remained a number of assumptions that significantly effected the cost calculations. It was assumed that device utility increased with each year of use. Costs were also estimated for those patients who failed to provide complete billing records. Actual billing data that was available demonstrated a wide range of costs associated with implantation; charges for the device ranged from approximately $14,000 to $37,000 while the cost of surgery itself ranged from $1274 to $11,094.

Any cost analysis performed in the United States is tainted by that country's dubious distinction as the most expensive healthcare market in the world. Similar cost analysis studies performed in other countries with significantly different healthcare financing structures have demonstrated the cost efficiency of implantation in adults. Work out of South Korea spanning a decade of implantation utilized a number of quality of life instruments to assess the cost per QALY.[26] Cochlear implantation costs ranged from $17,387/QALY to $40,474/QALY depending upon the quality of life instrument used. While these calculations are in line with those previously sited, they may represent a very conservative estimate of the true cost of implantation. In this South Korean study, there were no associated costs for battery replacement or processor upgrades. Other costs appeared quite low compared to their American counterparts; postoperative rehabilitation and audiologic follow-up cost a total of $124. Additional work from France further validates the cost efficiency of cochlear implantation.[27] Molinier and colleagues estimated the cost of adult implantation at €31,946. Although the total cost was not adjusted for QALY, this data from France indicates that cochlear implantation appears to be an efficient use of healthcare capital. Interestingly, this study, unlike many others examining the cost of implantation, included the familys' travel expenses.

Inclusion of additional expenses such as travel to and from the implantation center raises the question as to what expenses should be included when computing the total cost of the procedure. Costs are often divided between direct expenses, those directly resulting from the procedure such as physician fees, and indirect expenses. These indirect expenses could include costs such as education for deaf patients. Inclusion of indirect costs could perhaps provide a fuller picture of the total financial allocation for cochlear implantation. Inclusion of education costs (or savings depending upon the cost of deaf education) could more accurately determine if implantation wisely uses scarce healthcare resources. However, inclusion of these indirect costs could inject such variability that the cost estimates become practically useless. O'Neill and colleagues examined cochlear implantation costs in Great Britain and the associated indirect charges related to education.[28] Their work highlights the difficulty of accurately estimating indirect costs. In their work, geographic location and the governmental structure of educational funding greatly effected the QALY calculations for implantation. This effectively decreases or increases cost simply by inclusion of factors that have no pertinence to the cost of the procedure itself. Their articled raised the possibility that valid cost analysis data could be unduly influenced by unrelated factors such as the educational funding policy.

Cost analysis for younger patients suffers from many of the same limitations as calculations for their adult counterparts. Despite the difficulties associated with estimating the cost of numerous variables such as life expectancy and educational expenses, analysis has demonstrated that implantation in children is cost effective. Cheng et al utilized a number of instruments to determine the QALY associated with implantation in children.[29] Published in 2000, their work estimated costs based upon figures from the late 1990's until May 2000. Cost for implantation ranged from $5197/QALY to $9029/QALY.[29] By incorporating indirect costs such as reduced educational expenses, the authors estimated that implantation lead to a savings of over $53,000 per child. Colletti and colleagues also performed an expanded cost analysis that incorporated indirect cost such as education and family expenses. Their work examined the estimated cost savings of implantation compared to deaf children who did not undergo the procedure. The authors divided costs into those incurred by the health system, the family, and the educational system. They then subdivided the patients into three age cohorts. They estimated that the total cost to society to care for a six-year-old deaf child was approximately €161,000.[30] They then estimated that implanting children at age 1 resulted in a net cost savings to society of over €35,000 when compared to the oldest cohort of children. Cost savings for later implantation were less. While the difficulties of determining indirect costs have been discussed previously, their work add further evidence that cochlear implantation is a cost efficient use of healthcare resources.

While there appears to be a preponderance of evidence that unilateral, multichannel implantation in adults and children is cost efficient, bilateral implantation has not been as well studied. Lammers and colleagues performed a review examining the cost efficiency of bilateral cochlear implantation in adults and children.[31] Their analysis demonstrated a paucity of good data and the difficulties of determining the cost benefit of bilateral implantation. Only five studies qualified for inclusion in their review. Those studies demonstrated QALY calculations that varied over 4 fold. Additionally, the direct costs were considerably different between studies; manufacturer discounts granted for the second implant and simultaneous placement of the second implant greatly influenced cost.[31] Given these variations, cost calculations for adults ranged from adults $38,189 - $132,160 while pediatric costs were $30,973-$94,340.[31] Employing the WHO standard of three times annual income, bilateral implantation may not be cost efficient. Lammers et al employed a stricter standard of limiting cost to $48,300 for the second implant. Using this criterion, only one study demonstrated that bilateral implantation was likely to be cost effective.[32]

CONCLUSION

Widespread cochlear implantation has transformed the lives of deaf individuals and provided a powerful tool for the otolaryngologist. Despite the benefits of hearing restoration, controversy concerning the appropriate use of implantation remains. The vibrant and rich Deaf culture must adapt to the changes that this technology brings. Healthcare providers must understand the culture and historical issues surrounding Deaf culture and its early resistance to implantation in children. These same physicians must also critically examine the financial implications of widespread implementation of this costly technology. Rigorous financial analysis must continue to determine if bilateral implantation is a cost efficient allocation of scarce financial resources. Healthcare providers that work with cochlear implants must always be mindful of the vast consequences of their actions.

REFERENCES

[1] (1991) NS: National Association of the Deaf (NAD). Report of the task force on childhood cochlear implants. *NAD Broadcaster* 1991, 13:6-7.

[2] Silver A: Cochlear implants: Sure-fire prescription for long-term disaster. In *Book Cochlear implants: Sure-fire prescription for long-term disaster* (Editor ed.^eds.), vol. 53. pp. 4-5. City; 1992:4-5.

[3] Hladek GA: Cochlear implants, the deaf culture, and ethics: a study of disability, informed surrogate consent, and ethnocide. *Monash Bioeth Rev* 2002, 21:29-44.

[4] Mauldin L: Parents of deaf children with cochlear implants: a study of technology and community. *Sociol Health Illn* 2012, 34:529-543.

[5] Van Cleve JV, Crouch BA: A place of their own: Creating the deaf community in America. In *Book A place of their own: Creating the deaf community in America* (Editor ed.^eds.). City: Gallaudet University Press; 1989.

[6] Gannon JR: Deaf heritage: A narrative history of deaf America. In *Book Deaf heritage: A narrative history of deaf America* (Editor ed.^eds.). City: National Association of the Deaf; 1981.

[7] Pray JL, Jordan IK: The deaf community and culture at a crossroads: issues and challenges. . *J Soc Work Disabil Rehabil* 2010, 9:168-193.

[8] Johnston T: W(h)ither the deaf community? Population, genetics, and the future of Australian sign language. *Am Ann Deaf* 2004, 148:358-375.

[9] Byrd S, Shuman AG, Kileny S, Kileny PR: The right not to hear: the ethics of parental refusal of hearing rehabilitation. *Laryngoscope* 2011, 121:1800-1804.

[10] Crouch RA: Letting the deaf be deaf. Reconsidering the use of cochlear implants in prelingually deaf children. *Hastings Cent Rep* 1997, 27:14-21.

[11] Christiansen JB, Leigh IW: Children with cochlear implants: changing parent and deaf community perspectives. *Arch Otolaryngol Head Neck Surg* 2004, 130:673-677.

[12] Balkany TJ, Hodges AV: Misleading the deaf community about cochlear implantation in children. *Ann Otol Rhinol Laryngol Suppl* 1995, 166.

[13] NAD position statement on cochlear implants. [http://www.nad.org/issues/technology/assistive-listening/cochlear-implants]

[14] EuroQol--a new facility for the measurement of health-related quality of life. The EuroQol Group. *Health Policy* 1990, 16:199-208.

[15] Feeny D, Furlong W, Barr RD, Torrance GW, Rosenbaum P, Weitzman S: A comprehensive multiattribute system for classifying the health status of survivors of childhood cancer. *J Clin Oncol* 1992, 10:923-928.

[16] Wyatt JR, Niparko JK, Rothman ML, deLissovoy G: Cost effectiveness of the multichannel cochlear implant. *Am J Otol* 1995, 16:52-62.

[17] Sintonen H: The 15D instrument of health-related quality of life: properties and applications. *Ann Med* 2001, 33:328-336.

[18] Carter R, Hailey D: Economic evaluation of the cochlear implant. *Int J Technol Assess Health Care* 1999, 15:520-530.

[19] Health CoMa: Macroeconomics and health: investing in health for economic development. In *Book Macroeconomics and health: investing in health for economic development.* (Editor ed.^eds.). City: World Health Organization; 2001.

[20] DeNavas- Walt C, Proctor BD, Smith JC: Income, Poverty and Health Insurance Coverage in the United States: 2010. . In. US Census Bureau; 2011

[21] McMahon PM, Araki SS, Sandberg EA, Neumann PJ, Gazelle GS: Cost-effectiveness of PET in the diagnosis of Alzheimer disease. *Radiology* 2003, 228:515-522.

[22] Doyle LW: Evaluation of neonatal intensive care for extremely low birth weight infants in Victoria over two decades: I. Effectiveness. *Pediatrics* 2004, 113:505-509.

[23] Brown MM, Brown GC, Sharma S, Landy J: Health care economic analyses and value-based medicine. *Surv Ophthalmol* 2003, 48:204-223.

[24] Summerfield AQ, Marshall DH, Davis AC: Cochlear implantation: demand, costs, and utility. *Ann Otol Rhinol Laryngol Suppl* 1995, 166:245-248.

[25] Palmer CS, Niparko JK, Wyatt JR, Rothman M, de Lissovoy G: A prospective study of the cost-utility of the multichannel cochlear implant. *Arch Otolaryngol Head Neck Surg* 1999, 125:1221-1228.

[26] Lee HY, Park EC, Kim HJ, Choi JY, Kim HN: Cost-utility analysis of cochlear implants in Korea using different measures of utility. *Acta Otolaryngol* 2006, 126:817-823.

[27] Molinier L, Bocquet H, Bongard V, Fraysse B: The economics of cochlear implant management in France: a multicentre analysis. *Eur J Health Econ* 2009, 10:347-355.

[28] O'Neill C, Archbold SM, O'Donoghue GM, McAlister DA, Nikolopoulos TP: Indirect costs, cost-utility variations and the funding of paediatric cochlear implantation. *Int J Pediatr Otorhinolaryngol* 2001, 58:53-57.

[29] Cheng AK, Rubin HR, Powe NR, Mellon NK, Francis HW, Niparko JK: Cost-utility analysis of the cochlear implant in children. *Jama* 2000, 284:850-856.

[30] Colletti L, Mandala M, Shannon RV, Colletti V: Estimated net saving to society from cochlear implantation in infants: a preliminary analysis. *The Laryngoscope* 2011, 121:2455-2460.

[31] Lammers MJ, Grolman W, Smulders YE, Rovers MM: The cost-utility of bilateral cochlear implantation: a systematic review. *The Laryngoscope* 2011, 121:2604-2609.

[32] Summerfield AQ, Lovett RE, Bellenger H, Batten G: Estimates of the cost-effectiveness of pediatric bilateral cochlear implantation. *Ear Hear* 2010, 31:611-624.

[33] Brown GC, Brown MM, Sharma S, Tasman W, Brown HC: Cost-effectiveness of treatment for threshold retinopathy of prematurity. *Pediatrics* 1999, 104:e47.

[34] Busbee BG, Brown MM, Brown GC, Sharma S: Incremental cost-effectiveness of initial cataract surgery. *Ophthalmology* 2002, 109:606-612; discussion 612-603.

[35] Hayman JA, Hillner BE, Harris JR, Weeks JC: Cost-effectiveness of routine radiation therapy following conservative surgery for early-stage breast cancer. *J Clin Oncol* 1998, 16:1022-1029.

[36] Mushlin AI, Mooney C, Holloway RG, Detsky AS, Mattson DH, Phelps CE: The cost-effectiveness of magnetic resonance imaging for patients with equivocal neurological symptoms. *Int J Technol Assess Health Care* 1997, 13:21-34.

[37] Douzdjian V, Escobar F, Kupin WL, Venkat KK, Abouljoud MS: Cost-utility analysis of living-donor kidney transplantation followed by pancreas transplantation versus simultaneous pancreas-kidney transplantation. *Clin Transplant* 1999, 13:51-58.

[38] Brown MM, Brown GC, Sharma S: Cost-effective analysis. Central retinal artery obstruction. *Evidence-Based Eye Care* 2000, 1:243-247.

[39] Exploring perspectives on cochlear implants and language acquisition within the deafcommunity. Gale E. *J Deaf Stud Deaf Educ.* 2011 Winter;16(1):121-39. Epub 2010 Sep 29. PMID: 20881008

In: Inner Ear Development and Hearing Loss
Editors: Saima Riazuddin and Zubair Ahmed

ISBN: 978-1-62417-011-9

Chapter 7

HEREDITARY DEAFNESS AND COCHLEAR IMPLANTATION

Viet Pham, Rebecca Cook, Dayton Young and Tomoko Makishima
Department of Otolaryngology, University of Texas Medical Branch,
Galveston, Texas, US

ABSTRACT

A large amount of information regarding genetic hearing loss has become available over the past 20 years along with the identification of genetic loci and causative genes. Although many forms of hearing loss are thought to have a genetic etiology, in reality, many subjects do not undergo genetic testing. Cochlear implantation has become one of the mainstream treatment options for severe to profound hearing loss. Information and experience regarding cochlear implantation with genetic deafness is a valuable tool in considering treatment in any patient who might be a candidate for cochlear implantation. In this chapter, our intention was to review the literature on incidences of cochlear implantation in genetic deafness families and to determine if there were any characteristic findings regarding performance outcome. We reviewed reports in the literature (from 1994 to 2012) on patients with definitive diagnoses of genetic hearing loss who underwent cochlear implantation (total of 104 reports). The reports were limited to a fraction of the known loci or causative gene mutations, in which most cases had favorable results after cochlear implantation.

1. INTRODUCTION

Up to one half of congenital hearing deficits are attributed to a genetic etiology[1] with an incidence estimated at 1.2 - 1.7 in every 1000 births [2-5]. While genetic etiologies are commonly associated with childhood hearing loss, late-onset hearing loss has also been observed. Genetically-related hearing loss may be passed on from either affected parents or asymptomatic parents carrying a particular gene mutation. The hearing loss may be part of an underlying congenital syndrome, referred to as syndromic hearing loss, or as an isolated event denoted as non-syndromic hearing loss. Approximately 75 - 80% of genetic deafness is inherited through an autosomal recessive pattern, whereas 18 - 20% are autosomal dominant, and the small remainder include X-linked or mitochondrial forms of inheritance[6, 7].

The loci affiliated with autosomal dominant non-syndromic hearing loss are given the prefix DFNA, where DFN indicates deafness and A refers to an autosomal dominant inheritance pattern. Similarly, DFNB refers to an autosomal recessive non-syndromic hearing loss, and DFNX refers to X-linked non-syndromic hearing loss.

During the past two decades, there has been much progress in identifying genetic loci in hereditary deafness, leading to the characterization of its causative genes and its molecular mechanisms contributing to the deafness phenotype. To date, up to 64 DFNA loci with 27 genes, and up to 96 DFNB loci with 40 genes have been associated with genetic deafness[8].

Cochlear implantation has become one of the most utilized solutions to improve the hearing performance of people with severe to profound deafness in all age groups. Our goal was to review the literature regarding cochlear implantation in individual genetic deafness families, and to investigate if there were any differences in performance outcome.

2. Autosomal Recessive Non-syndromic Hearing Loss (DFNB)

Up to 80 % of genetic deafness is inherited through an autosomal recessive pattern, which also include patients who appear as "sporadic" cases. The characteristic DFNB hearing loss is a prelingual onset severe to profound hearing loss. The implementation of newborn screening has detected a larger number of children with hearing loss earlier. Among the children with severe to profound hearing loss, cochlear implantation is one of the definitive options for hearing improvement. Although more information on genetic deafness is available, in reality, most children with profound hearing loss who undergo surgery for cochlear implantation do not obtain genetic testing.

Reported cases of DFNB hearing loss with cochlear implantation and outcomes are summarized in Table 1. Characteristic phenotypes associated with specific loci are written in bold letters. Reports on sporadic cases within case series studies were included in the results.

DFNB1 is one of the earliest gene loci identified and contributes to approximately one half of autosomal recessive non-syndromic hearing loss cases [9]. The gene at this locus is *GJB2* which encodes the connexin 26 protein [1]. The connexin 26 protein plays a role in intercellular channels involved in potassium recycling from the outer hair cells to the stria vascularis [10] to facilitate resetting the mechanosensory transduction electrical gradients needed for auditory perception. Around 30 – 57 % of individuals with a *GJB2* mutation exhibit a profound hearing loss while another 26 – 30 % present with severe hearing loss [11]. A myriad of mutations can result in DFNB1-related hearing loss and specific mutations have been observed in higher frequency in certain ethnic groups including those of European descent, Ashkenazi Jews and Asians. Given its significant contribution to congenital hearing loss, genetic-testing for *GJB2*-related deafness is a vital tool by which genetic counseling and discussions about prognosis can be conducted. Regarding cochlear implantation reports, patients with *GJB2* mutations are the most frequently found in the literature. The performance outcome is generally good compared to patients without mutations.

Table 1. Cochlear Implantation Results in Autosomal Recessive Non-syndromic Hearing Loss

Locus	**Gene**	**Auditory phenotype and other characteristics**	**Cochlear Implant Results**
DFNB1	*GJB2* *GJB6*	Mild to profound prelingual SNHL	Better outcome in patients with mutations compared to those without mutations. [13, 30, 33, 36, 39, 42, 43, 45, 46, 68-73] Similar outcome in patients with mutations compared to those without mutations. [29, 35, 38, 40, 44, 74-77] Worse outcome in patients with mutations compared to those without mutations. [78] Improved function. [28, 79]
DFNB2	*MYO7A*	Severe to profound prelingual or postlingual SNHL	nr
DFNB3	*MYO15A*	Severe to profound prelingual SNHL	nr
DFNB4	*SLC26A4*	Progressive or non-progressive severe to profound prelingual or postlingual SNHL **Enlarged vestibular aqueduct**	Good outcome [80, 81] Better outcome in patients with mutations compared to those without mutations [13, 36]
DFNB5	*unknown*	Stable severe prelingual SNHL	nr
DFNB6	*TMIE*	Stable severe to profound prelingual SNHL	nr
DFNB7 DFNB11	*TMC1*	Stable severe to profound prelingual SNHL	nr
DFNB8 DFNB10	*TMPRSS3*	Stable or progressive prelingural or postlingual SNHL	Good outcome [82] Better outcome than without mutation[83]
DFNB9	*OTOF*	Stable severe to profound prelingual SNHL, **auditory neuropathy** in some patients	Better outcome in patients with mutations compared to those without mutations [13] Good results [84-87]
DFNB12	*CDH23*	Stable severe to profound prelingual SNHL	nr
DFNB13	*unknown*	Severe to profound progressive SNHL	nr
DFNB14	*unknown*	Profound prelingual SNHL	nr
DFNB15 DFNB72 DFNB95	*GIPC3*	Stable prelingual SNHL	CI done in one patient, but no information on outcome [88]

Table 1. (Continued)

Locus	Gene	Auditory phenotype and other characteristics	Cochlear Implant Results
DFNB16	*STRC*	Stable severe to profound prelingual SNHL more pronounced in higher frequencies	nr
DFNB17	*unknown*	SNHL not fully defined	nr
DFNB18	*USH1C*	Stable severe to profound prelingual SNHL	nr
DFNB19	*unknown*	Details unknown	
DFNB20	*unknown*	Postlingual moderate to severe SNHL	nr
DFNB21	*TECTA*	Stable severe to profound prelingual SNHL	nr
DFNB22	*OTOA*	Moderate to severe prelingual SNHL	nr
DFNB23	*PCDH15*	Stable severe to profound prelingual SNHL	nr
DFNB24	*RDX*	Stable severe to profound prelingual SNHL	nr
DFNB25	*GRXCR1*	Progressive moderate to profound prelingual SNHL	nr
DFNB26	*unknown*	SNHL, presence of **dominant modifier**	nr
DFNB27	*unknown*	Progressive variable SNHL	nr
DFNB28	*TRIOBP*	Stable severe to profound prelingual SNHL	nr
DFNB29	*CLDN14*	Stable severe to profound prelingual SNHL	nr
DFNB30	*MYO3A*	Progressive moderate to severe SNHL	nr
DFNB31	*WHRN*	Prelingual profound SNHL	nr
DFNB32	*unknown*	Stable severe to profound prelingual SNHL	nr
DFNB33	*unknown*	Profound prelingual SNHL	nr
DFNB35	*ESRRB*	Stable severe to profound SNHL	nr
DFNB36	*ESPN*	Profound prelingual SNHL	nr
DFNB37	*MYO6*	Severe to profound prelingual SNHL	nr
DFNB38	*unknown*	Profound prelingual SNHL in all frequencies	nr
DFNB39	*HGF*	Profound prelingual SNHL	nr
DFNB40	*unknown*	Profound prelingual SNHL	nr
DFNB42	*ILDR1*	Stable moderate to profound prelingual SNHL	nr
DFNB44	*unknown*	SNHL not fully defined	nr
DFNB45	*unknown*	Profound prelingual SNHL	nr
DFNB46	*unknown*	Profound SNHL	nr
DFNB47	*unknown*	SNHL not fully defined	nr
DFNB48	*unknown*	SNHL not fully defined	nr
DFNB49	*MARVELD2*	Stable moderate to profound prelingual SNHL	nr
DFNB51	*unknown*	Profound prelingual SNHL	nr
DFNB53	*COL11A2*	Stable severe to profound prelingual SNHL	nr

Locus	Gene	Auditory phenotype and other characteristics	Cochlear Implant Results
DFNB55	*unknown*	Profound prelingual SNHL in all frequencies	nr
DFNB59	*DFNB59*	Progressive severe to profound prelingual SNHL, **auditory neuropathy** in some patients	nr
DFNB60	*unknown*	SNHL not fully defined	nr
DFNB61	*SLC26A5*	Stable severe to profound prelingual SNHL	nr
DFNB62	*unknown*	Profound prelingual SNHL in all frequencies	nr
DFNB63	*LRTOMT*	Stable severe to profound prelingual SNHL	nr
DFNB65	*unknown*	Profound prelingual SNHL in all frequencies	nr
DFNB66	*unknown*	Profound SNHL	nr
DFNB67	*LHFPL5*	Stable severe to profound prelingual SNHL	nr
DFNB68	*unknown*	SNHL	nr
DFNB71	*unknown*	Profound prelingual SNHL in all frequencies	nr
DFNB73	*BSND*	Stable severe to profound prelingual SNHL	nr
DFNB74	*MSRB3*	profound prelingual SNHL	nr
DFNB77	*LOXHD1*	Progressive moderate to profound postlingual SNHL	nr
DFNB79	*TPRN*	Progressive severe to profound prelingual SNHL	nr
DFNB81	*unknown*	Profound prelingual SNHL	nr
DFNB82	*GPSM2*	Severe prelingual SNHL	nr
DFNB83	*unknown*	Prelingual SNHL not fully defined	nr
DFNB84	*PTPRQ*	Progressive moderate to profound prelingual SNHL	nr
DFNB85	*unknown*	Prelingual SNHL not fully defined	nr
DFNB86	*unknown*	Profound SNHL	nr
DFNB89	*unknown*	Prelingual moderate to severe SNHL	nr
DFNB90	*unknown*	Prelingual severe to profound SNHL	nr
DFNB91	*SERPINB6*	Progressive moderate to severe SNHL	nr
DFNB93	*unknown*	Moderate to severe SNHL	nr
DFNB96	*unknown*	Prelingual severe to profound SNHL	nr

SNHL – sensorineural hearing loss, nr – no reports. Some of the characteristic findings are written in bold letters.

For autosomal recessive non-syndromic hearing loss, the causative genes, in order of frequency, are *GJB2*, *SLC26A4*, *MYO15A*, *OTOF*, *CDH23*, and *TMC1* [12]. Among these, cochlear implantation reports were found in DFNB4 (*SLC26A4*) and DFNB9 (*OTOF*). Mutations in these genes are frequently found in patients who are cochlear implant candidates [13]. Each mutation has characteristic phenotypes which distinguish it from others: *SLC26A4* mutations are linked to enlarged vestibular aqueduct, and *OTOF* is linked to auditory neuropathy. Mutations in these genes have also been correlated with good performance outcome in cochlear implantation [13]. All of the cochlear implantation reports associated with *CDH23* mutations were those on Usher syndrome patients. Reports associated with *TMC1* mutation were those from DFNA36, and not DFNB7/11. These reports were not included in Table 1.

The majority of the DFNB loci and/or causative gene have been identified only recently. In addition, many of these families come from countries where cochlear implantation may not be readily available for treatment. With almost 100 DFNB loci identified in the literature, the large gap in the knowledge about their detailed clinical phenotype will hopefully become available with time.

3. Autosomal Dominant Non-syndromic Hearing Loss (DFNA)

Autosomal dominant deafness (DFNA) consists about 20% of all genetic deafness. Unlike DFNB hearing loss, most DFNA hearing loss has a postlingual onset and a milder degree of deafness. Thus, as expected, there were only a total of seven reports on cochlear implantation. Also of note is that as many of them present as a postlingual onset, there is a bias towards better outcome for post-implantation performance. The summary of the literature is shown in Table 2.

Within the DFNA group, reports of cochlear implantations were found in DFNA3 (*GJB2/GJB6*), DFNA9 (*COCH*), DFNA17 (*MYH9*), DFNA22 (*MYO6*) and DFNA36 (*TMC1*). The gene products of these genes have been shown to be present in the cochlea. Connexin 26 (*GJB2*) was expressed in many different cells within the cochlea [14], cochlin (*COCH*) was expressed in the spiral limbus, spiral ligament, and basilar membrane [15, 16], myosin VI (*MYO6*), and TMC1 protein (*TMC1*) was expressed in hair cells [17, 18]. While other genes were expressed mainly in areas without neural involvement, MYH9 protein (*MYH9*) was expressed in the spiral ligament, spiral limbus, hair cells and spiral ganglion [19, 20]. The expression patterns of the gene products suggest mostly a cochlear etiology of hearing loss and correlate with the good outcomes of cochlear implantation. Perhaps the neural involvement in *MYH9* expression explains the reason why some DFNA17 subjects had a poor response with cochlear implantation [21].

Due to limited cases reported, the clinical phenotypes may be somewhat biased by looking at a phenotype caused by a single mutation in the causative gene. In cases with multiple mutations identified in the same gene, the severity or spectrum of hearing loss may differ depending on the location of the mutation [12].

Moreover, some DFNB and DFNA share the same causative gene, which exhibit different phenotypes and further complicate the interpretation of genotype-phenotype correlation. Such examples include *GJB2/GJB6* (DFNA3 and DFNB1), *MYO7A* (DFNA11 and DFNB3), *MYO6* (DFNA22 and DFNB37), *COL11A2* (DFNA13 and DFNB53), *TECTA* (DFNA8/12 and DFNB21), and *TMC1* (DFNB7/11 and DFNA36). With the help of more genetic hearing loss cases being diagnosed and reported, these uncertainties will be clarified in the future.

Table 2. Cochlear Implantation Results in Autosomal Dominant Non-syndromic Hearing Loss

Locus	Gene	Auditory phenotype	Cochlear Implant Results
DFNA1	*DIAPH1*	Progressive **low-frequency** postlingual SNHL in first decade to profound deafness	nr
DFNA2	*KCNQ4*	Progressive high-frequency postlingual SNHL in second decade to profound deafness	nr
	GJB3	Progressive high-frequency postlingual SNHL in fourth decade to profound deafness	
DFNA3	*GJB2* *GJB6*	Progressive severe to profound high-frequency prelingual SNHL	Good outcome [89]
DFNA4	*MYH14*	Flat or gently downsloping postlingual SNHL to severe or profound deafness by fourth decade	nr
DFNA5	*ICERE-1*	Progressive high-frequency postlingual SNHL in first decade that gradually extends to low-frequency SNHL	nr
DFNA6 DFNA14 DFNA 38	*WFS1*	Progressive **low-frequency** prelingual SNHL to profound deafness by fourth decade	nr
DFNA8 DFNA12	*TECTA*	Stable moderate to severe prelingual SNHL in mid- to high-frequencies in first or second decade, some variants with progressive deafness	nr
DFNA9	*COCH*	High-frequency postlingual SNHL beginning in second decade progressing to anacusis by fourth or fifth decade, association with **vestibular dysfunction**	Good outcome [90]
DFNA10	*EYA4*	Flat or gently downsloping postlingual SNHL in third or fourth decade to severe or profound deafness	nr
DFNA11	*MYO7A*	Flat or gently downsloping mild to severe postlingual SNHL, some with **vestibular dysfunction**	nr
DFNA13	*COL11A2*	Progressive **mid-frequency** postlingual SNHL starting in second to fourth decade	nr
DFNA15	*POU4F3*	Progressive moderate to severe high-frequency postlingual SNHL	nr
DFNA16	*unknown*	**Fluctuating**, progressive, mild to severe SNHL	nr
DFNA17	*MYH9*	Progressive moderate to severe high-frequency postlingual SNHL	Good outcome [91] Poor outcome [21]
DFNA18	*unknown*	Progressive moderate to severe SNHL	
DFNA20 DFNA26	*ACTG1*	Progressive high-frequency postlingual SNHL to profound deafness in all frequencies	nr
DFNA21	*unknown*	Progressive, mid frequency, moderate to severe SNHL	nr

Table 2. (Continued)

Locus	Gene	Auditory phenotype	Cochlear Implant Results
DFNA22	*MYO6*	Progressive high-frequency postlingual SNHL in childhood to profound deafness, some association with **hypertrophic cardiomyopathy**	Good outcome [92]
DFNA23	*SIX1*	Downsloping mild to profound prelingual SNHL	nr
DFNA24	*unknown*	Prelingual, progressive, mid-high frequency, severe to profound SNHL	nr
DFNA25	*SLC17A8*	Progressive high-frequency postlingual SNHL between second and sixth decades	nr
DFNA27	*unknown*	Progressive, severe to profound SNHL	nr
DFNA28	*GRHL2*	Progressive flat or gently downsloping mild to moderate postlingual SNHL	nr
DFNA30	*unknown*	Mid to high frequency SNHL	nr
DFNA31	*unknown*	**Mid-frequency** moderate SNHL	nr
DFNA33	*unknown*	Progressive, moderate to severe SNHL	nr
DFNA36	*TMC1*	Postlingual downsloping rapidly progressive SNHL	Good outcome [93, 94]
DFNA39	*DSPP*	Progressive high-frequency postlingual SNHL in second or third decade, association with **dentinogenesis imperfecta**	nr
DFNA41	*unknown*	Progressive moderate to severe SNHL, **gender differences** in audiogram type	nr
DFNA42	*unknown*	Progressive, to profound SNHL	nr
DFNA43	*unknown*	Progressive, to severe SNHL	nr
DFNA44	*CCDC50*	Progressive **low- to mid-frequency** moderate postlingual SNHL in first decade to profound deafness by sixth decade	nr
DFNA47	*unknown*	Progressive, moderate to severe SNHL	nr
DFNA48	*MYO1A*	progressive moderate to severe postlingual SNHL	nr
DFNA49	*unknown*	Progressive, moderate to severe SNHL	nr
DFNA50	*MIR96*	Flat or progressive mild to moderate postlingual SNHL in second decade to severe or profound deafness	nr
DFNA51	*TJP2*	Progressive high-frequency postlingual SNHL in fourth decade to severe or profound deafness	nr
DFNA52	*unknown*	Progressive, to profound SNHL	nr
DFNA53	*unknown*	Progressive, to profound SNHL	nr
DFNA54	*unknown*	Progressive, **low frequency**, moderate SNHL	nr
DFNA58	*unknown*	Progressive, to severe SNHL	nr
DFNA59	*unknown*	Congenital, severe to profound SNHL	nr
DFNA64	*DIABLO*	Progressive moderate to severe postlingual SNHL in first to third decade	n/a

SNHL – sensorineural hearing loss, nr – no reports. Some of the characteristic findings are written in bold letters.

4. X-LINKED HEARING LOSS AND HEARING LOSS ASSOCIATED WITH MITOCHONDRIAL MUTATIONS

X-linked deafness and deafness due to mitochondrial mutations are rare, but distinctly recognizable because of the unique form of inheritance.

In X-linked deafness, the deafness phenotype is passed on maternally to the male patients. The loci affiliated with X-linked non-syndromic hearing loss are given the prefix DFNX (Table 3). Among the five loci identified, only DFNX2 has reports on cochlear implantation. Patients with DFNX2 (*POU3F4*) are associated with cochlear dysplasia and perilymphatic gusher and the performance outcome is variable [22-24].

In deafness due to mitochondrial mutations, the deafness phenotype is inherited maternally, affecting both males and females. The mutated mitochondria are distributed unevenly in each cell throughout the entire body, thus affecting some organs more than others. Different symptoms arise depending on the percentage of mutated mitochondria and the susceptibility of the specific organ within the body. Many patients with mitochondrial mutations develop a syndromic phenotype of progressive hearing loss accompanying diabetes, muscular dystrophy, and encephalopathy, among other symptoms. Hearing loss is often observed as one of the early symptoms in these patients. The association with susceptibility to aminoglycoside induced ototoxicity is a characteristic finding in some forms of mitochondrial mutations.

Table 3. Cochlear Implantation Results in X-Linked Non-syndromic Hearing Loss

Locus	Gene	Auditory phenotype and other characteristics	Cochlear Implant Results
DFNX1 (DFN2)	*PRPS1*	Progressive and non-progressive, prelingual and postlingual, moderate to profound SNHL	nr
DFNX2 (DFN3)	*POU3F4*	Prelingual, progressive, profound mixed hearing loss, **temporal bone abnormality**, **perilymph gusher**	Variable outcome, some good, some with minimal improvement [22] Gusher observed with surgery, limited improvement on functional outcome [23] Gusher observed with surgery, no mention on functional outcome [24]
DFNX3 (DFN4)	*unknown*	Stable prelingual profound SNHL	nr
DFNX4 (DFN6)	*SMPX*	Progressive severe to profound SNHL	nr
DFNX5 (AUNX1)	*unknown*	Progressive, severe to profound SNHL, **auditory neuropathy**	nr

SNHL – sensorineural hearing loss, nr – no reports. Some of the characteristic findings are written in bold letters.

Table 4. Cochlear Implantation Results in Mitochondrial Non-syndromic and Syndromic Hearing Loss

Gene	Phenotype	Cochlear Implant Results
MTRNR1	Highly variable SNHL with variable penetrance, **aminoglycoside ototoxicity**	Good outcome [95, 96] No change in auditory performance [97]
MTTS1	Highly variable SNHL with variable penetrance	nr
MTCO1	Severe to profound **aminoglycoside** associated SNHL	nr
MTTF	Progressive, severe to profound SNHL	Good outcome [98]
MTTL1	Progressive, severe to profound SNHL, MELAS	Good outcome [99-105]
Unknown Variable	Variable progressive, severe to profound SNHL	Overall good outcome, evaluation on 12 subjects from literature, with different mutations [106] Good outcome in subject with large rearrangement of mitochondrial DNA [107] Good outcome in subject with undefined mitochondrial cytopathy [108] Good outcome in subject with MNGIE [109] Good outcome in subject with KSS [110]

SNHL – sensorineural hearing loss, nr – no reports. Some of the characteristic findings are written in bold letters.

MELAS – mitochondrial encephalopathy, lactic acidosis, stroke-like episodes.

MNGIE – mitochondrial neurogastrointestinal encephalomyopathy.

KSS – Kearns-Sayre syndrome (oculocraniosomatic neuromuscular disease, cardiac conductive disturbance, deafness, and other symptoms).

Due to the progressive and syndromic nature of their phenotypes, outcomes of cochlear implantation vary depending on the overall condition of each individual. However, the majority of the patients with mitochondrial mutations performed well with cochlear implantation (Table 4).

5. Syndromic Hearing Loss (Table 5)

Some of the well-known syndromic conditions involving hearing loss are summarized in Table 5. The performance outcome of cochlear implantation depends largely on other anatomical, cognitive and overall condition affected by the different syndromes.

Different mutations in the same gene can manifest as non-syndromic or syndromic hearing loss. Such examples include *MYO7A* (Usher syndrome type 1, DFNB2, DFNA11), *CDH23* (Usher syndrome type 1, DFNB12), *PCDH15* (Usher syndrome type 1, DFNB23),

USH1C (Usher syndrome type 1, DFNB18), *WHRN* (Usher syndrome type 2, DFNB31), and *GJB2/GJB6* (KID syndrome, DFNB1, DFNA3).

Performance outcome of cochlear implantation is favorable overall, except for a few reports associated with CHARGE syndrome [25, 26] and Mohr-Tranebjaerg syndrome [27].

6. Gene Mutations and Cochlear Implant Outcome

There is no generalized method to evaluate the performance outcome across different languages. The reports originated from a wide variety of countries: USA, UK, Italy, Brazil, Iran, Turkey, Korea, China, Japan, Poland, Israel, Argentina, etc. Collectively, the outcome measures used in the reports differed largely, and was often modified to fit the individual languages. In addition, many reports consisted of small case reports/series. While some were objective, some were somewhat subjective. Thus, we were only able to assess the overall direction of the outcome. In the tables, we assigned the terms "good, better, worse, poor" to suit a wide range of outcome descriptions. Both objective and subjective results are included. For example, a "better" outcome may refer to a subject who may be able to use the phone, or a subject who still heavily depends on visual cues but had improved speech discrimination scores.

Table 5. Cochlear Implantation Results in Syndromic Hearing loss

Syndrome	Gene	Inheri-tance	Phenotype	Cochlear Implant Results
Branchio-oto-renal	*EYA1* *SIX5*	AD	Renal abnormalities, branchial fistula or cysts, structural defects of the ear, hearing loss	CI done, but no mention on outcome [111, 112]
CHARGE	*CHD7*	sporadic	Coloboma, atresia of the choanae, retardation of growth and/or development, gential and/or urinary abnormalities, and ear abnormalities and/or deafness	Venous malformation considerations during CI surgery, no mention on outcome [113] Variable outcome, some with good results, some with poor results [25, 26] Good outcome, improved performance [114-118]
Jervell and Lange-Nielsen	*KCNQ1* *KCNE1*	AR	Prolonged QT interval, congenital profound SNHL	Good outcome [112, 119-123]
Mohr-Tranebjaerg (deafness–dystonia–optic atrophy)	*TIMM8A*	X-linked	dystonia, optic atrophy, dementia, and progressive auditory neuropathy,	Marginal to poor outcome [27]
KID (Keratitis-ichthyosis-deafness)	*GJB2/GJB6*	AD, AR, sporadic	vascularizing keratitis, SNHL, erythrokeratoderma	Good outcome. Dermatological complications from surgery [124-128] Good outcome [129]
Pendred	*SLC26A4* *KCNJ10*	AR	Enlarged vestibular aqueduct, cochlear dysplasia, progressive SNHL, Thyroid dysfunction	Good outcome [130] Poor outcome due to unpredicted events [131]

Table 5. (Continued)

Syndrome		Gene	Inheritance	Phenotype	Cochlear Implant Results
Usher	Type I	*MYO7A* *USH1C* *CDH23* *PCDH15* *SANS*	AR	Congenital profound SNHL, vestibular dysfunction, retinitis pigmentosa	Better quality of life with cochlear implants [132] Improved performance if implanted early in life [133, 134] Good outcome with *PCDH15* mutation patients [135] Good outcome if CI performed by 3 years of age [136] Good outcome if CI performed by 3 years of age, not as good when implanted 14-17 years of age [137] Good outcome [138]
	Type II	*USH2A* *VLGR1* *WHRN*	AR	Congenital SNHL, normal vestibular function, retinitis pigmentosa	nr
	Type III	*CLRN1* *PDZD7*	AR	Progressive SNHL, variable vestibular dysfunction, retinitis pigmentosa	Good outcome [134, 139]
Waardenburg	Type I	*PAX3*	AD	heterochromia irides, white forelock, dystopia canthorum, SNHL	Improved performance with CI, but less so with behavioral disorders [140] Improved performance, but poorer outcome compared to pure SNHL patients with CI [141] Improved and comparable results with other CI patients [142] Good outcome in most patients. Patients with abnormal EABR perform poorly [143] Improved performance [112, 144-147]
	Type II	*MITF* *SNAI2*	AD	heterochromia irides and SNHL but dystopia canthorum and white forelock rare	Improved performance [145, 147-150]
	Type III	*PAX3*	AD	type 1 but with mental retardation and musculoskeletal abnormalities	Improved performance [145]
	Type IV	*EDN3* *EDNRB* *SOX10*	AD	association with Hirschsprung's disease	nr

AD – autosomal dominant, AR – autosomal recessive, SNHL – sensorineural hearing loss, nr – no report.

The majority of patients who receive cochlear implants are sporadic cases, without family history of profound hearing loss. In an effort to determine the causative gene mutation in these sporadic cases, several studies have screened deafness causing genes in cochlear implant recipients and have found novel and known mutations among this population [13, 28-46].

GJB2 mutations are the most frequent, which accounts for up to 50% of the causative mutatons [12]. Other frequently found causative genes include *SLC26A4*, *OTOF*, *CDH23*, and *TMC1*, which accounts for several percents combined. The remainder of the patients do not have mutations in tested genes. Thus, there are limited numbers of reports on cochlear implantation performance outcome other than those for *GJB2* mutations.

Overall, gene mutations with good cochlear implant performance outcomes were those with *GJB2*, *SLC26A4*, *OTOF*, *COCH*, *MYO6*, *TMC1* and mitochondrial mutations. Poor outcomes were reported only in a few reports associated with mutations of *GJB2*, *MYH9* and *POU3F4*. The causative genes for syndromic hearing loss are more frequently associated to poor outcome. *CHD7* (CHARGE syndrome), *TIMM8A* (Mohr-Tranebjaerg syndrome), and *PAX3* (Waardenburg syndrome) were reported with mixed or poor results.

7. Clinical Considerations for Cochlear Implantation in Hereditary Deafness

While there are some exceptions, hereditary hearing loss does not seem to result in significant aberrancy in the overall anatomical structure of the ear. Particularly in cases of hereditary sensorineural hearing loss, the specific anatomical structures thought to be defective are microscopic and occur at the level of individual cells within the cochlea, such as hair cells. Cochlear implants are engineered to bypass the intricate cellular microanatomy of the ear by stimulating the spiral ganglia of the cochlear nerve directly. As a result, it is speculated that most forms of severe to profound non-syndromic hereditary hearing loss can be rehabilitated by cochlear implantation with equal efficacy regardless of the specific gene responsible for the deafness.

In general, the cause of deafness does not affect the audiologic success with a cochlear implant, with a few exceptions [47]. One of the notable exceptions is the case of cochlear ossificans, which occurs as a result of an infectious etiology (meningitis) rather than a hereditary one. Post-infectious ossification of the cochlea can make placement of the implant difficult. In addition, cochlear ossificans has been shown to be associated with auditory neural depletion [47, 48]. Other exceptions include agenesis of the cochlea, malformation of the cochlea, absence of the auditory nerve, or loss of auditory nerve integrity [49-51]. While the latter causes of deafness may certainly have a genetic cause, they are more readily identified with imaging techniques such as computed tomography (CT) or magnetic resonance imaging (MRI) than by genetic testing. The above mentioned anatomical pathology should be assessed as part of the decision making process, as they may negatively affect a patient's chances of rehabilitation with cochlear implantation.

The primary factors which serve as predictors of success with cochlear implantation are: 1) duration of deafness, 2) age at implantation, and 3) whether the patient has a foundation of experience with hearing and understanding spoken language [52-59]. Simply put, the most successful outcomes are in those patients who lost their hearing after they had already developed speech and language skills (post-lingual deafness) and who are then implanted soon thereafter. The least successful outcomes are in those patients who were deaf before they had acquired speech and language skills (pre-lingual deafness) and who do not receive an implant until much later in life. Patients with pre-lingual or congenital deafness can have very successful outcomes, but that success is negatively correlated to the age at implantation. The earlier they are implanted, the better the outcome. Patients implanted before the age of two years do much better than those implanted later. Similarly, children or adults implanted after only a short duration of post-lingual deafness have better outcomes than those implanted many years after they lose their hearing.

The workup for cochlear implantation in hereditary hearing loss patients is not different from others. Candidacy for cochlear implantation is first assessed audiometrically. Cochlear implants are intended for patients who are deaf or nearly deaf (severe to profound sensorineural hearing loss). While surgeons go to great efforts to preserve residual natural hearing during surgical placement of the cochlear implant, a significant percentage of patients who are implanted lose some or all of the remaining natural hearing in the implanted ear. Therefore, if a patient can be better rehabilitated with amplification, cochlear implantation is not carried out and a hearing aid is prescribed. However, for those patients who can expect better speech recognition with cochlear implantation than with amplification, cochlear implantation is considered.

The audiometric criteria that define the point at which a cochlear implant is thought to be advantageous over traditional amplification have expanded over time to include patients with an increasing amount of residual hearing. To determine whether a patient has reached this point, a series of recorded speech recognition tests are conducted on patients who are already using a hearing aid at the time of testing. The hearing aid should already have been fitted and modified prior to testing, so that at the time of testing, it represents the "best aided" condition. Typically the "best-aided" condition occurs at sound amplification levels of 55 to 65 dB SPL (sound pressure level). Speech recognition tests are presented to the aided patient at intensity levels that reflect realistic listening levels in a normal environment. Patients who score less than or equal to 50% correct on speech recognition tests, under these "best aided "conditions, are more likely to have better understanding of speech with a cochlear implant than with traditional amplification using currently available technology [60].

In the United States, The Food and Drug Administration (FDA) guidelines prescribe that a prospective cochlear implant candidate be at least 12 months of age, first undergo a hearing aid trial, have a pure tone average (PTA) of 70 dB HL (hearing level) or greater, and have speech recognition scores no better than 50% in the ear to be implanted and no better than 60% in the opposite ear [61]. However, audiometric criteria have expanded in other parts of the world and will continue to expand. Experience in Europe and other countries have demonstrated successful outcomes in patients outside of the present criteria. For example, hybrid cochlear implants (both electrical and auditory stimulation) have been used successfully in ears with significantly more residual hearing than above criteria would prescribe [62, 63]. Also, patients with single sided deafness but good hearing in the opposite ear have been successfully implanted in Europe [64]. As techniques are refined and clinical trials continue to document success, the criteria will most likely be expanded to include patients with a lesser degree of hearing loss.

Patients who meet audiometric criteria are assessed by the medical team to determine whether they are healthy enough to undergo the surgical procedure without exceptional risk. Some patients with significant medical comorbidities may be declined because the risk of surgery is too great. Patients also undergo a cognitive and psychosocial evaluation to determine their level of cognitive function, ability to complete rehabilitation and to meet appropriate post-implant goals and expectations. Patients with multiple handicaps, such as cognitive impairment, visual impairment, psychological impairment or lack of a social network can be challenging, but with proper rehabilitative efforts, cochlear implantation in these patients can be successful, too [65, 66].

Radiographic imaging (CT, MRI) is carried out to determine any relative or absolute contraindications to implantation and to provide an assessment of the surgical anatomy to identify potential areas of risk. Imaging studies are important because approximately 20% of patients with congenital sensorineural hearing loss have radiographic abnormalities of the inner ear [67]. The only absolute contraindications for implantation are absence of the cochlear nerve and cochlear agenesis [49]. Other malformations such as Mondini dysplasia, common cavity deformity and cochlear ossificans are not contraindications, though they may portend a more difficult and potentially complicated surgery with a more limited hearing outcome [50, 67].

CONCLUSION

Cochlear implantation is a fascinating technology that is capable of providing significant rehabilitation to patients with severe to profound hereditary and non-hereditary forms of sensorineural hearing loss. In current medical practice, defining the specific gene causing hearing loss does not typically change the course of treatment. However, as most reports either show better or favorable performance outcomes in subjects with hereditary hearing loss, information on the causative gene can be used as positive information for treatment planning and counseling on cochlear implantation. As more complete information regarding the genetic and cellular mechanisms of hereditary hearing loss is compiled and as technology continues to advance, techniques to directly address the specific pathophysiology at a cellular level will undoubtedly be developed and will play an important role in treating hearing loss in the future.

REFERENCES

[1] Morton NE: Genetic epidemiology of hearing impairment. *Ann N Y Acad Sci* 1991, 630:16-31.

[2] Maki-Torkko EM, Lindholm PK, Vayrynen MR, Leisti JT, Sorri MJ: Epidemiology of moderate to profound childhood hearing impairments in northern Finland. Any changes in ten years? *Scand Audiol* 1998, 27:95-103.

[3] Fortnum HM, Summerfield AQ, Marshall DH, Davis AC, Bamford JM: Prevalence of permanent childhood hearing impairment in the United Kingdom and implications for universal neonatal hearing screening: questionnaire based ascertainment study. *Bmj* 2001, 323:536-540.

[4] Morton CC, Nance WE: Newborn hearing screening--a silent revolution. *N Engl J Med* 2006, 354:2151-2164.

[5] Kral A, O'Donoghue GM: Profound deafness in childhood. *N Engl J Med* 2010, 363:1438-1450.

[6] Cryns K, Van Camp G: Deafness genes and their diagnostic applications. *Audiol Neurootol* 2004, 9:2-22.

[7] Nance WE: The genetics of deafness. *Ment Retard Dev Disabil Res Rev* 2003, 9:109-119.

[8] Van Camp G, Smith RJH: *Hereditary Hearing Loss Homepage*:http://hereditary hearingloss.org

[9] Smith RJ, Robin NH: Genetic testing for deafness--GJB2 and SLC26A4 as causes of deafness. *J Commun Disord* 2002, 35:367-377.

[10] Steel KP: Perspectives: biomedicine. The benefits of recycling. *Science* 1999, 285:1363-1364.

[11] Cohn ES, Kelley PM: Clinical phenotype and mutations in connexin 26 (DFNB1/GJB2), the most common cause of childhood hearing loss. *Am J Med Genet* 1999, 89:130-136.

[12] Hilgert N, Smith RJ, Van Camp G: Forty-six genes causing nonsyndromic hearing impairment: which ones should be analyzed in DNA diagnostics? *Mutat Res* 2009, 681:189-196.

[13] Wu CC, Liu TC, Wang SH, Hsu CJ, Wu CM: Genetic characteristics in children with cochlear implants and the corresponding auditory performance. *Laryngoscope* 2011, 121:1287-1293.

[14] Lautermann J, ten Cate WJ, Altenhoff P, Grummer R, Traub O, Frank H, Jahnke K, Winterhager E: Expression of the gap-junction connexins 26 and 30 in the rat cochlea. *Cell Tissue Res* 1998, 294:415-420.

[15] Robertson NG, Resendes BL, Lin JS, Lee C, Aster JC, Adams JC, Morton CC: Inner ear localization of mRNA and protein products of COCH, mutated in the sensorineural deafness and vestibular disorder, DFNA9. *Hum Mol Genet* 2001, 10:2493-2500.

[16] Kommareddi PK, Nair TS, Raphael Y, Telian SA, Kim AH, Arts HA, El-Kashlan HK, Carey TE: Cochlin isoforms and their interaction with CTL2 (SLC44A2) in the inner ear. *J Assoc Res Otolaryngol* 2007, 8:435-446.

[17] Avraham KB, Hasson T, Sobe T, Balsara B, Testa JR, Skvorak AB, Morton CC, Copeland NG, Jenkins NA: Characterization of unconventional MYO6, the human homologue of the gene responsible for deafness in Snell's waltzer mice. *Hum Mol Genet* 1997, 6:1225-1231.

[18] Kurima K, Peters LM, Yang Y, Riazuddin S, Ahmed ZM, Naz S, Arnaud D, Drury S, Mo J, Makishima T, et al: Dominant and recessive deafness caused by mutations of a novel gene, TMC1, required for cochlear hair-cell function. *Nat Genet* 2002, 30:277-284.

[19] Lalwani AK, Goldstein JA, Kelley MJ, Luxford W, Castelein CM, Mhatre AN: Human nonsyndromic hereditary deafness DFNA17 is due to a mutation in nonmuscle myosin MYH9. *Am J Hum Genet* 2000, 67:1121-1128.

[20] Mhatre AN, Li Y, Atkin G, Maghnouj A, Lalwani AK: Expression of Myh9 in the mammalian cochlea: localization within the stereocilia. *J Neurosci Res* 2006, 84:809-818.

[21] Lalwani AK, Linthicum FH, Wilcox ER, Moore JK, Walters FC, San Agustin TB, Mislinski J, Miller MR, Sinninger Y, Attaie A, Luxford WM: A five-generation family with late-onset progressive hereditary hearing impairment due to cochleosaccular degeneration. *Audiol Neurootol* 1997, 2:139-154.

[22] Lee HK, Lee SH, Lee KY, Lim EJ, Choi SY, Park RK, Kim UK: Novel POU3F4 mutations and clinical features of DFN3 patients with cochlear implants. *Clin Genet* 2009, 75:572-575.

[23] Stankovic KM, Hennessey AM, Herrmann B, Mankarious LA: Cochlear implantation in children with congenital X-linked deafness due to novel mutations in POU3F4 gene. *Ann Otol Rhinol Laryngol* 2010, 119:815-822.

[24] Schild C, Prera E, Lublinghoff N, Arndt S, Aschendorff A, Birkenhager R: Novel mutation in the homeobox domain of transcription factor POU3F4 associated with profound sensorineural hearing loss. *Otol Neurotol* 2011, 32:690-694.

[25] Arndt S, Laszig R, Beck R, Schild C, Maier W, Birkenhager R, Kroeger S, Wesarg T, Aschendorff A: Spectrum of hearing disorders and their management in children with CHARGE syndrome. *Otol Neurotol* 2010, 31:67-73.

[26] Song MH, Cho HJ, Lee HK, Kwon TJ, Lee WS, Oh S, Bok J, Choi JY, Kim UK: CHD7 mutational analysis and clinical considerations for auditory rehabilitation in deaf patients with CHARGE syndrome. *PLoS One* 2011, 6:e24511.

[27] Brookes JT, Kanis AB, Tan LY, Tranebjaerg L, Vore A, Smith RJ: Cochlear implantation in deafness-dystonia-optic neuronopathy (DDON) syndrome. *Int J Pediatr Otorhinolaryngol* 2008, 72:121-126.

[28] Yoshikawa S, Kawano A, Hayashi C, Nishiyama N, Kawaguchi S, Furuse H, Ikeda K, Suzuki M, Nakagawa M: The clinical features of patients with the homozygous 235delC and the compound-heterozygous Y136X/G45E of the GJB2 mutations (Connexin 26) in cochlear implant recipients. *Auris Nasus Larynx* 2011, 38:444-449.

[29] Daneshi A, Hassanzadeh S, Emamdjomeh H, Mohammadi SH, Arzhangi S, Farhadi M, Najmabadi H: Prevalence of GJB2-associated deafness and outcomes of cochlear implantation in Iran. *J Laryngol Otol* 2011, 125:455-459.

[30] Chora JR, Matos TD, Martins JH, Alves MC, Andrade SM, Silva LF, Ribeiro CA, Antunes MC, Fialho MG, Caria MH: DFNB1-associated deafness in Portuguese cochlear implant users: prevalence and impact on oral outcome. *Int J Pediatr Otorhinolaryngol* 2010, 74:1135-1139.

[31] Hochman JB, Stockley TL, Shipp D, Lin VY, Chen JM, Nedzelski JM: Prevalence of Connexin 26 (GJB2) and Pendred (SLC26A4) mutations in a population of adult cochlear implant candidates. *Otol Neurotol* 2010, 31:919-922.

[32] Siem G, Fagerheim T, Jonsrud C, Laurent C, Teig E, Harris S, Leren TP, Fruh A, Heimdal K: Causes of hearing impairment in the Norwegian paediatric cochlear implant program. *Int J Audiol* 2010, 49:596-605.

[33] Reinert J, Honegger F, Gurtler N: High homogeneity in auditory outcome of pediatric CI-patients with mutations in Gap-Junction-Protein Beta2. *Int J Pediatr Otorhinolaryngol* 2010, 74:791-795.

[34] Fischer TC, Samanich J, Morrow BE, Chobot-Rodd J, Shanske A, Parikh SR: Genetic evaluation of American minority pediatric cochlear implant recipients. *Int J Pediatr Otorhinolaryngol* 2009, 73:195-203.

[35] Wrobel M, Magierska-Krzyszton M, Szyfter K, Mietkiewska D, Szyfter W, Rydzanicz M, Szyfter K, Karlik M: Comparison of rehabilitation results in deaf patients with and without genetically related hearing loss. *Cochlear Implants Int* 2008, 9:132-142.
[36] Wu CC, Lee YC, Chen PJ, Hsu CJ: Predominance of genetic diagnosis and imaging results as predictors in determining the speech perception performance outcome after cochlear implantation in children. *Arch Pediatr Adolesc Med* 2008, 162:269-276.
[37] Christiani TV, Alexandrino F, de Oliveira CA, Amantini RC, Bevilacqua MC, Filho OA, Porto P, Sartorato EL: Molecular study in Brazilian cochlear implant recipients. *Am J Med Genet A* 2007, 143A:1580-1582.
[38] Taitelbaum-Swead R, Brownstein Z, Muchnik C, Kishon-Rabin L, Kronenberg J, Megirov L, Frydman M, Hildesheimer M, Avraham KB: Connexin-associated deafness and speech perception outcome of cochlear implantation. *Arch Otolaryngol Head Neck Surg* 2006, 132:495-500.
[39] Propst EJ, Papsin BC, Stockley TL, Harrison RV, Gordon KA: Auditory responses in cochlear implant users with and without GJB2 deafness. *Laryngoscope* 2006, 116:317-327.
[40] Wiley S, Choo D, Meinzen-Derr J, Hilbert L, Greinwald J: GJB2 mutations and additional disabilities in a pediatric cochlear implant population. *Int J Pediatr Otorhinolaryngol* 2006, 70:493-500.
[41] Propst EJ, Stockley TL, Gordon KA, Harrison RV, Papsin BC: Ethnicity and mutations in GJB2 (connexin 26) and GJB6 (connexin 30) in a multi-cultural Canadian paediatric Cochlear Implant Program. *Int J Pediatr Otorhinolaryngol* 2006, 70:435-444.
[42] Sinnathuray AR, Toner JG, Clarke-Lyttle J, Geddis A, Patterson CC, Hughes AE: Connexin 26 (GJB2) gene-related deafness and speech intelligibility after cochlear implantation. *Otol Neurotol* 2004, 25:935-942.
[43] Sinnathuray AR, Toner JG, Geddis A, Clarke-Lyttle J, Patterson CC, Hughes AE: Auditory perception and speech discrimination after cochlear implantation in patients with connexin 26 (GJB2) gene-related deafness. *Otol Neurotol* 2004, 25:930-934.
[44] Lustig LR, Lin D, Venick H, Larky J, Yeagle J, Chinnici J, Polite C, Mhatre AN, Niparko JK, Lalwani AK: GJB2 gene mutations in cochlear implant recipients: prevalence and impact on outcome. *Arch Otolaryngol Head Neck Surg* 2004, 130:541-546.
[45] Green GE, Scott DA, McDonald JM, Teagle HF, Tomblin BJ, Spencer LJ, Woodworth GG, Knutson JF, Gantz BJ, Sheffield VC, Smith RJ: Performance of cochlear implant recipients with GJB2-related deafness. *Am J Med Genet* 2002, 109:167-170.
[46] Fukushima K, Sugata K, Kasai N, Fukuda S, Nagayasu R, Toida N, Kimura N, Takishita T, Gunduz M, Nishizaki K: Better speech performance in cochlear implant patients with GJB2-related deafness. *Int J Pediatr Otorhinolaryngol* 2002, 62:151-157.
[47] Nadol JB, Jr.: Histological considerations in implant patients. *Arch Otolaryngol* 1984, 110:160-163.
[48] Nadol JB, Jr., Hsu WC: Histopathologic correlation of spiral ganglion cell count and new bone formation in the cochlea following meningogenic labyrinthitis and deafness. *Ann Otol Rhinol Laryngol* 1991, 100:712-716.
[49] Shelton C, Luxford WM, Tonokawa LL, Lo WW, House WF: The narrow internal auditory canal in children: a contraindication to cochlear implants. *Otolaryngol Head Neck Surg* 1989, 100:227-231.

[50] Miyamoto RT, Robbins AJ, Myres WA, Pope ML: Cochlear implantation in the Mondini inner ear malformation. *Am J Otol* 1986, 7:258-261.

[51] Jackler RK, Luxford WM, House WF: Sound detection with the cochlear implant in five ears of four children with congenital malformations of the cochlea. *Laryngoscope* 1987, 97:15-17.

[52] Tyler RS, Summerfield AQ: Cochlear implantation: relationships with research on auditory deprivation and acclimatization. *Ear Hear* 1996, 17:38S-50S.

[53] Friedland DR, Venick HS, Niparko JK: Choice of ear for cochlear implantation: the effect of history and residual hearing on predicted postoperative performance. *Otol Neurotol* 2003, 24:582-589.

[54] Kileny PR, Zwolan TA, Ashbaugh C: The influence of age at implantation on performance with a cochlear implant in children. *Otol Neurotol* 2001, 22:42-46.

[55] Zwolan TA, Ashbaugh CM, Alarfaj A, Kileny PR, Arts HA, El-Kashlan HK, Telian SA: Pediatric cochlear implant patient performance as a function of age at implantation. *Otol Neurotol* 2004, 25:112-120.

[56] Bollard PM, Chute PM, Popp A, Parisier SC: Specific language growth in young children using the CLARION cochlear implant. *Ann Otol Rhinol Laryngol Suppl* 1999, 177:119-123.

[57] Robbins AM, Osberger MJ, Miyamoto RT, Kessler KS: Language development in young children with cochlear implants. *Adv Otorhinolaryngol* 1995, 50:160-166.

[58] Rubinstein JT, Parkinson WS, Tyler RS, Gantz BJ: Residual speech recognition and cochlear implant performance: effects of implantation criteria. *Am J Otol* 1999, 20:445-452.

[59] Moog JS, Geers AE: Speech and language acquisition in young children after cochlear implantation. *Otolaryngol Clin North Am* 1999, 32:1127-1141.

[60] Criteria of candidacy for unilateral cochlear implantation in postlingually deafened adults III: prospective evaluation of an actuarial approach to defining a criterion. *Ear Hear* 2004, 25:361-374.

[61] FDA:http://www.fda.gov/MedicalDevices/ProductsandMedicalProcedures/ImplantsandProsthetics/CochlearImplants/ucm062882.htm.

[62] Van de Heyning P, Vermeire K, Diebl M, Nopp P, Anderson I, De Ridder D: Incapacitating unilateral tinnitus in single-sided deafness treated by cochlear implantation. *Ann Otol Rhinol Laryngol* 2008, 117:645-652.

[63] Gantz BJ, Turner C, Gfeller KE: Acoustic plus electric speech processing: preliminary results of a multicenter clinical trial of the Iowa/Nucleus Hybrid implant. *Audiol Neurootol* 2006, 11 Suppl 1:63-68.

[64] Gifford RH, Dorman MF, McKarns SA, Spahr AJ: Combined electric and contralateral acoustic hearing: word and sentence recognition with bimodal hearing. *J Speech Lang Hear Res* 2007, 50:835-843.

[65] Lesinski A, Hartrampf R, Dahm MC, Bertram B, Lenarz T: Cochlear implantation in a population of multihandicapped children. *Ann Otol Rhinol Laryngol Suppl* 1995, 166:332-334.

[66] Waltzman SB, Scalchunes V, Cohen NL: Performance of multiply handicapped children using cochlear implants. *Am J Otol* 2000, 21:329-335.

[67] Jackler RK, Luxford WM, House WF: Congenital malformations of the inner ear: a classification based on embryogenesis. *Laryngoscope* 1987, 97:2-14.

[68] Motta LH, Felix TM, Souza LT, Lavinsky-Wolff M, Costa-Motta FM, Faria MR, Lavinsky L: Prevalence of the 35delG mutation in deaf South Brazilian infants submitted to cochlear implantation. *Int J Pediatr Otorhinolaryngol* 2012, 76:287-290.

[69] Connell SS, Angeli SI, Suarez H, Hodges AV, Balkany TJ, Liu XZ: Performance after cochlear implantation in DFNB1 patients. *Otolaryngol Head Neck Surg* 2007, 137:596-602.

[70] Bauer PW, Geers AE, Brenner C, Moog JS, Smith RJ: The effect of GJB2 allele variants on performance after cochlear implantation. *Laryngoscope* 2003, 113:2135-2140.

[71] Matsushiro N, Doi K, Fuse Y, Nagai K, Yamamoto K, Iwaki T, Kawashima T, Sawada A, Hibino H, Kubo T: Successful cochlear implantation in prelingual profound deafness resulting from the common 233delC mutation of the GJB2 gene in the Japanese. *Laryngoscope* 2002, 112:255-261.

[72] Kawasaki A, Fukushima K, Kataoka Y, Fukuda S, Nishizaki K: Using assessment of higher brain functions of children with GJB2-associated deafness and cochlear implants as a procedure to evaluate language development. *Int J Pediatr Otorhinolaryngol* 2006, 70:1343-1349.

[73] Angeli SI, Suarez H, Lopez A, Balkany TJ, Liu XZ: Influence of DFNB1 status on expressive language in deaf children with cochlear implants. *Otol Neurotol* 2011, 32:1437-1443.

[74] Karamert R, Bayazit YA, Altinyay S, Yilmaz A, Menevse A, Gokdogan O, Gokdogan C, Ant A: Association of GJB2 gene mutation with cochlear implant performance in genetic non-syndromic hearing loss. *Int J Pediatr Otorhinolaryngol* 2011, 75:1572-1575.

[75] Dalamon V, Lotersztein V, Lipovsek M, Beheran A, Mondino ME, Diamante F, Pallares N, Diamante V, Elgoyhen AB: Performance of speech perception after cochlear implantation in DFNB1 patients. *Acta Otolaryngol* 2009, 129:395-398.

[76] Cullen RD, Buchman CA, Brown CJ, Copeland BJ, Zdanski C, Pillsbury HC, 3rd, Shores CG: Cochlear implantation for children with GJB2-related deafness. *Laryngoscope* 2004, 114:1415-1419.

[77] Mesolella M, Tranchino G, Nardone M, Motta S, Galli V: Connexin 26 mutations in nonsyndromic autosomal recessive hearing loss: speech and hearing rehabilitation. *Int J Pediatr Otorhinolaryngol* 2004, 68:995-1005.

[78] Lalwani AK, Budenz CL, Weisstuch AS, Babb J, Roland JT, Jr., Waltzman SB: Predictability of cochlear implant outcome in families. *Laryngoscope* 2009, 119:131-136.

[79] Pagarkar W, Bitner-Glindzicz M, Knight J, Sirimanna T: Late postnatal onset of hearing loss due to GJB2 mutations. *Int J Pediatr Otorhinolaryngol* 2006, 70:1119-1124.

[80] de Wolf MJ, Honings J, Joosten FB, Hoefsloot L, Mylanus EA, Cremers CW: Two siblings with progressive, fluctuating hearing loss after head trauma, treated with cochlear implantation. *J Laryngol Otol* 2010, 124:86-89.

[81] Kim S, Song DG, Bae JW, Choi SY, Kim UK, Choi YJ, Lee KY, Lee SH, Lee JR: A Family of H723R Mutation for SLC26A4 Associated with Enlarged Vestibular Aqueduct Syndrome. *Clin Exp Otorhinolaryngol* 2009, 2:100-102.

[82] Elbracht M, Senderek J, Eggermann T, Thurmer C, Park J, Westhofen M, Zerres K: Autosomal recessive postlingual hearing loss (DFNB8): compound heterozygosity for two novel TMPRSS3 mutations in German siblings. *J Med Genet* 2007, 44:e81.

[83] Weegerink NJ, Schraders M, Oostrik J, Huygen PL, Strom TM, Granneman S, Pennings RJ, Venselaar H, Hoefsloot LH, Elting M, et al: Genotype-phenotype correlation in DFNB8/10 families with TMPRSS3 mutations. *J Assoc Res Otolaryngol* 2011, 12:753-766.

[84] Rouillon I, Marcolla A, Roux I, Marlin S, Feldmann D, Couderc R, Jonard L, Petit C, Denoyelle F, Garabedian EN, Loundon N: Results of cochlear implantation in two children with mutations in the OTOF gene. *Int J Pediatr Otorhinolaryngol* 2006, 70:689-696.

[85] Rodriguez-Ballesteros M, del Castillo FJ, Martin Y, Moreno-Pelayo MA, Morera C, Prieto F, Marco J, Morant A, Gallo-Teran J, Morales-Angulo C, et al: Auditory neuropathy in patients carrying mutations in the otoferlin gene (OTOF). *Hum Mutat* 2003, 22:451-456.

[86] Varga R, Avenarius MR, Kelley PM, Keats BJ, Berlin CI, Hood LJ, Morlet TG, Brashears SM, Starr A, Cohn ES, et al: OTOF mutations revealed by genetic analysis of hearing loss families including a potential temperature sensitive auditory neuropathy allele. *J Med Genet* 2006, 43:576-581.

[87] Zadro C, Ciorba A, Fabris A, Morgutti M, Trevisi P, Gasparini P, Martini A: Five new OTOF gene mutations and auditory neuropathy. *Int J Pediatr Otorhinolaryngol* 2010, 74:494-498.

[88] Charizopoulou N, Lelli A, Schraders M, Ray K, Hildebrand MS, Ramesh A, Srisailapathy CR, Oostrik J, Admiraal RJ, Neely HR, et al: Gipc3 mutations associated with audiogenic seizures and sensorineural hearing loss in mouse and human. *Nat Commun* 2011, 2:201.

[89] Weegerink NJ, Pennings RJ, Huygen PL, Hoefsloot LH, Cremers CW, Kunst HP: Phenotypes of two Dutch DFNA3 families with mutations in GJB2. *Ann Otol Rhinol Laryngol* 2011, 120:191-197.

[90] Vermeire K, Brokx JP, Wuyts FL, Cochet E, Hofkens A, De Bodt M, Van de Heyning PH: Good speech recognition and quality-of-life scores after cochlear implantation in patients with DFNA9. *Otol Neurotol* 2006, 27:44-49.

[91] Hildebrand MS, de Silva MG, Gardner RJ, Rose E, de Graaf CA, Bahlo M, Dahl HH: Cochlear implants for DFNA17 deafness. *Laryngoscope* 2006, 116:2211-2215.

[92] Sanggaard KM, Kjaer KW, Eiberg H, Nurnberg G, Nurnberg P, Hoffman K, Jensen H, Sorum C, Rendtorff ND, Tranebjaerg L: A novel nonsense mutation in MYO6 is associated with progressive nonsyndromic hearing loss in a Danish DFNA22 family. *Am J Med Genet A* 2008, 146A:1017-1025.

[93] Makishima T, Kurima K, Brewer CC, Griffith AJ: Early onset and rapid progression of dominant nonsyndromic DFNA36 hearing loss. *Otol Neurotol* 2004, 25:714-719.

[94] Kitajiri S, Makishima T, Friedman TB, Griffith AJ: A novel mutation at the DFNA36 hearing loss locus reveals a critical function and potential genotype-phenotype correlation for amino acid-572 of TMC1. *Clin Genet* 2007, 71:148-152.

[95] Ulubil SA, Furze AD, Angeli SI: Cochlear implantation in a patient with profound hearing loss with the A1555G mitochondrial DNA mutation and no history of aminoglycoside exposure. *J Laryngol Otol* 2006, 120:230-232.

[96] Tono T, Ushisako Y, Kiyomizu K, Usami S, Abe S, Shinkawa H, Komune S: Cochlear implantation in a patient with profound hearing loss with the A1555G mitochondrial mutation. *Am J Otol* 1998, 19:754-757.

[97] Bitner-Glindzicz M, Osei-Lah V, Colvin I, Sirimanna T, Lucas D, Mac Ardle B, Webb D, Shankar A, Kingston J, Jenkins L, Rahman S: Aminoglycoside-induced deafness during treatment of acute leukaemia. *Arch Dis Child* 2010, 95:153-155.

[98] Sudo A, Takeichi N, Hosoki K, Saitoh S: Successful cochlear implantation in a patient with mitochondrial hearing loss and m.625G>A transition. *J Laryngol Otol* 2011, 125:1282-1285.

[99] Mancuso M, Filosto M, Forli F, Rocchi A, Berrettini S, Siciliano G, Murri L: A non-syndromic hearing loss caused by very low levels of the mtDNA A3243G mutation. *Acta Neurol Scand* 2004, 110:72-74.

[100] Howes T, Madden C, Dasgupta S, Saeed S, Das V: Role of mitochondrial variation in maternally inherited diabetes and deafness syndrome. *J Laryngol Otol* 2008, 122:1249-1252.

[101] Sue CM, Lipsett LJ, Crimmins DS, Tsang CS, Boyages SC, Presgrave CM, Gibson WP, Byrne E, Morris JG: Cochlear origin of hearing loss in MELAS syndrome. *Ann Neurol* 1998, 43:350-359.

[102] Karkos PD, Anari S, Johnson IJ: Cochlear implantation in patients with MELAS syndrome. *Eur Arch Otorhinolaryngol* 2005, 262:322-324.

[103] Yasumura S, Aso S, Fujisaka M, Watanabe Y: Cochlear implantation in a patient with mitochondrial encephalopathy, lactic acidosis and stroke-like episodes syndrome. *Acta Otolaryngol* 2003, 123:55-58.

[104] Rosenthal EL, Kileny PR, Boerst A, Telian SA: Successful cochlear implantation in a patient with MELAS syndrome. *Am J Otol* 1999, 20:187-190; discussion 190-181.

[105] Hill D, Wintersgill S, Stott L, Cadge B, Graham J: Cochlear implantation in a profoundly deaf patient with MELAS syndrome. *J Neurol Neurosurg Psychiatry* 2001, 71:281.

[106] Sinnathuray AR, Raut V, Awa A, Magee A, Toner JG: A review of cochlear implantation in mitochondrial sensorineural hearing loss. *Otol Neurotol* 2003, 24:418-426.

[107] Counter PR, Hilton MP, Webster D, Wardell T, Taylor RW, Besley G, Turnbull DM, Robinson PJ: Cochlear implantation of a patient with a previously undescribed mitochondrial DNA defect. *J Laryngol Otol* 2001, 115:730-732.

[108] Cullington HE: Cochlear implantation of a deaf blind patient with mitochondrial cytopathy. *J Laryngol Otol* 1999, 113:353-354.

[109] Li JN, Han DY, Ji F, Chen AT, Wu N, Xi X, Shen WD, Yang SM: Successful cochlear implantation in a patient with MNGIE syndrome. *Acta Otolaryngol* 2011, 131:1012-1016.

[110] Pijl S, Westerberg BD: Cochlear implantation results in patients with Kearns-Sayre syndrome. *Ear Hear* 2008, 29:472-475.

[111] Ikezono T, Sugizaki K, Shindo S, Sekiguchi S, Pawankar R, Baba S, Yagi T: CTP (Cochlin-tomoprotein) detection in the profuse fluid leakage (gusher) from cochleostomy. *Acta Otolaryngol* 2010, 130:881-887.

[112] Yogesh B, Nick G, Kathryn F, Ben H, Chris J, Nico J, David A, Martin B, Michelle W, Lesley C: Surgical aspects of cochlear implantation in syndromic children. *Cochlear Implants Int* 2011.

[113] Friedmann DR, Amoils M, Germiller JA, Lustig LR, Glastonbury CM, Pramanik BK, Lalwani AK: Venous malformations of the temporal bone are a common feature in CHARGE syndrome. *Laryngoscope* 2012.

[114] Southwell KE, Bird PA, Murray DP: Cochlear Implantation in children with CHARGE syndrome. *Cochlear Implants Int* 2010, 11:170-183.

[115] Meinzen-Derr J, Wiley S, Grether S, Choo DI: Language performance in children with cochlear implants and additional disabilities. *Laryngoscope* 2010, 120:405-413.

[116] Lanson BG, Green JE, Roland JT, Jr., Lalwani AK, Waltzman SB: Cochlear implantation in Children with CHARGE syndrome: therapeutic decisions and outcomes. *Laryngoscope* 2007, 117:1260-1266.

[117] Bauer PW, Wippold FJ, 2nd, Goldin J, Lusk RP: Cochlear implantation in children with CHARGE association. *Arch Otolaryngol Head Neck Surg* 2002, 128:1013-1017.

[118] Warren FM, 3rd, Wiggins RH, 3rd, Pitt C, Harnsberger HR, Shelton C: Apparent cochlear nerve aplasia: to implant or not to implant? *Otol Neurotol* 2010, 31:1088-1094.

[119] Chorbachi R, Graham JM, Ford J, Raine CH: Cochlear implantation in Jervell and Lange-Nielsen syndrome. *Int J Pediatr Otorhinolaryngol* 2002, 66:213-221.

[120] Yanmei F, Yaqin W, Haibo S, Huiqun Z, Zhengnong C, Dongzhen Y, Shankai Y: Cochlear implantation in patients with Jervell and Lange-Nielsen syndrome, and a review of literature. *Int J Pediatr Otorhinolaryngol* 2008, 72:1723-1729.

[121] Daneshi A, Ghassemi MM, Talee M, Hassanzadeh S: Cochlear implantation in children with Jervell, Lange-Nielsen syndrome. *J Laryngol Otol* 2008, 122:314-317.

[122] Green JD, Schuh MJ, Maddern BR, Haymond J, Helffrich RA: Cochlear implantation in Jervell and Lange-Nielsen syndrome. *Ann Otol Rhinol Laryngol Suppl* 2000, 185:27-28.

[123] Siem G, Fruh A, Leren TP, Heimdal K, Teig E, Harris S: Jervell and Lange-Nielsen syndrome in Norwegian children: aspects around cochlear implantation, hearing, and balance. *Ear Hear* 2008, 29:261-269.

[124] Arndt S, Aschendorff A, Schild C, Beck R, Maier W, Laszig R, Birkenhager R: A novel dominant and a de novo mutation in the GJB2 gene (connexin-26) cause keratitis-ichthyosis-deafness syndrome: implication for cochlear implantation. *Otol Neurotol* 2010, 31:210-215.

[125] Smyth CM, Sinnathuray AR, Hughes AE, Toner JG: Cochlear implantation in keratitis-ichthyosis-deafness syndrome - 10-year follow-up of two patients. *Cochlear Implants Int* 2012, 13:54-59.

[126] Barker EJ, Briggs RJ: Cochlear implantation in children with keratitis-ichthyosis-deafness (KID) syndrome: outcomes in three cases. *Cochlear Implants Int* 2009, 10:166-173.

[127] Cushing SL, MacDonald L, Propst EJ, Sharma A, Stockley T, Blaser SL, James AL, Papsin BC: Successful cochlear implantation in a child with Keratosis, Icthiosis and Deafness (KID) Syndrome and Dandy-Walker malformation. *Int J Pediatr Otorhinolaryngol* 2008, 72:693-698.

[128] Hampton SM, Toner JG, Small J: Cochlear implant extrusion in a child with keratitis, ichthyosis and deafness syndrome. *J Laryngol Otol* 1997, 111:465-467.
[129] Choung YH, Shin YR, Kim HJ, Kim YC, Ahn JH, Choi SJ, Jeong SY, Park K: Cochlear implantation and connexin expression in the child with keratitis-ichthyosis-deafness syndrome. *Int J Pediatr Otorhinolaryngol* 2008, 72:911-915.
[130] Kontorinis G, Lenarz T, Lesinski-Schiedat A, Neuburger J: Cochlear implantation in Pendred syndrome. *Cochlear Implants Int* 2011, 12:157-163.
[131] Sanei-Moghaddam A, Wilson T, Kumar S, Gray R: An unfortunate case of Pendred syndrome. *J Laryngol Otol* 2011, 125:965-967.
[132] Damen GW, Pennings RJ, Snik AF, Mylanus EA: Quality of life and cochlear implantation in Usher syndrome type I. *Laryngoscope* 2006, 116:723-728.
[133] Pennings RJ, Damen GW, Snik AF, Hoefsloot L, Cremers CW, Mylanus EA: Audiologic performance and benefit of cochlear implantation in Usher syndrome type I. *Laryngoscope* 2006, 116:717-722.
[134] Loundon N, Marlin S, Busquet D, Denoyelle F, Roger G, Renaud F, Garabedian EN: Usher syndrome and cochlear implantation. *Otol Neurotol* 2003, 24:216-221.
[135] Brownstein Z, Ben-Yosef T, Dagan O, Frydman M, Abeliovich D, Sagi M, Abraham FA, Taitelbaum-Swead R, Shohat M, Hildesheimer M, et al: The R245X mutation of PCDH15 in Ashkenazi Jewish children diagnosed with nonsyndromic hearing loss foreshadows retinitis pigmentosa. *Pediatr Res* 2004, 55:995-1000.
[136] Liu XZ, Angeli SI, Rajput K, Yan D, Hodges AV, Eshraghi A, Telischi FF, Balkany TJ: Cochlear implantation in individuals with Usher type 1 syndrome. *Int J Pediatr Otorhinolaryngol* 2008, 72:841-847.
[137] Blanchet C, Roux AF, Hamel C, Ben Salah S, Artieres F, Faugere V, Uziel A, Mondain M: [Usher type I syndrome in children: genotype/phenotype correlation and cochlear implant benefits]. *Rev Laryngol Otol Rhinol (Bord)* 2007, 128:137-143.
[138] Hinderlink JB, Brokx JP, Mens LH, van den Broek P: Results from four cochlear implant patients with Usher's syndrome. *Ann Otol Rhinol Laryngol* 1994, 103:285-293.
[139] Pietola L, Aarnisalo AA, Abdel-Rahman A, Vastinsalo H, Isosomppi J, Lopponen H, Kentala E, Johansson R, Valtonen H, Vasama JP, et al: Speech recognition and communication outcomes with cochlear implantation in Usher syndrome type 3. *Otol Neurotol* 2012, 33:38-41.
[140] Kontorinis G, Lenarz T, Giourgas A, Durisin M, Lesinski-Schiedat A: Outcomes and special considerations of cochlear implantation in waardenburg syndrome. *Otol Neurotol* 2011, 32:951-955.
[141] Amirsalari S, Ajallouyean M, Saburi A, Haddadi Fard A, Abed M, Ghazavi Y: Cochlear implantation outcomes in children with Waardenburg syndrome. *Eur Arch Otorhinolaryngol* 2011.
[142] Deka RC, Sikka K, Chaturvedy G, Singh CA, Venkat Karthikeyan C, Kumar R, Agarwal S: Cochlear implantation in Waardenburg syndrome: The Indian scenario. *Acta Otolaryngol* 2010, 130:1097-1100.
[143] Pau H, Gibson WP, Gardner-Berry K, Sanli H: Cochlear implantations in children with Waardenburg syndrome: an electrophysiological and psychophysical review. *Cochlear Implants Int* 2006, 7:202-206.
[144] Cullen RD, Zdanski C, Roush P, Brown C, Teagle H, Pillsbury HC, 3rd, Buchman C: Cochlear implants in Waardenburg syndrome. *Laryngoscope* 2006, 116:1273-1275.

[145] Daneshi A, Hassanzadeh S, Farhadi M: Cochlear implantation in children with Waardenburg syndrome. *J Laryngol Otol* 2005, 119:719-723.

[146] Loundon N, Rouillon I, Munier N, Marlin S, Roger G, Garabedian EN: Cochlear implantation in children with internal ear malformations. *Otol Neurotol* 2005, 26:668-673.

[147] Migirov L, Henkin Y, Hildesheimer M, Muchnik C, Kronenberg J: Cochlear implantation in Waardenburg's syndrome. *Acta Otolaryngol* 2005, 125:713-717.

[148] Kaufmann L, Sauter TB, Lee DJ: Dysplasia of the cerebellum in Waardenburg syndrome: outcomes following cochlear implantation. *Int J Pediatr Otorhinolaryngol* 2010, 74:93-96.

[149] Moon SK, Choi HS, Lee SJ, Choung YH, Park K: Cochlear implantation in a case with Waardenburg syndrome. *Cochlear Implants Int* 2004, 5 Suppl 1:212-214.

[150] Sugii A, Iwaki T, Doi K, Takahashi Y, Yamamoto K, Fuse Y, Kobayashi R, Kubo T: Cochlear implant in a young child with Waardenburg syndrome. *Adv Otorhinolaryngol* 2000, 57:215-219.

In: Inner Ear Development and Hearing Loss
Editors: Saima Riazuddin and Zubair Ahmed
ISBN: 978-1-62417-011-9

Chapter 8

DEAFNESS GENE DISCOVERY IN THE GENOMIC ERA

Tal Elkan-Miller* and Karen B. Avraham

Department of Human Molecular Genetics and Biochemistry,
Sackler Faculty of Medicine and Sagol School of Neuroscience,
Tel Aviv University, Tel Aviv, Israel

ABSTRACT

Hereditary deafness is a genetically heterogeneous disease, with wide variation in clinical symptoms displayed, including age of onset, frequencies affected, and changes in hearing threshold. As a result, there are some common and many more rare forms of deafness, each represented by mutations in different genes. The major challenge and goal in the field has been to identify the genes containing mutations leading to deafness, and to elucidate the auditory and vestibular pathways the proteins they encode are involved in. A remarkable amount of data has accumulated over the years to address the mechanisms associated with normal hearing and pathology of the inner ear. To date, there are 60 genes known to be involved in non-syndromic hearing loss (NSHL), and 34 genes known to be associated with 10 forms of syndromic hearing loss (SHL). Nevertheless, it is estimated that there are many more genes to be found implicated in human deafness. Furthermore, there are countless small families that remain unsolved with respect to the cause of their sensory loss. The difficulties of obtaining large pedigrees, the laborious process of genotyping, linkage analysis, positional cloning, and sequencing of dozens of genes in a critical region has hindered the process of further gene discovery. Clinically, this has limited carrier testing of deafness-causing mutations only to the most common ones, or to a specific mutation having been found previously found in the same ethnic population. Therefore the reality is that despite there being over 60 known genes, only one to four genes can be examined for each patient. Since the completion of the Human Genome Project (HGP) and the appearance of Next Generation Sequencing (NGS), or Massively Parallel Sequencing (MPS) and Deep Sequencing, technologies, rapid high-throughput identification of new deafness genes and mutations has been greatly streamlined. A single deep sequencing experiment can be completed within a few days and lead to the identification of new mutations. While the computational analysis and validation of variants still remains the bottleneck for finding new mutations, as more

* Tel: 03-640-6642, Fax: 03-640-9360

genes are discovered and bioinformatics tools developed, this process will become much easier. The application of genomic analysis for early clinical diagnosis of deafness will enable prediction of abnormal phenotypes that might arise later, improve rehabilitation of deaf children and simplify decisions for subsequent treatment. Identification of more genes involved in the auditory and vestibular pathways will help elucidate pathways and mechanisms of inner ear function. In this chapter we will review the advances deep sequencing is having on the discovery of new deafness genes and pathogenic mutations in these genes.

INTRODUCTION

Defining genetic mutations in human genes is unequivocally the first step to determine the pathways involved in a disease, so that targeted therapy may be developed. The general approach to human disease gene identification has been to take a positional cloning approach in order to identify an approximate chromosomal location, and follow with a candidate cloning approach in order to screen relevant genes in the region that might be suitable candidates based on the known phenotype of the disease. Until recently, identification of deafness loci was performed mainly by one of two ways: candidate gene analysis and genome-wide linkage analysis in family members with shared genetic relationships using genetic markers such as microsatellites or single nucleotide polymorphisms (SNPs). As many deafness-associated mutations have been previously identified, an initial strategy is to examine these genes and if they are excluded, to work towards discovery of a new gene. When no known gene is deemed as a potential candidate or when the candidate gene analysis strategy has failed, genome-wide segregation analysis is performed in order to determine the chromosomal region that segregates with a trait. The genetic linkage data obtained could be analyzed by various methods, such as parametric multipoint linkage analysis and, in the case of autosomal recessive disorders, homozygosity mapping, particularly in consanguineous families [1, 2]. As the next step, the causative gene within the genetic linkage data is obtained by various methods. When the size of the linked region is relatively small the conventional strategy has been to utilize Sanger sequencing to sequence the coding regions of each gene in the linked interval one by one in an order based on candidate genes prioritization. For large intervals this technique is costly and time-consuming, making it more necessary to focus on genes known to be expressed in the inner ear. Such methods can be impractical, especially in the case of large intervals as the risk of missing the causative mutation is high.

Over the years the linkage analysis approach has led to the identification of many deafness genes (Hereditary Hearing Loss Homepage, http://hereditaryhearingloss.org/). Deafness may be isolated, as in non-syndromic hearing loss (NSHL), or in conjunction with other abnormalities, as in syndromic hearing loss (SHL). The first NSHL locus was mapped to chromosome 5q31 in 1992 by using linkage analysis in a large Costa Rican family [3]. Mutations in the gene leading to hearing loss (HL), diaphanous 1, were found five years later [4]. The first NSHL recessive locus was mapped in 1994 [5] and three years later, mutations were found in *GJB2* encoding connexin 26 [6]. This gene has turned out to be the most common form of genetic deafness, responsible for 30-50% of congenital HL [7]. Since then, the progress in the identification of new genes has been remarkable, with new genes reported at a monthly rate. However, the list of unresolved human loci linked with HL remains longer than the list of cloned genes (Hereditary Hearing Loss Homepage). This is due to the

limitation of linkage methods and the length and cost required for gene identification. Limitations in using linkage methods include the need for relatively large families with multiply affected individuals and a two-step process of determining the chromosomal region of the disease locus and then searching through genes in the region for the causative mutation. Several large-scale screening technologies have emerged that increase facilitated disease gene identification for deafness. One such example is the use of array comparative genomic hybridization (array CGH) for the identification of chromosomal imbalances such as genomic deletions and duplications. Using this method, an inverted genomic duplication of the *TJP2* gene was discovered to be the cause of progressive NSHL in *DFNA51* [8]. A second example is the Hereditary Hearing Loss Arrayed Primer Extension microarray that enables an analysis of 198 mutations across eight prevalent genes in a single test (*GJB2, GJB6, GJB3, GJA1, SLC26A4, SLC26A5, MTRNR1* and *MTTS1*) [9]. Such a tool can be useful in the clinic; however it does not detect new mutations or mutations within genes not previously associated with deafness. Though the advances in deafness gene discovery have been considerable, the great limitations that are still encountered indicate a need for large-scale techniques that will screen a larger number of genes in a reasonable amount of time and more cost-effective manner, and that can detect all types of mutations underlying deafness.

The Emergence of NGS Technology

Sequencing of the first human genome was performed using the chain-terminator method, also known as Sanger sequencing [10]. The first diploid sequence of an individual was reported in 2008, that of J. Craig Venter, the founder of Celera Genomics, with 1.5 gigabase (Gb) of sequence, performed at an estimated cost of 200 million dollars [11]. However, Sanger sequencing has limitations, as it is time- and cost-consuming to perform. The number of large genes involved in HL has made complete sequencing on a regular basis impractical, even for research purposes, and the costs of identifying new deafness genes are tremendous. Next Generation Sequencing (NGS), also named Massively Parallel Sequencing (MPS) or Deep Sequencing, enables large scale screening of a wide variety of genes and in addition, identification of mutations in non-coding regions that may affect gene expression. While Sanger sequencing yields an output of 120,000 bp per day for a cost of approximately $4000 per Mb sequenced [12], with a cost of $200,000 to sequence 3.2 Gb of a single human genome, the output of a single MPS machine stood at 30 Gb per day in 2011 [13], with the costs coming down almost daily. The genome of James Watson, winner of the 1962 Nobel Prize in Physiology or Medicine for his co-discovery of the molecular structure of nucleic acids (http://www.nobelprize.org/nobel_prizes/medicine/laureates/1962/), was sequenced using this newer technology and ran at a cost of approximately $1 million, a far cry from the cost by Sanger sequencing [14]. When compared to Sanger sequencing, MPS has an increased error rate, due to the increased output [15], but this problem is overcome by repeated sequencing to achieve greater coverage or read depth. Currently there are three commonly used commercial MPS platforms. These include the 454 Sequencing System (454 Life Sciences, a Roche company), the first MPS platform introduced, using pyrosequencing [16]; the Illumina platform (Illumina, Inc.), the most widely used platform, using cyclic reversible termination (CRT) technology [17]; and the SOLiD™ System (Life Technologies, Applied Biosystems) using sequence-by-ligation (SBL) technology [18]. Each of the technologies mentioned has advantages and disadvantages (for a comprehensive review, see [13, 19]). One of the major challenges of the NGS technology is the formidable amount of data generated, thus making it necessary to develop bioinformatic filtering techniques, data analysis tools and storage solutions. Adding a genomic enrichment step to isolate a selected region of the genome can greatly reduce the costs and bioinformatic infrastructure necessary for data analysis. Narrowing the studied genomic region can be done by either targeted genomic capture or by whole exon (exome) sequencing. In targeted genomic capture, any region of interest in the genome can be targeted including disease-associated linkage intervals or the exons of genes that are known to be associated with a specific disease or organ. There are two main methods for targeted capture, solid-phase targeted enrichment, based on a DNA microarray technology, and liquid-based targeted enrichment, using RNA or DNA based complementary probes (for a comprehensive review of targeted capture, see [20]). Whole exon sequencing enriches all the exons of the genes within the genome for NGS. One of its major advantages is that it does not limit the genes analyzed to ones already associated with the disease, thus allowing for the identification of new disease genes.

NGS technologies have revolutionized the field of gene discovery and genetic testing by enabling the detection of genomic variations within millions and even billions of base pairs. In many cases these variations are benign polymorphisms with no clinical significance. One of the challenges of analyzing data generated by NGS technology is to define the significance of the variants detected and decide which are SNPs and which are disease-causing mutations. Approaches to rule out SNPs include searching large sequencing projects (such as the 1000 Genomes Project, http://1000genomes.org), the NHLBI Exome Sequencing Project (http://evs.gs.washington.edu/EVS/), and databases of known polymorphisms (such as the dbSNP, http://www.ncbi.nlm.nih.gov/projects/SNP/), applying computational prediction of the potential effect of the variation on protein function, and sequencing the gene containing the variation in a large set of control population from a similar genetic background. Such a step is extremely important to detect the variants most likely to be disease-causing mutations.

NGS in Hearing Loss Research

NGS offers an ideal solution for the many challenges in the identification of causative mutations in heterogenic diseases such as deafness. Since its emergence, NGS has had an important impact on both research and clinical diagnosis in many diseases including cancer [21-24], inflammatory bowel disease [25], and cognitive disorders [26], as it enables screening of a large number of genes in one test. The many advantages of this system to deafness research include parallel analysis all known deafness genes; identification of mutations in genes previously not implicated in deafness; detection of all types of mutations; screening of large genes that have previously been largely untested; parallel processing of a large number of samples; and the fact that it can be used in cases of isolated deafness. It is therefore not surprising that in the last two years this technology has begun to play a pivotal role in elucidating the molecular genetic basis underlying deafness. To date, the two methods used in this field have been targeted gene capture and multiple parallel sequencing or homozygosity mapping prior to exome sequencing (for an example of an experiment scheme see Figure 1).

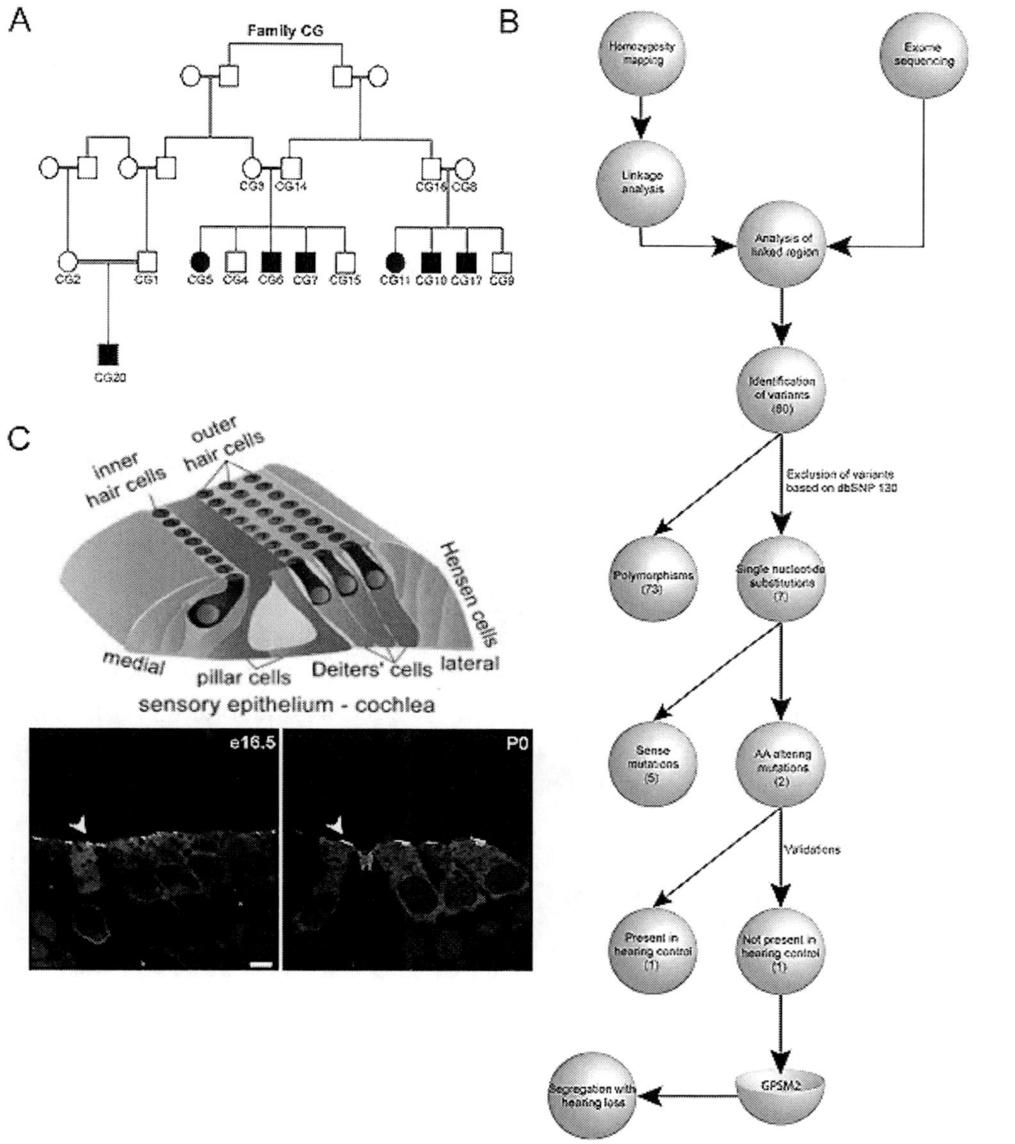

Figure 1. A representative scheme of a NGS experiment. This scheme illustrates the workflow utilized to identify *GPSM2* as the cause of deafness. (A) The investigated Family CG with inheritance of a mutation in *GPSM2* and hearing loss (filled symbols). (B) A diagram illustrating the workflow used to identify *GPSM2* as the causative mutation in Family CG. A combined homozygosity mapping and whole exome sequencing approach was utilized in order to narrow down the data that needed to be analyzed. In the region analyzed, 80 variants were detected, 73 of which appeared to be known SNPs. Of the seven variants previously unidentified, five were sense mutations and two were amino acid (AA)-altering mutations, within the *MYBPHL* and *GPSM2* genes. The two variants were analyzed in a large control population. While the variant in the *MYBPHL* gene was identified in one percent of the control population, the substitution in the *GPSM2* gene was not present in the control population. Further analysis found that the mutation in *GPSM2* segregates with deafness in Family CG. (C) Immunohistochemistry staining for *Gpsm2* within the e16.5 and P0 mouse inner ear. *Gpsm2* is expressed at the apical surface of the hair and supporting cells of the cochlea, utricle, saccule and cristae. Expression in the cochlea is shown. Adapted from [46].

This more targeted approach is due to the current bioinformatics limitations, as well as time and budget constraints. However, in the near future such restrictions will surely decrease, thus allowing a more widespread use of whole-exome or whole-genome sequencing. Within the field of human deafness research, to date, NGS has been predominantly used for two major applications: the discovery of new deafness causative genes and new mutations within known genes; and large-scale screening of affected individuals and generation of clinical diagnosis platforms. These two approaches enable both the expansion of the understanding of deafness genetics, as well as clinical application of the current knowledge of genes underlying deafness.

NGS for Discovery of New Deafness-Causative Genes and Pathogenic Mutations

NGS can be a powerful tool in the detection of new deafness-causing mutations, both in previously known genes, as well as in genes not previously implied in HL. This technology helps overcome the serious drawbacks of linkage analysis, the most widely used method to search for genetic disease mutations in the genomic era. Indeed, since this technology entered the market, its use to identify causative genes and mutations in deaf individuals has grown tremendously. Targeted capture and MPS appears to be the ideal tool for this task as it limits the analysis to a manageable subset of the whole genome, thus reducing the cost, time and bioinformatics infrastructure necessary for the analysis of large-scale data.

Combined Targeted Capture and MPS Approach

The first study utilizing targeted genomic capture and MPS within the field of HL research identified the *C9orf75* (*TPRN*) gene, encoding taperin, as the mutated gene in NSHL *DFNB79* [27]. Targeted capture was conducted on a refined region containing 108 genes, with 870 protein-coding exons of the previously identified *DFNB79* linkage region [28]. Protein-coding sequences, as well as untranslated regions (UTRs), introns and noncoding genes were analyzed. The genomic DNA (gDNA) of a single affected individual from a Pakistani consanguineous *DFNB79*-linked family was analyzed, revealing a nonsense mutation in the *TPRN* gene. Subsequently, mutations within the additional three *DFNB79*-linked families were identified as frameshift mutations within the *TPRN* gene. Furthermore, using immunolocalization, within the mouse cochlea, the mouse Taperin orthologue was localized at the taper region at the base of the hair cell stereocilia, thus providing the gene's descriptive name. In addition, taperin was localized to the supporting cells and to a lesser extent to Reissner's membrane and spiral ligament. These findings led to the speculation that taperin may modulate actin dynamics through direct or indirect interaction with pointed ends of actin filaments.

Two studies followed that utilized targeted genomic capture and MPS technology to identify the X-linked gene *SMPX*, encoding small muscle protein, as the causative gene for DFNX4 nonsyndromic hearing impairment. Genome-wide linkage analysis was utilized on 11 affected individuals from a large German family with X-linked NSHL to reveal linkage to a

17.5 MB region on chromosome *Xp22*.12 overlapping the *DFNX4* locus previously identified in a study of a Spanish family [29, 30]. Targeted genomic capture with enrichment of all exons and 1 kb of the promoter regions of the 88 coding genes within the linked interval was conducted followed by NGS. Six variants located in exons that were not annotated as SNPs were identified. The nonsense mutation in the *SMPX* gene was considered the best candidate and was validated using Sanger sequencing. Subsequent investigation of the *DFNX4*-linked Spanish family led to the discovery of a nonsense mutation within the *SMPX* gene that segregates with HL in the family. In parallel, linkage analysis for the known X-chromosomal NSHL loci, *DFNX1-5* led to the identification of a critical linkage interval overlapping the *DFNX4* locus [29, 31]. Using NGS and filtering for predicted sequence variants against dbSNP, the 1000 Genome Project and 200 Danish controls, a single variant within the linkage interval, a nonsense mutation in the *SMPX* gene that co-segregated with hearing impairment in the family, was detected. Subsequent Sanger sequencing-based screening of 26 individuals from small families for which X-linked NSHL was not excluded revealed a frameshift mutation in the *SMPX* gene in one of the screened individuals. *SMPX* was initially cloned from human muscle [32], where it localizes to costamere structures that protect the sarcolemmal plasma membrane from damage generated by the mechanical stress caused by the contraction of muscle cells [33]. Using both quantitative PCR on fetal human inner ear [31] and immunohistochemistry of the adult mouse inner ear [30], the expression of SMPX was verified within the mammalian inner ear. Within the organ of Corti, SMPX was localized to different cell types, including Böttcher cells, root cells, pillar cells, and interdental cells of the spiral limbus, with low levels of expression in the hair cells [30].

In addition to its use in the discovery of deafness genes causing NSHL, a combined approach using targeted capture and MPS has been used to identify causative mutations leading to SHL. To date, mutations leading to SHL were identified in 36 genes leading to 10 syndromes (Hereditary Hearing Loss Homepage). These mutations are both in nuclear and mitochondrial DNA. Though quite a few mutations have been identified thus far, there are still many families with SHL for whom the causative gene mutated gene is still unknown. In an attempt to uncover the genetic basis of Perrault syndrome, in a non-consanguineous European family, a combined linkage analysis and Sanger sequencing approach together with NGS was undertaken [34]. Perrault syndrome is a genetically heterogeneous recessive disorder characterized by sensorineural hearing loss and ovarian dysgenesis, as well as neurological manifestation in some families [35-37]. Genome wide linkage analysis identified a 4.142 Mb interval on chromosome 5 containing 58 genes. The exons of these genes, as well as the flanking regulatory regions, were analyzed using Sanger sequencing and missense mutations were found in the *HARS2* gene in affected individuals. In order to rule out additional candidate mutations within the linked region, target capture and MPS were conducted and *HARS2* was identified as the only gene in the regions with variants leading to a predicted functional affect. In addition to the missense mutation, in one of the two alleles the nucleotide substitution created an alternative splice site, leading to a 12 codon deletion. *HARS2* encodes a mitochondrial histidyl tRNA synthetase [38] that catalyzes the covalent linkage between tRNAs and specific amino acids, a process necessary for the translation of mitochondrial-encoded proteins [39]. Analyzing the mutations in yeast and *Caenorhabditis elegans*, Pierce et al. were able to conclude that Perrault syndrome was caused by a reduction in HARS2 activity in the family studied.

Mutations in the *DNMT1* gene were identified in two separate studies using NGS technology for two distinct syndromes that include HL in their phenotype. *DNMT1* encodes the DNA methyltransferase 1 protein, a widely expressed protein that maintains methylation patterns in development, and mediates transcriptional repression [40]. Utilizing linkage analysis and exome sequencing, a form of hereditary sensory and autonomic neuropathy type 1 (HSAN1) syndrome, a neurodegenerative disorder with central and peripheral involvement including dementia and hearing loss [41], was studied. The form investigated in the study showed early onset dementia and sensorineural hearing loss, followed by sensory neuropathy. Four kindreds with similar phenotypes were investigated, two American, one Japanese and one European. In all cases one of two nonsense mutations were identified in exon 20 of the *DNMT1* gene within the target-sequencing domain that regulates DNMT1 binding to chromatin, leading to premature degradation of the mutant protein. Using *in vitro* studies, the mutations were demonstrated to disrupt proper folding of the protein, preventing it from entering the nuclei, as well as an effect on the stability and enzymatic activity of the full length protein, leading to global hypomethylation and local sight-specific hypermethylation. Another study performed whole exome sequencing in five affected individuals from three different kindreds with autosomal dominant cerebellar ataxia, deafness and narcolepsy (ADCA-DN) characterized by late onset sensory neuronal deafness, narcolepsy or cataplexy, cerebellar ataxia and dementia [42]. The studied population included an American family, a Swedish family and Italian kindred. After filtering for SNPs, only a single gene, *DNMT1*, was mutated in all five individuals studied, with two different mutations detected. In all cases the mutations were in exon 21. Sanger sequencing confirmed the mutations and showed cosegregation for the American and Swedish mutations with affected individuals. Sanger sequencing was also used to identify an additional mutation within exon 21 of the *DNMT1* gene in an ADCA-DN Italian family.

Whole Exome Sequencing in HL Research

Whole exome sequencing screens the exons of all genes in the human genome, thus enabling the discovery of novel deafness genes. It is estimated that approximately 60% of genes for Mendelian disease could be discovered using this technology [43]. This method can be extremely useful in cases involving small or non-consanguineous pedigrees where neither linkage analysis nor homozygosity mapping would be informative. In one study, whole exome sequencing of genomic DNA from one of two sisters with Perrault syndrome identified two rare functional variants in the *HSD17B4* gene, leading to a compound heterozygote genotype [44]. *HSD17B4* encodes 17b-hydroxysteroid dehydrogenase type 4, a peroxisomal enzyme involved in steroid metabolism and fatty acid β-oxidation. In this study showed that one of the two variants uncovered, a missense mutation, is predicted to destabilize the HSD17B4 dehydrogenase domain, whereas the second, a nonsense mutation, leads to very low levels of the HSD17B4 transcript. Furthermore, they were able to show that expression of mutant HSD17B4 protein in a compound heterozygote was severely reduced. Thus using NGS, this study was able to discover mutations in two separate genes, *HSD17B4* and *HARS2*, as the cause of Perrault syndrome in two families [34, 44]. These are the only two genes thus far linked to Perrault syndrome and without the NGS technology these mutations would most probably have not been identified. The authors analyzed *HSD17B4* and *HARS2* were analyzed in six additional families and another study analyzed these genes in eight Perrault syndrome families [45]. However, no additional mutations were detected, indicating that other critical genes remain to be identified.

The major limitation of whole exome sequencing is in the vast bioinformatics infrastructure necessary for data analysis. One approach to reduce this limitation is to compare variants within the exome after filtering for known SNPs, as utilized to identify mutations in *DNMT1* [42]. Another approach is to perform a whole exome sequencing experiment along with homozygosity mapping for recessive families in order to narrow down the regions to analyze. Three studies utilized such a method, the first of which was a study that identified a mutation in the gene *GPSM2* as the cause of NSHL *DFNB82* in a consanguineous Palestinian family (Figure 1A-B) [46]. The *DFNB82* region, located on chromosome 1, spanned 50 annotated protein-coding genes and one microRNA. Whole exome sequencing was conducted on genomic DNA from a single affected individual. By focusing on exonic and flanking intronic variants within the linked region, the data generated was narrowed down (Figure 1). To further define the potential role of Gpsm2 in the inner ear, immunohistochemistry staining for Gpsm2 was performed, revealing its expression in a pattern characteristic for proteins involved in the planar cell polarity pathway. A second truncating mutation was found in the *GPSM2* gene in a consanguineous Turkish family [47]. A subsequent study revealed that these patients previously diagnosed with NSHL also had Chudley-McCullough syndrome (CMS), with frontal polymicrogyria, abnormal corpus callosum and gray matter heterotopia [48]. Homozygosity mapping was also used to narrow down the data generated by whole exome sequencing for three individuals from two consanguineous Turkish families with phenotypes resembling the Carnevale, Malpuech, Michels and oculo-skeletal-abdominal (OSA) syndromes, including distinctive facial features, skeletal anomalies, developmental delay, periumbilical defects and mixed hearing loss [48]. Whole exome sequencing of one proband and analysis of the mapped region revealed a missense mutation in the *MASP1* gene, encoding mannan-binding lectin serine protease 1, which co-segregated with the phenotype. In the second family a nonsense mutation in the *MASP1* gene was identified using Sanger sequencing. As the two mutations occur in a *MASP1* isoform previously reported to process insulin-like growth factor binding protein (IGFBP5) [49], the authors concluded that MASP1 most probably plays a critical role in insulin growth factor availability during craniofacial and muscle development.

A third study combining homozygosity mapping and whole exome sequencing identified two novel missense variants in *GIPC3*, encoding a protein that localized to the inner ear hair cells, and *ZNF57*, a zinc finger gene, [50]. Both variant co-segregated in affected individuals with NSHL born to a consanguineous Turkish family. An initial analysis of the exome sequencing data using a read depth filter of ≥8x identified only the mutation in *ZNF57*. However, while the study was ongoing, reports of two missense mutations in *GIPC3* in two small families with sensorineural HL and an association between a mutation in *GIPC3* and age-related sensorineural HL in mice were published. The authors re-analyzed their data using a less stringent read depth filter of ≥4x. This analysis detected two additional variants within the autozygous region with only one, in exon 3 of the *GIPC3* gene, confirmed by Sanger sequencing. The authors concluded that the HL in the family they describe is caused by a novel missense mutation in *GIPC3,* as such mutations have been described in other families with NSHL. They speculated that it is possible that the mutation in *ZNF57* may contribute to the phenotype or to susceptibility to another phenotype that was not considered in their study. This work is a clear example of a major challenge of using NGS technology for the discovery of causative mutations in Mendelian diseases. It shows that even when a whole exome study attains the expected quality standards for the number of reads, the amount of DNA generated, the target coverage and the average depth across the intended target, a marked unevenness of capture of one region may occur, influencing the results.

One common approach used to identify disease-causing mutations within a genetically linked region is to search for variations in genes within this region that were previously shown to either cause deafness or to be expressed within the inner ear. In such a case one must exclude additional potential disease-causing variants within the linked region. In the past, this approach has been done using Sanger sequencing. However, such a method is extremely time- and cost-consuming, especially in the case of a relatively large linked region. NGS was used to verify that a mutation in *CEACAM16* is the cause of autosomal dominant NSHL in an American family linked to the *DFNA4* locus [51]. CECAM16 is a member of the carcinoembryonic antigen-related cell adhesion family of adhesion molecules [52]. CECAM16 was shown to be expressed in the cochlear outer hair cells, the tips of the tallest stereocilia and the tectorial membrane, and to interact with α-tectorin, a major component of the tectorial membrane. Thus it was a candidate for a deafness gene based on chromosomal location and predicted function. Indeed, mutation screening of its coding exons revealed a heterozygous missense mutation. This mutation co-segregated with the phenotype within the family and was not identified in ethnically-matched controls. The *DFNA4* interval contains 715 genes, therefore, in an attempt to exclude variants in other genes within this region, whole exome sequencing was performed on genomic DNA from a single affected individual. After filtering for documented SNPs, the authors identified 12 additional variants within the linked interval. However, as these were either not verified by Sanger sequencing or did not co-segregate with HL, they were excluded, providing strong evidence that the mutation in *CECAM16* is the cause of HL within this family.

NGS for Screening and Clinical Diagnosis Platforms

To date, PCR, restriction enzyme analysis and Sanger sequencing are the most widely used technologies for the detection of genetic mutations in the clinics. Routine clinical use of NGS technologies in the clinical setting is appealing as it has the potential to decrease sequencing costs and increase throughput. However, translational use in clinical care mandates high accuracy, simple assays, inexpensive instruments, short run times and easy data analysis. In a few cases, NGS has been used clinically for diagnostic purposes, especially in cancer [53, 54]. Hereditary HL can be predicted by genetic testing with high accuracy as the cause is monogenic in most cases, thus making it an ideal candidate for genetic screening using NGS. Indeed, in the last two years, a number of studies have set out to create platforms for diagnostic mutation detection of focused panels of deafness genes.

The feasibility of target enrichment and MPS technologies was used to examine the exons of 54 genes associated with human NSHL [55]. The genes analyzed included Usher syndrome genes since the Usher syndrome phenotype is not always distinguished from NSHL in children. The platform and diagnostic pipeline was named OtoSCOPE (Otologic Sequence Capture Of Pathogenic Exons). The study compared two platforms, the SureSelect-Illumina (solution-based) and NimbleGen-454 (solid-phase) platforms, in an effort to determine the most efficient method for identifying deafness genes for screening towards clinical diagnosis. They tested nine individuals diagnosed with genetic HL, including three positive controls diagnosed by Sanger sequencing prior to the study. Pathogenetic mutations in the *STRC, CDH23, MYO6, KCNQ4* and *MYH14* genes were found in six probands. While both platforms provided high specificity and sensitivity, the authors concluded that under their conditions the SureSelect-Illumina platform was preferable with regards to scalability, sensitivity, and cost. In a further effort to develop clinical diagnosis platforms, a combined targeted genomic capture and MPS on a cohort of Israeli Jewish and Palestinian Arab hearing impaired probands was performed [56]. In this study, a custom cRNA oligonucleotide design containing 246 genes responsible for syndromic and NSHL in humans and mice was constructed. Targets were 82 human-protein coding genes, 2 human microRNAs and the human orthologues of 162 mouse deafness genes, based on the fact that many of the human deafness genes also cause deafness in mice. Using this array, samples from 11 probands of families with HL were sequenced. After filtering for reported SNPs, rare single base pair and insertion/deletion (indel) variants were identified. Using this approach, critical mutations were identified in six of the original probands and their families. These include mutations in the *TMC1, CDH23, MYO15A, TECTA* and *WFS1* genes. These mutations were found to co-segregate with HL in the affected families. A novel mutation identified in *TMC1* was further shown to contribute to 38% of hereditary HL in the Moroccan Jewish population, solving the cause of HL in an additional 20 families. This approach exploits the high-throughput nature of targeted MPS to make a single fully comprehensive test for all known deafness genes. The approach had the added benefit of including genes associated with deafness in mice, thereby having the potential to discover additional human deafness genes.

One of the main limitations of an NGS-based platform for clinical application is the high per-sample cost. In an attempt to reduce costs, in-house cDNA-based probes were produced for targeted gene enrichment [57]. As proof of principle, PCR amplicons from cDNA clones of five genes known to cause deafness (*GJB2, GJB3, GJB6, SLC26A4* and *MYO15A*) were used as bait probes in hybridization for capturing human genomic DNA (gDNA) fragments. The captured gDNA fragments were then sequenced using the Illumina GAII platform. The authors used gDNA samples from two normal hearing human subjects and ten individuals previously shown to have genetic mutations in *GJB2* by Sanger sequencing. The results were confirmed by Sanger sequencing in all cases. The authors concluded that their approach achieves the necessary specificity, depth of coverage, multiplexicity and uniformity for accurate sequencing by a NGS platform, as well as significantly reduces per-patient cost.

CONCLUSION

NGS has transformed genomic research by decreasing the costs of sequencing and increasing throughput. Its impact on the auditory field is in its infancy and will no doubt increase by many fold in the near future. Applications of NGS technology have recently begun to transition into clinical care. Such applications will surely enable rapid pathogenic mutation screening that will be widely used, thus reducing the need for multiple parallel diagnostic approaches. In addition, there is great hope that NGS will greatly advance patient tailored therapeutics. The advances made so far are encouraging, but for wide and routine use in the clinic, additional improvements will need to be made, including reduction in costs, simple assays and easy data analysis. A number of NGS systems recently launched have some of these characteristics, but still face a number of challenges [58]. In addition, ethical issues will need to be addressed; including the possibility that this new technology may exacerbate the ambivalence society has towards physical differences and anomalies [59]. Furthermore, the likelihood of unintended discoveries as a by-product of the technology complicates matters even further. Therefore the issue of an individual's genomic privacy is of utmost importance and invites questions such as, who has accessibility to the data generated and how is it stored and disposed of, which must be promptly addressed [60]. Finally, the impact deep sequencing has had on the hearing and deafness field is dramatic. The ethical implications described above play a role in this field as well. Furthermore, there is the added issue that termination of pregnancy was controversial in this area [61], and once genetic diagnosis is available to all, the option of using it for prenatal diagnosis and family planning is a reality. In addition, deep sequencing may identify more than one variant that appears to be a mutation without a sufficient number of affected family members to provide validation, making it difficult to conclusively determine which is the causative mutation and complicating genetic counseling. Nonetheless, the ability to diagnose and define a mutation has become much more amenable for the hearing impaired population. This has and continues to pave the way for elucidation of pathways and mechanisms of genetic hearing loss, with the impending development of therapeutics.

ACKNOWLEDGMENTS

Research in the Avraham laboratory for human genomics is funded by the National Institutes of Health (NIDCD) R01DC011835; Israeli Centers of Research Excellence (I-CORE), Gene Regulation in Complex Human Disease, Center No 41/11; and the Hedrich Charitable Trust. We thank Shaked Shivatzki for help with figures.

REFERENCES

[1] J.E. Bailey-Wilson and A.F. Wilson, *Hum. Hered.* 72, 228 (2001).

[2] E.S. Lander and D. Botstein, *Science*, 236, 1567 (1987).

[3] P.E. Leon, H. Raventos, E. Lynch, J. Morrow, and M.C. King, *Proc. Natl. Acad. Sci. U S A.* 89, 5181 (1992).

[4] E.D. Lynch, M.K. Lee, J.E. Morrow, P.L. Welcsh, P.E. Leon, and M.C. King, *Science*, 278, 1315 (1997).

[5] H. Chaib, G. Lina-Granade, P. Guilford, H. Plauchu, J. Levilliers, A. Morgon, and C. Petit, *Hum. Mol. Genet.* 3, 2219 (1994).

[6] D.P. Kelsell, J. Dunlop, H.P. Stevens, N.J. Lench, J.N. Liang, G. Parry, R.F. Mueller, and I.M. Leigh, *Nature*, 387, 80 (1997).

[7] F. Denoyelle, S. Marlin, D. Weil, L. Moatti, P. Chauvin, E.N. Garabedian, and C. Petit, *Lancet*, 353, 1298 (1999).

[8] T. Walsh, S.B. Pierce, D.R. Lenz, Z. Brownstein, O. Dagan-Rosenfeld, H. Shahin, W. Roeb, S. McCarthy, A.S. Nord, C.R. Gordon, Z. Ben-Neriah, J. Sebat, M. Kanaan, M.K. Lee, M. Frydman, M.C. King, and K.B. Avraham, *Am. J. Hum. Genet.* 87, 101 (2010).
[9] J. Rodriguez-Paris, L. Pique, T. Colen, J. Roberson, P. Gardner, and I. Schrijver, *PLoS One*, 5, e11804 (2010).
[10] F. Sanger, S. Nicklen, and A.R. Coulson, *Proc. Natl. Acad. Sci. USA.* 74, 5463 (1977).
[11] S. Levy, G. Sutton, P.C. Ng, L. Feuk, A.L. Halpern, B.P. Walenz, N. Axelrod, J. Huang, E.F. Kirkness, G. Denisov, Y. Lin, J.R. MacDonald, A.W. Pang, M. Shago, T.B. Stockwell, A. Tsiamouri, V. Bafna, V. Bansal, S.A. Kravitz, D.A. Busam, K.Y. Beeson, T.C. McIntosh, K.A. Remington, J.F. Abril, J. Gill, J. Borman, Y.H. Rogers, M.E. Frazier, S.W. Scherer, R.L. Strausberg, and J.C. Venter, *PLoS Biol.* 5, e254 (2007).
[12] M.L. Metzker, *Nat. Rev. Genet.* 11, 31 (2010).
[13] A.E. Shearer, M.S. Hildebrand, C.M. Sloan, and R.J. Smith, *Hear. Res.* 282, 1 (2011).
[14] D.A. Wheeler, M. Srinivasan, M. Egholm, Y. Shen, L. Chen, A. McGuire, W. He, Y.J. Chen, V. Makhijani, G.T. Roth, X. Gomes, K. Tartaro, F. Niazi, C.L. Turcotte, G.P. Irzyk, J.R. Lupski, C. Chinault, X.Z. Song, Y. Liu, Y. Yuan, L. Nazareth, X. Qin, D.M. Muzny, M. Margulies, G.M. Weinstock, R.A. Gibbs, and J.M. Rothberg, *Nature*, 452, 872 (2008).
[15] T.C. Glenn, *Mol. Ecol. Resour.* 11, 759 (2011).
[16] M. Margulies, M. Egholm, W.E. Altman, S. Attiya, J.S. Bader, L.A. Bemben, J. Berka, M.S. Braverman, Y.J. Chen, Z. Chen, S.B. Dewell, L. Du, J.M. Fierro, X.V. Gomes, B.C. Godwin, W. He, S. Helgesen, C.H. Ho, G.P. Irzyk, S.C. Jando, M.L. Alenquer, T.P. Jarvie, K.B. Jirage, J.B. Kim, J.R. Knight, J.R. Lanza, J.H. Leamon, S.M. Lefkowitz, M. Lei, J. Li, K.L. Lohman, H. Lu, V.B. Makhijani, K.E. McDade, M.P. McKenna, E.W. Myers, E. Nickerson, J.R. Nobile, R. Plant, B.P. Puc, M.T. Ronan, G.T. Roth, G.J. Sarkis, J.F. Simons, J.W. Simpson, M. Srinivasan, K.R. Tartaro, A. Tomasz, K.A. Vogt, G.A. Volkmer, S.H. Wang, Y. Wang, M.P. Weiner, P. Yu, R.F. Begley, and J.M. Rothberg, *Nature*, 437, 376 (2005).
[17] J. Ju, D.H. Kim, L. Bi, Q. Meng, X. Bai, Z. Li, X. Li, M.S. Marma, S. Shi, J. Wu, J.R. Edwards, A. Romu, and N.J. Turro, *Proc. Natl. Acad. Sci. USA.* 103, 19635 (2006).
[18] A. Valouev, J. Ichikawa, T. Tonthat, J. Stuart, S. Ranade, H. Peckham, K. Zeng, J.A. Malek, G. Costa, K. McKernan, A. Sidow, A. Fire, and S.M. Johnson, *Genome Res.* 18, 1051 (2008).
[19] E.R. Mardis, *Trends Genet.* 24, 133 (2008).
[20] X. Lin, W. Tang, S. Ahmad, J. Lu, C.C. Colby, J. Zhu, and Q. Yu, *Hear. Res.* in press (2012).
[21] W. Lee, Z. Jiang, J. Liu, P.M. Haverty, Y. Guan, J. Stinson, P. Yue, Y. Zhang, K.P. Pant, D. Bhatt, C. Ha, S. Johnson, M.I. Kennemer, S. Mohan, I. Nazarenko, C. Watanabe, A.B. Sparks, D.S. Shames, R. Gentleman, F.J. de Sauvage, H. Stern, A. Pandita, D.G. Ballinger, R. Drmanac, Z. Modrusan, S. Seshagiri, and Z. Zhang, *Nature*, 465, 473 (2010).
[22] S. Turajlic, S.J. Furney, M.B. Lambros, C. Mitsopoulos, I. Kozarewa, F.C. Geyer, A. Mackay, J. Hakas, M. Zvelebil, C.J. Lord, A. Ashworth, M. Thomas, G. Stamp, J. Larkin, J.S. Reis-Filho, and R. Marais, *Genome Res.* 22, 196 (2012).

[23] T. Walsh, S. Casadei, M.K. Lee, C.C. Pennil, A.S. Nord, A.M. Thornton, W. Roeb, K.J. Agnew, S.M. Stray, A. Wickramanayake, B. Norquist, K.P. Pennington, R.L. Garcia, M.C. King, and E.M. Swisher, *Proc. Natl. Acad. Sci. USA.* 108, 18032 (2011).

[24] T. Walsh, M.K. Lee, S. Casadei, A.M. Thornton, S.M. Stray, C. Pennil, A.S. Nord, J.B. Mandell, E.M. Swisher, and M.C. King, *Proc. Natl. Acad. Sci. USA.* 107, 12629 (2010).

[25] E.A. Worthey, A.N. Mayer, G.D. Syverson, D. Helbling, B.B. Bonacci, B. Decker, J.M. Serpe, T. Dasu, M.R. Tschannen, R.L. Veith, M.J. Basehore, U. Broeckel, A. Tomita-Mitchell, M.J. Arca, J.T. Casper, D.A. Margolis, D.P. Bick, M.J. Hessner, J.M. Routes, J.W. Verbsky, H.J. Jacob, and D.P. Dimmock, *Genet. Med.* 13, 255 (2011).

[26] H. Najmabadi, H. Hu, M. Garshasbi, T. Zemojtel, S.S. Abedini, W. Chen, M. Hosseini, F. Behjati, S. Haas, P. Jamali, A. Zecha, M. Mohseni, L. Puttmann, L.N. Vahid, C. Jensen, L.A. Moheb, M. Bienek, F. Larti, I. Mueller, R. Weissmann, H. Darvish, K. Wrogemann, V. Hadavi, B. Lipkowitz, S. Esmaeeli-Nieh, D. Wieczorek, R. Kariminejad, S.G. Firouzabadi, M. Cohen, Z. Fattahi, I. Rost, F. Mojahedi, C. Hertzberg, A. Dehghan, A. Rajab, M.J. Banavandi, J. Hoffer, M. Falah, L. Musante, V. Kalscheuer, R. Ullmann, A.W. Kuss, A. Tzschach, K. Kahrizi, and H.H. Ropers, *Nature*, 478, 57 (2011).

[27] A.U. Rehman, R.J. Morell, I.A. Belyantseva, S.Y. Khan, E.T. Boger, M. Shahzad, Z.M. Ahmed, S. Riazuddin, S.N. Khan, and T.B. Friedman, *Am. J. Hum. Genet.* 86, 378 (2010).

[28] S.Y. Khan, S. Riazuddin, M. Shahzad, N. Ahmed, A.U. Zafar, A.U. Rehman, R.J. Morell, A.J. Griffith, Z.M. Ahmed, and T.B. Friedman, *Eur. J. Hum. Genet.* 18, 125 (2010).

[29] I. del Castillo, M. Villamar, M. Sarduy, L. Romero, C. Herraiz, F.J. Hernandez, M. Rodriguez, I. Borras, A. Montero, J. Bellon, M.C. Tapia, and F. Moreno, *Hum. Mol. Genet.* 5, 1383 (1996).

[30] A.K. Huebner, M. Gandia, P. Frommolt, A. Maak, E.M. Wicklein, H. Thiele, J. Altmuller, F. Wagner, A. Vinuela, L.A. Aguirre, F. Moreno, H. Maier, I. Rau, S. Giesselmann, G. Nurnberg, A. Gal, P. Nurnberg, C.A. Hubner, I. del Castillo, and I. Kurth, *Am. J. Hum. Genet.* 88, 621 (2011).

[31] M. Schraders, S.A. Haas, N.J. Weegerink, J. Oostrik, H. Hu, L.H. Hoefsloot, S. Kannan, P.L. Huygen, R.J. Pennings, R.J. Admiraal, V.M. Kalscheuer, H.P. Kunst, and H. Kremer, *Am. J. Hum. Genet.* 88, 628 (2011).

[32] D. Patzak, O. Zhuchenko, C.C. Lee, and M. Wehnert, *Hum. Genet.* 105, 506 (1999).

[33] S. Palmer, N. Groves, A. Schindeler, T. Yeoh, C. Biben, C.C. Wang, D.B. Sparrow, L. Barnett, N.A. Jenkins, N.G. Copeland, F. Koentgen, T. Mohun, and R.P. Harvey, *J. Cell Biol.* 153, 985 (2001).

[34] S.B. Pierce, K.M. Chisholm, E.D. Lynch, M.K. Lee, T. Walsh, J.M. Opitz, W. Li, R.E. Klevit, and M.C. King, *Proc. Natl. Acad. Sci. U S A.* 108, 6543 (2011).

[35] A. Fiumara, G. Sorge, A. Toscano, E. Parano, L. Pavone, and J.M. Opitz, *Am. J. Med. Genet. A.* 128A, 246 (2004).

[36] C. Kobe, L.W. Kracht, L. Timmermann, J. Bachmann, and M.C. Schmidt, *Clin. Nucl. Med.* 33, 922 (2008).

[37] M. Perrault, B. Klotz, and E. Housset, *Bull. Mem. Soc. Med. Hop. Paris*, 67, 79 (1951).

[38] T.P. O'Hanlon, N. Raben, and F.W. Miller, *Bioch. Biophys. Res. Commun.* 210, 556 (1995).

[39] A. Antonellis and E.D. Green, *Annu. Rev. Genomics Hum. Genet.* 9, 87 (2008).
[40] Z.M. Svedruzic, *Prog. Mol. Biol. Transl. Sci.* 101, 221 (2011).
[41] C.J. Klein, M.V. Botuyan, Y. Wu, C.J. Ward, G.A. Nicholson, S. Hammans, K. Hojo, H. Yamanishi, A.R. Karpf, D.C. Wallace, M. Simon, C. Lander, L.A. Boardman, J.M. Cunningham, G.E. Smith, W.J. Litchy, B. Boes, E.J. Atkinson, S. Middha, B.D. PJ, J.E. Parisi, G. Mer, D.I. Smith, and P.J. Dyck, *Nat. Genet.* 43, 595 (2011).
[42] J. Winkelmann, L. Lin, B. Schormair, B.R. Kornum, J. Faraco, G. Plazzi, A. Melberg, F. Cornelio, A.E. Urban, F. Pizza, F. Poli, F. Grubert, T. Wieland, E. Graf, J. Hallmayer, T.M. Strom, and E. Mignot, *Hum. Mol. Genet.* 21, 2205 (2012).
[43] C. Gilissen, A. Hoischen, H.G. Brunner, and J.A. Veltman, *Eur. J. Hum. Genet.* 20, 490 (2012).
[44] S.B. Pierce, T. Walsh, K.M. Chisholm, M.K. Lee, A.M. Thornton, A. Fiumara, J.M. Opitz, E. Levy-Lahad, R.E. Klevit, and M.C. King, *Am. J. Hum. Genet.* 87, 282 (2010).
[45] E.M. Jenkinson, J. Clayton-Smith, S. Mehta, C. Bennett, W. Reardon, A. Green, S.H. Pearce, G. De Michele, G.S. Conway, D. Cilliers, N. Moreton, J.R. Davis, D. Trump, and W.G. Newman, *J. Neurol.* in press (2011).
[46] T. Walsh, H. Shahin, T. Elkan-Miller, M.K. Lee, A.M. Thornton, W. Roeb, A. Abu Rayyan, S. Loulus, K.B. Avraham, M.C. King, and M. Kanaan, *Am. J. Hum. Genet.* 87, 90 (2010).
[47] K.O. Yariz, T. Walsh, H. Akay, D. Duman, A.C. Akkaynak, M.C. King, and M. Tekin, *Clin. Genet.* 81, 289 (2012).
[48] A. Sirmaci, T. Walsh, H. Akay, M. Spiliopoulos, Y.B. Sakalar, A. Hasanefendioglu-Bayrak, D. Duman, A. Farooq, M.C. King, and M. Tekin, *Am. J. Hum. Genet.* 87, 679 (2010).
[49] C.L. Cortesio and W. Jiang, *Arch. Bioch. Biophys.* 449, 164 (2006).
[50] A. Sirmaci, Y.J. Edwards, H. Akay, and M. Tekin, *PLoS One*, 7, e32000 (2012).
[51] J. Zheng, K.K. Miller, T. Yang, M.S. Hildebrand, A.E. Shearer, A.P. DeLuca, T.E. Scheetz, J. Drummond, S.E. Scherer, P.K. Legan, R.J. Goodyear, G.P. Richardson, M.A. Cheatham, R.J. Smith, and P. Dallos, *Proc. Natl. Acad. Sci. U S A.* 108, 4218 (2011).
[52] K. Kuespert, S. Pils, and C.R. Hauck, *Curr. Opin. Cell. Biol.* 18, 565 (2006).
[53] D.C. Link, L.G. Schuettpelz, D. Shen, J. Wang, M.J. Walter, S. Kulkarni, J.E. Payton, J. Ivanovich, P.J. Goodfellow, M. Le Beau, D.C. Koboldt, D.J. Dooling, R.S. Fulton, R.H. Bender, L.L. Fulton, K.D. Delehaunty, C.C. Fronick, E.L. Appelbaum, H. Schmidt, R. Abbott, M. O'Laughlin, K. Chen, M.D. McLellan, N. Varghese, R. Nagarajan, S. Heath, T.A. Graubert, L. Ding, T.J. Ley, G.P. Zambetti, R.K. Wilson, and E.R. Mardis, *JAMA*, 305, 1568 (2011).
[54] J.S. Welch, P. Westervelt, L. Ding, D.E. Larson, J.M. Klco, S. Kulkarni, J. Wallis, K. Chen, J.E. Payton, R.S. Fulton, J. Veizer, H. Schmidt, T.L. Vickery, S. Heath, M.A. Watson, M.H. Tomasson, D.C. Link, T.A. Graubert, J.F. DiPersio, E.R. Mardis, T.J. Ley, and R.K. Wilson, *JAMA*, 305, 1577 (2011).
[55] A.E. Shearer, A.P. DeLuca, M.S. Hildebrand, K.R. Taylor, J. Gurrola, 2nd, S. Scherer, T.E. Scheetz, and R.J. Smith, *Proc. Natl. Acad. Sci. U S A.* 107, 21104 (2010).

[56] Z. Brownstein, L.M. Friedman, H. Shahin, V. Oron-Karni, N. Kol, A.A. Rayyan, T. Parzefall, D. Lev, S. Shalev, M. Frydman, B. Davidov, M. Shohat, M. Rahile, S. Lieberman, E. Levy-Lahad, M.K. Lee, N. Shomron, M.C. King, T. Walsh, M. Kanaan, and K.B. Avraham, *Genome Biol.* 12, R89 (2011).

[57] W. Tang, D. Qian, S. Ahmad, D. Mattox, N.W. Todd, H. Han, S. Huang, Y. Li, Y. Wang, H. Li, and X. Lin, *Genet. Test Mol. Biomarkers* in press (2012).

[58] A. Desai and A. Jere, *Clin. Genet.* 81, 503 (2012).

[59] J.L. Scully, *Nat. Rev. Genet.* 9, 797 (2008).

[60] F.S. Ong, W.W. Grody, and J.L. Deignan, *Expert Rev. Mol. Diagn.* 11, 457 (2011).

[61] S.J. Stern, K.S. Arnos, L. Murrelle, K.O. Welch, W.E. Nance, and A. Pandya, *J. Med. Genet.* 39, 449 (2002).

In: Inner Ear Development and Hearing Loss
Editors: Saima Riazuddin and Zubair Ahmed
ISBN: 978-1-62417-011-9

Chapter 9

NONSYNDROMIC HEARING IMPAIRMENT: THE UTILITY OF FAMILIES FOR THE IDENTIFICATION OF HEARING IMPAIRMENT GENES, VARIANTS AND PHENOTYPES

Regie Lyn P. Santos-Cortez and Suzanne M. Leal*
Center for Statistical Genetics, Department of Molecular and Human Genetics,
Baylor College of Medicine, Houston, Texas, US

ABSTRACT

Genetic hearing impairment accounts for more than 60% of congenital hearing impairment, and at least 80% of genetic hearing impairment is nonsyndromic. Nonsyndromic hearing impairment (NSHI) is characterized by locus, allelic and phenotypic heterogeneity. Inheritance is usually monogenic with complete penetrance. Extended and consanguineous families play an important role in the identification of genes and variants and the description of genotype-phenotype correlations. In order to localize NSHI genes, linkage mapping, haplotype reconstruction, and in the case of autosomal recessive (AR)NSHI genes, homozygosity mapping, are performed using marker genotypes from informative family members. After the mapping of a NSHI locus there are many genes in which the causal variant can lie. Until recently a positional candidate gene approach was used to identify the causal gene. In recent years next-generation sequencing (NGS), in particular exome sequencing, has greatly aided the identification of NSHI genes. Even with this advanced technology, families with linkage information paired with NGS are highly beneficial in facilitating NSHI gene identification. NGS should also greatly facilitate diagnostic screening for NSHI patients. However experiences in variant detection using NGS data from NSHI families foreshadow some difficulties in diagnosis and genetic counseling of sporadic NSHI patients using NGS data.

---

* E-mail address: sleal@bcm.edu

INTRODUCTION

Hearing impairment affects nearly 300 million people worldwide, and can place a significant socio-economic burden on both individuals and societies [1]. While universal newborn hearing screening in the United States has identified hearing impairment in 1.4 of 1000 babies [2], prevalence data from 2001 to 2008 show that for individuals aged 12 and older, 1 in 5 people in the US had bilateral or unilateral hearing loss [3]. The prevalence of hearing impairment increases per decade of life, from 2.3% in adolescents to 89% in individuals older than 80 years of age [3]. At any age, hearing impairment reduces quality of life [4-5]. While timely habilitation improves socio-emotional status and communication skills [6-7], in children, in particular, early diagnosis and intervention for hearing impairment has a major impact on language, cognitive and overall development [8].

Although previous studies have estimated that the congenital hearing impairment in about half of newborns are due to genetic risk factors, the availability of newborn screening for both genetic and environmental risk factors have shed new information on the etiology of hearing loss. In a study of more than 300 Japanese infants with abnormal hearing tests, of those that underwent additional testing, about 30% had mutations which are putatively causal for hearing impairment in the *GJB2* gene, 17% were positive for cytomegalovirus (CMV) DNA in umbilical cord blood and a large proportion of infants had temporal bone anomalies by high-resolution CT scan, namely middle ear fluid (39%), external and middle ear anomalies (12%) and abnormalities in the inner ear and internal auditory meatus (17%) [9]. In a few cases, other perinatal factors such as neonatal asphyxia (n=13), cranial anomalies (n=9), very low birth weight (n=7), hyperbilirubinemia (n=2), and rubella (n=1) were documented, additionally 23% (n=31) had a family history of hearing loss [9]. On the other hand, a study of 268 babies with impaired hearing in the Netherlands showed that 20% were conductive in nature, mostly from otitis media with effusion and 3% were due to middle and/or external ear defects [10]. Of those children with sensorineural hearing loss, the etiology was unknown in 43% of the cases, due to intrauterine viral infection (rubella, CMV) in 2% of the cases, and due to genetic etiology in 13% of the cases (6% syndromic based on clinical exam and 7% nonsyndromic based on a positive genetic test or family history of early-onset hearing impairment) [10]. In another study of 87 hearing-impaired infants from Belgium, an etiologic diagnosis can only be confirmed in 55%, while 33% had *GJB2* mutations, syndromes, chromosomal aberrations or a family history of hearing loss [11]. In a fourth study, of 500 US children with sensorineural hearing loss, 14% had syndromes, while 12.6% were *GJB2*-positive [12]. Additionally temporal bone CT findings were present in 18% of those screened, while 32% of those who were tested for *GJB2* were heterozygous or negative for mutations but had close relatives with hearing loss [12]. In these four populations, assuming that a large proportion of children with temporal bone anomalies and hearing loss of unknown etiology actually have a genetic cause, the current estimate for the prevalence of genetic etiology among newborns with congenital hearing impairment may well be in excess of 60%. These four studies were conducted in high-income countries, but in middle- and low-income countries, genetic and CT studies may not be readily available for newborn infants. Despite documentation of craniofacial anomalies (2%), family history of deafness (5-7%) or consanguinity (14%) as risk factors, in hearing-impaired infants in countries of lower income, perinatal, neonatal and maternal factors continue to predominate [13-15]. Based on these studies, the newborn prevalence of syndromic hearing impairment including those due to chromosomal abnormalities is within the range of 10-14%.

In childhood, the increase in proportion of infectious causes of hearing impairment, such as otitis media and meningitis, decreases the prevalence of genetic hearing impairment. In adolescents and adults, however, hearing impairment is usually noise-induced or age-related. Although recent studies have identified genetic factors that confer susceptibility to otitis media [16], noise-induced hearing loss [17] and presbycusis [18], and for less common causes of hearing impairment such as otosclerosis [19] and ototoxicity from chemotherapy [20], the rest of this chapter will concentrate on nonsyndromic hearing impairment (NSHI).

NONSYNDROMIC HEARING IMPAIRMENT AS A HETEROGENEOUS TRAIT

Hearing impairment is one of the most genetically heterogeneous traits known to man. It is estimated that more than a thousand genes may be implicated in the etiology of NSHI. However to date less than 200 genes have been localized in the genome, and only about 60 NSHI genes have been identified (Hereditary Hearing Loss Homepage, http://hereditary hearingloss.org). For NSHI loci that have been mapped, inheritance is autosomal recessive (AR) in 91, autosomal dominant (AD) in 57, X-linked in one locus and Y-linked in one locus. Additionally there are 2 modifier loci and one locus for auditory neuropathy (AUNA). Of the known NSHI genes, inheritance for 32 genes is AR, 17 genes AD, for 8 genes both AR and AD inheritance have been observed, and for 3 genes X-linked. The vast majority of these genes and loci were identified in families segregating NSHI. An early study found that 77% of cases of NSHI in newborns and early childhood are of AR inheritance, 22% display AD inheritance and ~1% are X-linked [21]. A more recent study in the Brazilian population which examined both children and adults showed an almost equal proportion of NSHI patients with AD or AR inheritance [22]. Many would indicate sporadic cases of unknown inheritance to be AR, however, this does not take into account other causes such as de novo mutations [23-25]. Depending on the study population, NSHI due to mitochondrial DNA mutations are seen in 2-4% of sporadic cases [26-27].

Almost all of the genes that have thus far been identified are monogenic, where only one gene causes the hearing impairment. There have been a few exceptions. Compound heterozygosity for two different ARNSHI genes can cause hearing impairment, for example, for *GJB2* and *GJB6* [28], for *CDH23* and *PCDH15* [29] and for *KCNJ10* and *SLC26A4* [30]. Studies in mice suggest that digenic inheritance can cause Usher syndrome [31], although only a few human cases of Usher syndrome have been found with digenic inheritance [29, 32-34]. Compound heterozygosity for *KCNJ10* and *SLC26A4* has been reported in two families [30]. In the case of *GJB2* and *GJB6*, two genes that are both within the *DFNB1/DFNA3* locus, more examples of digenic inheritance have been found although only at low frequencies in select populations, thus it still considered a rare occurrence [28, 35-42].

Incomplete penetrance based on age and sex has been reported for ADNSHI loci or genes and less frequently for ARNSHI [43]. Also phenotypic modifiers have been identified for various loci, such as: (1) the dominant modifier *DFNM1* which suppresses profound hearing loss due to *DFNB26* [44]; and (2) the p.Met34Thr and p.Val37Ile variants in the *GJB2* gene which have much lower penetrance than most *GJB2* variants and are predicted to cause a milder form of hearing impairment later in life [45]. In the latter case, however, the pathogenicity of these variants remains controversial due to their high allele frequencies in controls [45].

As multiple genes cause NSHI within populations, the gene-specific prevalence rates are expected to be different between populations. Table 1 shows a comparison of the reported frequencies of mutations in selected NSHI genes in three family-based cohorts from different populations. Most notably although the *GJB2* gene is a major cause of NSHI in European patient populations [46-47], it has low or zero frequencies in several countries, including Pakistan [48-50].

NSHI genes may also display extreme allelic heterogeneity with a large number of alleles or variants causing NSHI. Each of the *GJB2* and *SLC26A4* genes has >200 known variants (The Human Gene Mutation Database, http://www.hgmd.cf.ac.uk/ac/). On the other hand, specific variants may be prevalent within the population. For *GJB2* the c.35delG mutation is prevalent in Europeans [46], the c.167delT mutation in Ashkenazi Jews [56] and the c.235delC variant is common in East Asian populations [57]. For >90% of Pakistani families with an *HGF* variant, hearing impairment is due to the same 3bp deletion, which was observed to occur within the same haplotype in families from different ethno-linguistic groups of Pakistan and from India [58].

Table 1. Comparison of frequencies of selected NSHI genes with mutations in family-based cohorts

Gene	Palestinian consanguineous families (N=286, %)	Pakistani consanguineous families/ Leal cohort [1] (N=579, %)	UK Caucasian sibpairs (N=142, %)
GJB2	23 (8.0) [51]	32 (5.5)	47 (33.1) [47]
HGF	0 [52]	26 (4.5)	Not Available
SLC26A4	2 (0.7) [51,53]	21 (3.6)	5 (3.5) [47]
TMC1	2 (0.7) [52]	12 (2.1)	Not Available
TMPRSS3	5 (1.7) [51,54]	10 (1.7)	1 (0.7) [47]
TRIOBP	9 (3.1) [55]	1 (0.2)	Not Available

[1] Unpublished frequencies

NSHI is also characterized by phenotypic heterogeneity. *WFS1* is a relatively frequent cause of progressive, low-frequency sensorineural ADNSHI [59], while *TECTA* mutations cause mid-frequency NSHI [60], although within the same gene variability in age-of-onset and progression occurs. Because many ADNSHI genes are found only in a few families, inter- and intra-familial variability in severity and progression of hearing impairment may be expected. Likewise for ARNSHI genes, the occurrence of enlarged vestibular aqueducts for *SLC26A4* [61] and of truncating mutations for *GJB2* [62] have been associated with more severe hearing impairment. It has been demonstrated that there is wide variation for severity even with the same genotype. For example, patients who are homozygous for the *GJB2* c.35delG mutation have a wide range of severity of hearing impairment [62]. In searching for modifiers that modulate severity due to the same *GJB2* genotype, no association has been found between the c.35delG mutation and environmental factors [63]. A genome-wide association study did not identify a major modifier gene that influences the *GJB2* phenotype due to the c.35delG variant, however there was evidence that a few common variants with weak effects act as modifiers [64].

Different mutations within the same gene can cause either AD or AR NSHI (e.g. *TMC1* for *DFNA36* or *DFNB7/11*), and either syndromic or NSHI (e.g. *WFS1* and *SLC26A4*). Missense mutations in the C-terminal domain of the *WFS1* gene cause low-frequency ADNSHI, while most stop, frameshift, insertion and deletion mutations result in autosomal recessive Wolfram syndrome or DIDMOAD (diabetes insipidus, diabetes mellitus, optic atrophy and deafness) [65]. AR mutations in the *SLC26A4* gene can cause either NSHI, nonsyndromic enlargement of the vestibular aqueduct (EVA) or Pendred syndrome (goiter and deafness with inner ear anomalies such as EVA or Mondini's dysplasia) [66]. However there is still controversy whether the structural cochlear anomalies in this spectrum of disorders are directly caused by *SLC26A4* variants [67].

Despite the predominance of peripheral vestibular deficits in mouse models for NSHI genes, only the *COCH* gene is well-known as a cause of ADNSHI with balance dysfunction [68]. However recent findings suggest that vestibular dysfunction in NSHI patients may have been underdiagnosed. To illustrate, vertigo symptoms were shown to occur more in patients with *GJB2* and *GJB6* mutations compared to non-carrier deaf individuals [69-70]. In addition, balance impairment has been described in families with mutations in NSHI genes *MYO6* [71], *ESPN* [72], *ACTG1* [73], *MYO7A* [74], *POU4F3* [75], *GRXCR1* [76] and *PTPRQ* [77]. Future studies would require routine objective assessment of vestibular function using a battery of balance tests in order to fully understand the impact of NSHI gene mutations on the human vestibular system.

LARGE AND CONSANGUINEOUS FAMILIES AS A RICH RESOURCE FOR NSHI GENE IDENTIFICATION

Due to the extreme genetic heterogeneity and the Mendelian pattern of inheritance, NSHI gene identification has been highly successful using consanguineous families and/or large extended pedigrees with multiple affected individuals. In particular, the Pakistani population is a rich resource for ARNSHI gene identification because most marriages (~60%) are consanguineous [78]. Studies using Pakistani families have led to the identification of ~30 ARNSHI genes, and the mapping of at least 20 additional loci for which the NSHI genes have not been identified.

For NSHI gene identification, established and proven methods are used to ascertain families with NSHI, perform whole-genome genotyping, and analyze pedigree structures and genotype data using linkage analysis, haplotype reconstruction, and for ARNSHI families, homozygosity mapping. These methods require the ascertainment of consanguineous and/or extended pedigrees with both hearing and hearing-impaired family members that are genotyped for polymorphic markers across the genome, and then testing for the co-segregation of the causal variant with the alleles of a marker or set of markers. The availability of multiple families for study is a great advantage because: (1) having multiple families with linkage to the same region, if they segregate variants in the same gene, aids in refining the NSHI locus to the smallest genetic interval; and (2) identification of putatively causal variants in multiple families linked to the same locus helps to strengthen evidence that a specific gene is involved in NSHI etiology.

Due to phenotypic heterogeneity, it is very important to adequately describe the hearing impairment phenotype during family ascertainment, not only to delineate syndromes like Usher or Pendred, but also to alert the investigator to the possibility of intra-familial heterogeneity, which may be due to phenocopies from either genetic or environmental causes. It is possible to have two different NSHI genes as the cause of hearing impairment within a family, or to have hearing impairment that is due to an environmental cause but the cause is unknown to the family or person involved. For linkage analysis, the maximum LOD score is based upon hearing-impaired family members being homozygous or compound heterozygous (ARNSHI) or heterozygous (ADNSHI) for the same causal variant(s). Misclassification of hearing-impaired individuals as affected when the individual is a phenocopy will result in a deflated LOD score, and linkage to the region containing the causal variant can remain unidentified. Haplotype reconstruction can help to elucidate individuals who are phenocopies as non-carriers of the haplotype that segregates with the NSHI trait.

In previous studies, genome-wide genotyping has been carried out using short tandem repeat or single nucleotide polymorphism (SNP) markers that are approximately equally spaced across the genome. After linkage analysis and haplotype reconstruction are performed using the marker genotypes, candidate genes can be selected and Sanger sequencing performed within the region of homozygosity and/or 3-unit support interval to elucidate putatively causal variants. This process can be laborious, time-consuming and expensive. With the advent of next-generation sequencing (NGS) technology, it is now possible to perform whole-genome or whole-exome sequencing, which at a single-base pair resolution, is a more cost-effective way of detecting variants in all the genes within a locus. Although it is also possible to design custom capture arrays to sequence the entire 3-unit support interval and/or region of homozygosity, this strategy may not be cost-effective. NGS can also facilitate gene identification in smaller families. At least 8 genes have been identified for syndromic and NSHI using NGS [79].

If linkage information is available, identification of the causal variant is made even easier and faster because the search will be limited to the genomic region within the linkage interval. Genome scans can also help to prioritize which families to select to undergo exome sequencing. Some families are problematic and segregate more than one NSHI locus. Sometimes these issues can be resolved from information from the genome scan while at other times these issues cannot be resolved and it is questionable if exome sequencing will reveal the causal variants. Additionally phenocopies can be elucidated from genome scans and the selection of these individuals for exome sequencing can be avoided. Therefore if genome scan data is not available it is highly advisable that it is obtained and analyzed before embarking on NGS.

When studying consanguineous ARNSHI families, a single hearing-impaired individual with the smallest region of homozygosity can be selected to undergo NGS. For ADNSHI families, identification of heterozygous variants in at least two hearing-impaired individuals with NGS data can markedly reduce the search space within the genome. These hearing-impaired individuals can be selected based upon the smallest overlapping haplotype if a genome scan has been previously performed or the two individuals who are most distantly related.

Several criteria have been used in the analysis of NGS data for identification of causal variants, most commonly are the following: (1) the variant(s) must be in the homozygous or compound heterozygous state in the individual with ARNSHI, or heterozygous if ADNSHI; (2) loss-of-function filter, such that frameshift, splice-site, nonsense or missense mutations and indels are prioritized over synonymous SNPs and variants in untranslated, regulatory or intergenic/intronic regions; and (3) the variant must not occur at high frequencies in databases such as dbSNP (http://www.ncbi.nlm.nih.gov/projects/SNP/), 1000 Genomes (http://www.1000genomes.org/) and the NHLBI Exome Variant Server (http://evs.gs. washington.edu/EVS/). Once variants are shown to meet these criteria it can be determined if they segregate with the phenotype within the family by sequencing the variant region in all informative family members with and without hearing impairment. Additionally because some populations such as the Pakistani population are not well represented in databases, controls should be sequenced to determine whether or not the variant is present within the control population.

Bioinformatic tools are useful for prediction of the functional effect of identified variants, particularly for nonsynonymous SNPs, for which multiple software (e.g. PolyPhen-2 [80], SIFT [81]) are available. However when each program is used alone the sensitivity or specificity may be low, thus the use of multiple programs is recommended. Although there are synonymous SNPs that have been reported to alter splicing [82], this mechanism has so far not been seen in NSHI genes. This possibility can be considered in the very rare case when no other loss-of-function types of variants are found within the NSHI locus. For all variant types within coding regions, other prediction tools for protein motifs (e.g. PROSITE [83]), topology prediction for transmembrane proteins (e.g. TMHMM 2.0 [84]) and protein modeling software (e.g. SWISS-MODEL [85]) may be used depending on the availability of database information on similar protein structures. There is still a dearth of prediction tools for non-coding regions, although several programs that estimate evolutionary constraint at the nucleotide level (i.e. GERP [86], phastCons [87], phyloP [88]) are widely used. Note that the specificity and sensitivity of prediction tools rely on what is known about the protein structure and the availability of gene sequences from multiple phylogenies, thus bioinformatic results for specific variants may have an inherent bias.

When looking at minor allele frequencies (MAF) for each variant site in databases, for causal variants ideally the MAF equals zero. However because the vast majority of study populations that are annotated in databases may be markedly different from a case population that is not well-represented in databases, MAF=0 may not imply causality but rather would be reflective of population differences, i.e. the variant may not be prevalent in populations that are well-described in databases but are prevalent within the case population. On the other hand, if a variant is found to have a high MAF in databases, given that most of the included subjects were studied for phenotypes other than NSHI or are healthy control individuals, it is likely that such a variant is non-causal. Because in some cases the individuals that are included in databases may actually be a carrier for an ARNSHI gene, a causal variant may be falsely eliminated based on its presence in database genotypes. Thus it is advisable that non-zero frequencies in databases will not be used to exclude a variant as non-causal, instead variants with sufficiently low MAF (e.g. $\leq$2%) will be considered for further evaluation although given a lower priority. Additionally, as more NGS data from each ethnic population become available, the establishment of population-specific repositories for NGS data would be helpful in identifying many more common variants that would be useful for excluding non-causal variants for individuals from both within and from other populations. More importantly segregating variants that are predicted to be functional and have low MAF in databases should be followed up by sequencing in unrelated, ethnically matched control individuals.

Despite variant screening based on bioinformatic tools and genotypes from control individuals, due to linkage disequilibrium several variants within a linkage region in the same or different genes can be identified to segregate with the hearing impairment. It is more likely that only one of these variants is truly causing the hearing impairment phenotype, rather than having variants in multiple interacting genes. Identification of one of these variants or other putatively causal variants in the same gene, in families displaying linkage to the same region, can help to pinpoint the correct gene. If there is more than one putatively causal variant in the same gene, it becomes more difficult to determine which variant is causal particularly if additional families with NSHI that segregate a variant within the same gene cannot be found. Even if within a family, after screening databases and controls a single variant is identified, identification of the same variant as well as additional putatively causal variants in the same gene in other families adds evidence to support involvement of the gene in hearing impairment etiology. Additionally, functional studies may be designed to check whether the genes are expressed in the inner ear or if animal knock-out models have inner ear defects. This step of the research process can be expensive and time-consuming.

There are a few caveats in using NGS data. Other genetic causes such as cytogenetic aberrations, complex rearrangements and epigenetic mechanisms or regulatory elements may not be detected properly with sequencing, specifically if the causal variants lie within poorly captured or poorly annotated exons (e.g. in genes overlapping with segmental duplications). Very few of these types of mutations have been identified for NSHI, such as a tandem inverted duplication for *TJP2* [89] and a point mutation in miR-96 [90], which may either be because they are rare or they are not easily detected by commonly used techniques. If whole-exome sequences are used, a variant that lies outside the exome definition, such as those within intronic regions, will be missed. For example, a 3bp deletion within intron 4 of the *HGF* gene was found to be prevalent in Pakistani families with NSHI [58]. As the cost and technology of NGS continue to improve at the current pace, accurate detection of complex variants in whole-genome sequences can be easily attained. The only difficulty that remains would be the interpretation of which variants are truly causal of NSHI based on current limitations in knowledge of gene function, especially outside coding regions.

Implications for Genetic Screening in the General Population

Without available pedigree, phenotype and genotype data from extended pedigrees, it can be difficult to determine which among the variants in NSHI genes that segregate with the phenotype within a family is causal. We already encounter this problem even in families with suggestive linkage in which LOD scores >1.5 can be obtained in multiple genomic regions. Thus the problem of identifying the correct causal variant due to multiple hits across the genome is much greater when screening variants for individuals with sporadic NSHI.

Although there are many success stories of NGS, it often does not lead to the identification of the causal locus. These failures are usually not reported in the literature.

Because current analysis of NGS data relies on functional annotation or prediction and allele frequency estimates in non-NSHI individuals, it is possible to identify a variant as functional but it is not necessarily causal of NSHI. Due to the rarity of causal variants and the extreme genetic heterogeneity for NSHI, comparison of allele frequencies between population cases and non-cases is not enough to detect causal variants. As databases become inundated with NGS variants, an increase in variant MAF may be due to individuals who have normal hearing and are heterozygous for an ARNSHI variant or due to individuals with an unreported hearing impairment phenotype. We already see this problem with *GJB2* variants p.Met34Thr and p.Val37Ile, which remain controversial due to the findings of milder hearing impairment in NSHI individuals, proof of pathogenicity from in vitro studies, but MAF of >10% in non-case populations [45]. Reduced penetrance has been proposed to explain the data inconsistencies for these variants [45]. However it should be stated that although screened databases can be beneficial in helping to identify the causal variant, lack of a variant within a database is not conclusive evidence that a variant is causal.

The use of NGS technology for diagnostic screening of NSHI is readily available, but the major hurdles for genetic counseling remain. Although de novo events have been reported in NSHI genes [23-25], repeated validation would be required to ensure that the occurrence of de novo variants are not due to genotyping error, and for that matter, the same careful attention to validation must be given for all potentially causal variants that are detected by NGS. At the individual level, for a case of sporadic NSHI, aside from difficulties in discriminating which variant is truly causal of NSHI, when multiple variants in known NSHI genes are identified across the genome, patient advice will also be guarded for variants that cause later-onset hearing impairment or have reduced penetrance. Because of great inter- and intra-familial variability in hearing impairment phenotypes, predicting the severity and progression of hearing impairment based solely on genotype is not straightforward. It was previously predicted that if an NSHI gene variant is found, the patient saves on cost for additional testing for syndromic or balance phenotypes. Although this might still be true for a good number of NSHI genes, more recent evidence points toward underdiagnosis of vestibular dysfunction in NSHI patients, and over the years more NSHI genes have been found to also cause syndromic or other non-cochlear disease. Recently *LOXHD1*, which was initially identified as an ARNSHI gene, was also shown to cause corneal dystrophy [91].

Most importantly, the main driver for the usability of NGS in diagnostic screening for NSHI would be the availability of genotype-guided therapy for general clinical use. Associations between mutations in NSHI genes and cochlear implant outcomes have been confounded by length of implant use [92] and many of such studies also suffer from lack of power to detect association due to small sample size. Some progress in development of inner ear gene therapy and hair cell regeneration techniques has been made [93] but would still require further research prior to clinical application for patients with NSHI.

REFERENCES

[1] World Health Organization, Deafness and hearing impairment, Fact sheet N°300 (2012), http://www.who.int/mediacentre/factsheets/fs300/en/.

[2] Centers for Disease Control and Prevention,http://www.cdc.gov/ncbddd/hearingloss /data.

[3] F. R. Lin, J. K. Niparko, and L. Ferrucci, *Arch. Intern. Med.* 171, 1851 (2011).

[4] J. Fellinger, D. Holzinger, H. Sattel, and M. Laucht, *Eur. Child Adolesc. Psychiatry* 17, 414 (2008).

[5] E. M. Chia, J. J. Wang, E. Rochtchina, R. R. Cumming, P. Newall, and P. Mitchell, *Ear Hear.* 28, 187 (2007).

[6] C. Yoshinaga-Itano, *Ment. Retard. Dev. Disabil. Res. Rev.* 9, 252 (2003).

[7] P. B. Kricos, S. Erdman, G. W. Bratt, D. W. Williams, *J. Am. Acad. Audiol.* 18, 304 (2007).

[8] A. M. Korver, S. Konings, F. W. Dekker, M. Beers, C. C. Wever, J. H. Frijns, A. M. Oudesluys-Murphy, and DECIBEL Collaborative Study Group, *JAMA* 304, 1701 (2010).

[9] N. Adachi, K. Ito, H. Sakata, and T. Yamasoba, *Otolaryngol. Head Neck Surg.* 143, 97 (2010).

[10] I. L. Holster, L. J. Hoeve, M. H. Wieringa, R. M. Willis-Lorrier, and H. H. de Gier, *J. Pediatr.* 155, 646 (2009).

[11] F. Declau, A. Boudewyns, J. Van den Ende, A. Peeters, and P. van den Heyning, *Pediatrics* 121, 1119 (2008).

[12] D. Yaeger, J. McCallum, K. Lewis, L. Soslow, U. Shah, W. Potsic, C. Stolle, and I. D. Krantz, *Am. J. Med. Genet. A* 140, 827 (2006).

[13] B. O. Olusanya, and A. A. Okolo, *Paediatr. Perinat. Epidemiol.* 20, 366 (2006).

[14] J. Attias, M. Al-Masri, L. AbuKader, G. Cohen, P. Merlov, H. Pratt, R. Othman-Jebara, P. Aber, F. Raad, and A. Noyek, *Int. J. Audiol.* 45, 528 (2006).

[15] M. A. Musani, A. Rauf, M. Ahsan, and F. A. Khan, *J. Pak. Med. Assoc.* 61, 141 (2011).

[16] M. S. Rye, J. M. Blackwell, and S. E. Jamieson, *Laryngoscope* 122, 665 (2012).

[17] M. Pawelczyk, L. Van Laer, E. Fransen, E. Rajkowska, A. Konings, P. I. Carlsson, E. Borg, G. Van Camp, and M. Sliwinska-Kowalska, *Ann. Hum. Genet.* 73, 411 (2009).

[18] R. A. Friedman, L. Van Laer, M. J. Huentelman, S. S. Sheth, E. Van Eyken, J. J. Corneveaux, W. D. Tembe, R. F. Halperin, A. Q. Thorburn, S. Thys, S. Bonneux, E. Fransen, J. Huyghe, I. Pyykko, C. W. Cremers, H. Kremer, I. Dhooge, D. Stephens, E. Orzan, M. Pfister, M. Bille, A. Parving, M. Sorri, P. H. Van de Heyning, L. Makmura, J. D. Ohmen, F. H. Linthicum Jr, J. N. Fayad, J. V. Pearson, D. W. Craig, D. A. Stephan, and G. Van Camp, *Hum. Mol. Genet.* 18, 785 (2009).

[19] I. Schrauwen, M. Ealy, M. J. Huentelman, M. Thys, N. Homer, K. Vanderstraeten, E. Fransen, J. J. Corneveaux, D. W. Craig, M. Claustres, C. W. Cremers, I. Dhooge, P. Van de Heyning, R. Vincent, E. Offeciers, R. J. Smith, and G. Van Camp, *Am. J. Hum. Genet.* 84, 328 (2009).

[20] C. J. Ross, H. Katzov-Eckert, M. P. Dube, B. Brooks, S. R. Rassekh, A. Barhdadi, Y. Feroz-Zada, H. Visscher, A. M. Brown, M. J. Rieder, P. C. Rogers, M. S. Phillips, B. C. Carleton, M. R. Hayden, and CPNDS Consortium, *Nat. Genet.* 41, 1345 (2009).

[21] M. Cohen, and R. Gorlin, Chapter 3: Epidemiology, etiology, and genetic patterns. In: R. Gorlin, H. Toriello, and M. Cohen, *Hereditary hearing loss and its syndromes*, Oxford University Press, New York (1995).
[22] N. M. Kokitsu-Nakata, M. L. Guion-Almeida, and A. Richieri-Costa, *Am. J. Audiol.* 13, 99 (2004).
[23] A. Pera, M. Villamar, A. Vinuela, M. Gandia, C. Meda, F. Moreno, and C. Hernandez-Chico, *Eur. J. Hum. Genet.* 16, 888 (2008).
[24] P. Primignani, L. Trotta, P. Castorina, F. Lalatta, D. Cuda, A. Murri, U. Ambrosetti, A. Cesarani, C. Curcio, D. Coviello, and M. Travi, *Laryngoscope* 117, 821 (2007).
[25] F. Donaudy, R. Snoeckx, M. Pfister, H. P. Zenner, N. Blin, M. Di Stazio, A. Ferrara, C. Lanzara, R. Ficarella, F. Declau, C. M. Pusch, P. Nurnberg, S. Melchionda, L. Zelante, E. Ballana, X. Estivill, G. Van Camp, P. Gasparini, and A. Savoia, *Am. J. Hum. Genet.* 74, 770 (2004).
[26] S. Usami, S. Nishio, M. Nagano, S. Abe, T. Yamaguchi, and Deafness Gene Study Consortium, *PLoS One* 7, e31276 (2012).
[27] M. Ealy, K. A. Lynch, N. C. Meyer, and R. J. Smith, *Laryngoscope* 121, 1184 (2011).
[28] I. Lerer, M. Sagi, Z. Ben-Neriah, T. Wang, H. Levi, and D. Abeliovich, *Hum. Mutat.* 18, 460 (2001).
[29] Q. Y. Zheng, D. Yan, X. M. Ouyang, L. L. Du, H. Yu, B. Chang, K. R. Johnson, and X. Z. Liu, *Hum. Mol. Genet.* 14, 103 (2005).
[30] T. Yang, J. G. Gurrola 2nd, H. Wu, S. M. Chiu, P. Wangemann, P. M. Snyder, and R. J. Smith, *Am. J. Hum. Genet.* 84, 651 (2009).
[31] Q. Y. Zheng, J. D. Scarborough, Y. Zheng, H. Yu, D. Choi, and P. G. Gillespie, *Hum. Mol. Genet.* 21, 2588 (2012).
[32] I. Ebermann, J. B. Phillips, M. C. Liebau, R. K. Koenekoop, B. Schermer, I. Lopez, E. Schafer, A. F. Roux, C. Dafinger, A. Bernd, E. Zrenner, M. Claustres, B. Blanco, G. Nurnberg, R. Ruland, M. Westerfield, T. Benzing, and H. J. Bolz, *J. Clin. Invest.* 120, 1812 (2010).
[33] D. Vozzi, A. Aaspollu, E. Athanasakis, A. Berto, A. Fabretto, D. Licastro, M. Kulm, F. Testa, P. Trevisi, M. Vahter, C. Ziviello, A. Martini, F. Simonelli, S. Banfi, and P. Gasparini, *Mol. Vis.* 17, 1662 (2011).
[34] P. Le Quesne Stabej, Z. Saihan, N. Rangesh, H. B. Steele-Stallard, J. Ambrose, A. Coffey, J. Emmerson, E. Haralambous, Y. Hughes, K. P. Steel, L. M. Luxon, A. R. Webster, and M. Bitner-Glindzicz, *J. Med. Genet.* 49, 27 (2011).
[35] del Castillo, M. Villamar, M. A. Moreno-Pelayo, F. J. del Castillo, A. Alvarez, D. Telleria, I. Menendez, and F. Moreno, *N. Engl. J. Med.* 346, 243 (2002).
[36] N. Pallares-Ruiz, P. Blanchet, M. Mondain, M. Claustres, and A. F. Roux, *Eur. J. Hum. Genet.* 10, 72 (2002).
[37] H. Bolz, G. Schade, S. Ehmer, C. Kothe, M. Hess, and A. Gal, *Hear. Res.* 188, 42 (2004).
[38] R. Utrera, V. Ridaura, Y. Rodriguez, M. J. Rojas, L. Mago, S. Angeli, and O. Henriquez, *Genet. Test.* 11, 347 (2007).
[39] N. Gurtler, C. Egenter, N. Bosch, and M. Plasilova, *Acta Otolaryngol.* 128, 1056 (2008).
[40] E. Cama, S. Melchionda, T. Palladino, M. Carella, R. Santarelli, E. Genovese, F. Benettazzo, L. Zelante, and E. Arslan, *Int. J. Audiol.* 48, 12 (2009).

[41] S. M. da Silva-Costa, F. T. Martins, T. Pereira, M. C. Pomilio, A. P. Marques-de-Faria, and E. L. Sartorato, *Genet. Test. Mol. Biomarkers* 15, 849 (2011).
[42] A. Asma, A. Ashwaq, A. G. Norzana, A. M. Atmadini, B. H. Ruszymah, L. Saim, and I. F. Wahida, *Med. J. Malaysia* 66, 124 (2011).
[43] A. S. Thirlwall, D. J. Brown, P. M. McMillan, S. E. Barker, and M. M. Lesperance, *Arch. Otolaryngol. Head Neck Surg.* 129, 830 (2003).
[44] S. Riazuddin, C. M. Castelein, Z. M. Ahmed, A. K. Lalwani, M. A. Mastroianni, S. Naz, T. N. Smith, N. A. Liburd, T. B. Friedman, A. J. Griffith, S. Riazuddin, and E. R. Wilcox, *Nat. Genet.* 26, 431 (2000).
[45] A. Pollak, A. Skorka, M. Mueller-Malesinska, G. Kostrzewa, B. Kisiel, J. Waligora, P. Krajewski, M. Oldak, L. Korniszewski, H. Skarzynski, and R. Ploski, *Am. J. Med. Genet. A* 143A, 2534 (2007).
[46] X. Estivill, P. Fortina, S. Surrey, R. Rabionet, S. Melchionda, L. D'Agruma, E. Mansfield, E. Rappaport, N. Govea, M. Mila, L. Zelante, and P. Gasparini, *Lancet* 351, 394 (1998).
[47] T. Hutchin, N. N. Coy, H. Conlon, E. Telford, K. Bromelow, D. Blaydon, G. Taylor, E. Coghill, S. Brown, R. Trembath, X. Z. Liu, M. Bitner-Glindzicz, and R. Mueller, *Clin. Genet.* 68, 506 (2005).
[48] R. L. Santos, M. Wajid, T. L. Pham, J. Hussan, G. Ali, W. Ahmad, and S. M. Leal, *Clin. Genet.* 67, 61 (2005).
[49] N. M. Gasmelseed, M. Schmidt, M. M. Magzoub, M. Macharia, O. M. Elmustafa, B. Ototo, E. Winkler, G. Ruge, R. D. Horstmann, and C. G. Meyer, *Hum. Mutat.* 23, 206 (2004).
[50] R. I. Kabahuma, X. Ouyang, L. L. Du, D. Yan, T. Hutchin, M. Ramsay, C. Penn, and X. Z. Liu, *Int. J. Pediatr. Otorhinolaryngol.* Epub ahead of print (2011).
[51] H. Shahin, T. Walsh, A. Abu Rayyan, M. K. Lee, J. Higgins, D. Dickel, K. Lewis, J. Thompson, C. Baker, A. S. Nord, S. Stray, D. Gurwitz, K. B. Avraham, M. C. King, and M. Kanaan, *Eur. J. Hum. Genet.* 18, 407 (2010).
[52] Z. Brownstein, L. M. Friedman, H. Shahin, V. Oron-Karni, N. Kol, A. Abu Rayyan, T. Parzefall, D. Lev, S. Shalev, M. Frydman, B. Davidov, M. Shohat, M. Rahile, S. Lieberman, E. Levy-Lahad, M. K. Lee, N. Shomron, M. C. King, T. Walsh, M. Kanaan, and K. B. Avraham, *Genome Biol.* 12, R89 (2011).
[53] Z. N. Brownstein, A. A. Dror, D. Gilony, L. Migirov, K. Hirschberg, and K. B. Avraham, *Arch. Otolaryngol. Head Neck Surg.* 134, 403 (2008).
[54] T. Walsh, A. Abu Rayyan, J. Abu Sa'ed, H. Shahin, J. Shepshelovich, M. K. Lee, K. Hirschberg, M. Tekin, W. Salhab, K. B. Avraham, M. C. King, and M. Kanaan, *Hum. Genomics* 2, 203 (2006).
[55] H. Shahin, T. Walsh, T. Sobe, J. Abu Sa'ed, A. Abu Rayyan, E. D. Lynch, M. K. Lee, K. B. Avraham, M. C. King, and M. Kanaan, *Am. J. Hum. Genet.* 78, 144 (2006).
[56] R. J. Morell, H. J. Kim, L. J. Hood, L. Goforth, K. Friderici, R. Fisher, G. Van Camp, C. I. Berlin, C. Oddoux, H. Ostrer, B. Keats, and T. B. Friedman, *N. Engl. J. Med.* 339, 1500 (1998).
[57] D. Yan, H. J. Park, X. M. Ouyang, A. Pandya, K. Doi, R. Erdenetungalag, L. L. Du, N. Matsushiro, W. E. Nance, A. J. Griffith, and X. Z. Liu, *Hum. Genet.* 114, 44 (2003).

[58] J. M. Schultz, S. N. Khan, Z. M. Ahmed, S. Riazuddin, A. M. Waryah, D. Chhatre, M. F. Starost, B. Ploplis, S. Buckley, D. Velasquez, M. Kabra, K. Lee, M. J. Hassan, G. Ali, M. Ansar, M. Ghosh, E. R. Wilcox, W. Ahmad, G. Merlino, S. M. Leal, S. Riazuddin, T. B. Friedman, and R. J. Morell, *Am. J. Hum. Genet.* 85, 25 (2009).

[59] H. Fukuoka, Y. Kanda, S. Ohta, and S. Usami, *J. Hum. Genet.* 52, 510 (2007).

[60] M. S. Hildebrand, M. Morin, N. C. Meyer, F. Mayo, S. Modamio-Hoybjor, A. Mencia, L. Olavarrieta, C. Morales-Angulo, C. J. Nishimura, H. Workman, A. P. DeLuca, I. del Castillo, K. R. Taylor, B. Tompkins, C. W. Goodman, I. Schrauwen, M. Van Wesemael, K. Lachlan, A. E. Shearer, T. A. Braun, P. L. M. Huygen, H. Kremer, G. Van Camp, F. Moreno, T. L. Casavant, R. J. H. Smith, and M. A. Moreno-Pelayo, *Hum. Mutat.* 32, 825 (2011).

[61] Q. Gopen, G. Zhou, K. Whittemore, and M. Kenna, *Laryngoscope* 121, 1971 (2011).

[62] R. L. Snoeckx, P. L. Huygen, D. Feldmann, S. Marlin, F. Denoyelle, J. Waligora, M. Mueller-Malesinska, A. Pollak, R. Ploski, A. Murgia, E. Orzan, P. Castorina, U. Ambrosetti, E. Nowakowska-Szyrwinska, J. Bal, W. Wiszniewski, A. R. Janecke, D. Nekahm-Heis, P. Seeman, O. Bendova, M. A. Kenna, A. Frangulov, H. L. Rehm, M. Tekin, A. Incesulu, H. H. Dahl, D. du Sart, L. Jenkins, D. Lucas, M. Bitner-Glindzicz, K. B. Avraham, Z. Brownstein, I. del Castillo, F. Moreno, N. Blin, M. Pfister, I. Sziklai, T. Toth, P. M. Kelley, E. S. Cohn, L. Van Maldergem, P. Hilbert, A. F. Roux, M. Mondain, L. H. Hoefsloot, C. W. Cremers, T. Lopponen, H. Lopponen, A. Parving, K. Gronskov, I. Schrijver, J. Roberson, F. Gualandi, A. Martini, G. Lina-Granade, N. Pallares-Ruiz, C. Correia, G. Fialho, K. Cryns, N. Hilgert, P. Van de Heyning, C. J. Nishimura, R. J. Smith, and G. Van Camp, *Am. J. Hum. Genet.* 77, 945 (2005).

[63] E. Van Eyken, L. Van Laer, E. Fransen, V. Topsakal, J. J. Hendrickx, K. Demeester, P. Van de Heyning, E. Maki-Torkko, S. Hannula, M. Sorri, M. Jensen, A. Parving, M. Bille, M. Baur, M. Pfister, A. Bonaconsa, M. Mazzoli, E. Orzan, A. Espeso, D. Stephens, K. Verbruggen, J. Huyghe, I. Dhooge, P. Huygen, H. Kremer, C. Cremers, S. Kunst, M. Manninen, I. Pyykko, E. Rajkowska, M. Pawelczyk, M. Sliwinska-Kowalska, M. Steffens, T. Wienker, and G. Van Camp, *Otol. Neurotol.* 28, 970 (2007).

[64] N. Hilgert, M. J. Huentelman, A. Q. Thorburn, E. Fransen, N. Dieltjens, M. Mueller-Malesinska, A. Pollak, A. Skorka, J. Waligora, R. Ploski, P. Castorina, P. Primignani, U. Ambrosetti, A. Murgia, E. Orzan, A. Pandya, K. Arnos, V. Norris, P. Seeman, P. Janousek, D. Feldmann, S. Marlin, F. Denoyelle, C. J. Nishimura, A. Janecke, D. Nekahm-Heis, A. Martini, E. Mennucci, T. Toth, I. Sziklai, I. del Castillo, F. Moreno, M. B. Petersen, V. Iliadou, M. Tekin, A. Incesulu, E. Nowakowska, J. Bal, P. Van de Heyning, A. F. Roux, C. Blanchet, C. Goizet, G. Lancelot, G. Fialho, H. Caria, X. Z. Liu, O, Xiaomei, P. Govaerts, K. Gronskov, K. Hostmark, K. Frei, I. Dhooge, S. Vlaeminck, E. Kunstmann, L. Van Laer, R. J. H. Smith, and G. Van Camp, *Eur. J. Hum. Genet.* 17, 517 (2009).

[65] K. Cryns, T. A. Sivakumaran, J. M. W. Van den Ouweland, R. J. E. Pennings, C. W. R. J. Cremers, K. Flothmann, T. L. Young, R. J. H. Smith, M. M. Lesperance, and G. Van Camp, *Hum. Mutat.* 22, 275 (2003).

[66] S. P. Pryor, A. C. Madeo, J. C. Reynolds, N. J. Sarlis, K. S. Arnos, W. E. Nance, Y. Yang, C. K. Zalewski, C. C. Brewer, J. A. Butman, and A. J. Griffith, *J. Med. Genet.* 42, 159 (2005).

[67] B. Y. Choi, A. C. Madeo, K. A. King, C. K. Zalewski, S. P. Pryor, J. A. Muskett, W. E. Nance, J. A. Butman, C. C. Brewer, and A. J. Griffith, *J. Med. Genet.* 46, 856 (2009).

[68] N. G. Robertson, L. Lu, S. Heller, S. N. Merchant, R. D. Eavey, M. McKenna, J. B. Nadol Jr, R. T. Miyamoto, F. H. Linthicum Jr, J. F. Lubianca Neto, A. J. Hudspeth, C. E. Seidman, C. C. Morton, and J. G. Seidman, *Nat. Genet.* 20, 299 (1998).

[69] K. M. Dodson, S. H. Blanton, K. O. Welch, V. W. Norris, R. L. Nuzzo, J. A. Wegelin, R. S. Marin, W. E. Nance, A. Pandya, and K. S. Arnos, *Am. J. Med. Genet. A* 155, 993 (2011).

[70] M. Kasai, C. Hayashi, T. Iizuka, A. Inoshita, K. Kamiya, H. Okada, Y. Nakajima, K. Kaga, and K. Ikeda, *Acta Otolaryngol.* 130, 990 (2010).

[71] Z. M. Ahmed, R. J. Morell, S. Riazuddin, A. Gropman, S. Shaukat, M. M. Ahmad, S. A. Mohiddin, L. Fananapazir, R. C. Caruso, T. Husnain, S. N. Khan, S. Riazuddin, A. J. Griffith, T. B. Friedman, and E. R. Wilcox, *Am. J. Hum. Genet.* 72, 1315 (2003).

[72] S. Naz, A. J. Griffith, S. Riazuddin, L. Hampton, J. Battey, S. Khan, S. Riazuddin, E. Wilcox, and T. Friedman, *J. Med. Genet.* 41, 591 (2004).

[73] M. H. Kemperman, E. M. De Leenheer, P. L. Huygen, E. van Wijk, G. van Duijnhoven, F. P. Cremers, H. Kremer, and C. W. Cremers, *Arch. Otolaryngol. Head Neck Surg.* 130, 281 (2004).

[74] A. M. Bischoff, R. J. Pennings, P. L. Huygen, M. W. Luijendijk, E. Van Wijk, J. R> Cruysberg, H. Kremer, and C. W. Cremers, *Otol. Neurotol.* 27, 323 (2006).

[75] F. J. van Drunen, R. J. Pauw, R. W. Collin, H. Kremer, P. L. Huygen, and C. W. Cremer, *Audiol. Neurootol.* 14, 303 (2009).

[76] M. Schraders, K. Lee, J. Oostrik, P. L. M. Huygen, G. Ali, L. H. Hoefsloot, J. A. Veltman, F. P. M. Cremers, S. Basit, M. Ansar, C. W. R. J. Cremers, H. P. M. Kunst, W. Ahmad, R. J. C. Admiraal, S. M. Leal, and H. Kremer, *Am. J. Hum. Genet.* 86, 138 (2010).

[77] M. Schraders, J. Oostrik, P. L. M. Huygen, T. M. Strom, E. van Wijk, H. P. M. Kunst, L. H. Hoefsloot, C. W. R. J. Cremers, R. J. C. Admiraal, and H. Kremer, *Am. J. Hum. Genet.* 86, 604 (2010).

[78] M. Sajjad, A. A. Khattak, J. E. G. Bunn, and I. Mackenzie, *J. Laryngol. Otol.* 122, 1057 (2008).

[79] A. E. Shearer, M. S. Hildebrand, C. M. Sloan, and R. J. H. Smith, *Hear. Res.* 282, 1 (2011).

[80] I. A. Adzhubei, S. Schmidt, L. Peshkin, V. E. Ramensky, A. Gerasimova, P. Bork, A. S. Kondrashov, and S. R. Sunyaev, *Nat. Methods* 7, 248 (2010).

[81] P. C. Ng, and S. Henikoff, *Genome Res.* 11, 863 (2001).

[82] A. Woolfe, J. C. Mullikin, and L. Elnitski, *Genome Biol.* 11, R20 (2010).

[83] C. J. Sigrist, L. Cerutti, E. de Castro, P. S. Langendijk-Genevaux, V. Bulliard, A. Bairoch, and N. Hulo, *Nucleic Acids Res.* 28, D161 (2010).

[84] A. Krogh, B. Larsson, G. von Heijne, and E. L. L. Sonnhammer, *J. Mol. Biol.* 305, 567 (2001).

[85] K. Arnold, L. Bordoli, J. Kopp, and T. Schwede, *Bioinformatics* 22, 195 (2006).

[86] G. M. Cooper, E. A. Stone, G. Asimenos, NISC Comparative Sequencing Program, E. D. Green, S. Batzoglou, and A. Sidow, *Genome Res.* 15, 901 (2005).

[87] A. Siepel, G. Bejerano, J. S. Pedersen, A. S. Hinrichs, M. Hou, K. Rosenbloom, H. Clawson, J. Spieth, L. W. Hillier, S. Richards, G. M. Weinstock, R. K. Wilson, R. A. Gibbs, W. J. Kent, W. Miller, and D. Haussler, *Genome Res.* 15, 1034 (2005).

[88] K. S. Pollard, M. J. Hubisz, K. R. Rosenbloom, and A. Siepel, *Genome Res.* 20, 110 (2010).

[89] T. Walsh, S. B. Pierce, D. R. Lenz, Z. Brownstein, O. Dagan-Rosenfeld, H. Shahin, W. Roeb, S. McCarthy, A. S. Nord, C. R. Gordon, Z. Ben-Neriah, J. Sebat, M. Kanaan, M. K. Lee, M. Frydman, M. C. King, and K. B. Avraham, *Am. J. Hum. Genet.* 87, 101 (2010).

[90] A. Mencia, S. Modamio-Høybjør, N. Redshaw, M. Morín, F. Mayo-Merino, L. Olavarrieta, L. A. Aguirre, I. del Castillo, K. P. Steel, T. Dalmay, F. Moreno, and M. A. Moreno-Pelayo, *Nat. Genet.* 41, 609 (2009).

[91] S. A. Riazuddin, D. S. Parker, E. J. McGlumphy, E. C. Oh, B. W. Iliff, T. Schmedt, U. Jurkunas, R. Schleif, N. Katsanis, and J. D. Gottsch, *Am. J. Hum. Genet.* 90, 533 (2012).

[92] S. S. Connell, S. I. Angeli, H. Suarez, A. V. Hodges, T. J. Balkany, and X. Z. Liu, *Otolaryngol. Head Neck Surg.* 137, 596 (2007).

[93] L. R. Lustig, and O. Akil, *Curr. Opin. Neurol.* 25, 57 (2012).

In: Inner Ear Development and Hearing Loss
Editors: Saima Riazuddin and Zubair Ahmed
ISBN: 978-1-62417-011-9

Chapter 10

Interpretation of Variants of Uncertain Clinical Significance (VUCS): The Paradigm of Usher Syndrome

***D. Baux*[1], *C. Vaché*[1], *S. Malcolm*[2], *M. Claustres*[1,3,4] *and A-F. Roux*[1,3]**

[1]Laboratoire de génétique moléculaire, CHU Montpellier, Montpellier, France
[2]Clinical and Molecular Genetics, Institute of Child Health, University College London, UK
[3]INSERM, U827, Montpellier, France
[4]University Montpellier I, Montpellier, France

Abstract

Since the beginning of the molecular genetics era as routine sequencing of disease genes has become established, the chance of identifying Variants of Uncertain Clinical Significance (VUCS) has massively increased. Proper assessment of these variants has become a major issue in many human diseases, such as Cystic Fibrosis or Breast Cancer. This is also a well-identified problem in Usher syndrome, an autosomal recessive disorder involving both deafness and blindness, and in which the major genes are particularly prone to VUCS. This chapter deals with molecular diagnosis of Usher syndrome. We point out relevant clinical and genetic features, the range and type of mutations found, and focus on a simple methodology that has been designed to assess the potential clinical impact of VUCS identified in Usher genes. This method has been tested on hundreds of variants, has proven its efficiency, and is progressively integrated in the reference set of Locus-Specific DataBases dedicated to Usher syndrome, LOVD-USHbases.

INTRODUCTION

Usher syndrome is an autosomal recessive disorder which affects both hearing and vision. This is the major cause of deaf blindness in man, and the prevalence has recently been estimated around 1/6,000 [1]. The syndrome is clinically and genetically heterogeneous with three clinical types and nine causative genes identified. Among these, at least five can be considered to be large genes (> 7kb coding sequence), and sequencing of these genes produces a substantial number of DNA variations. Most pathogenic mutations in Usher syndrome are private, and missense and other Variants of Uncertain Clinical Significance (VUCS) are often encountered. Altogether, these observations explain the necessity to use a robust and efficient approach to assess the potential effect of the variants.

DEFINITION OF VUCSS

VUCS are variations at the DNA level that cannot definitively be considered to be neutral or pathogenic. While this can be the case for virtually all types of variations, in practice these variants are for the majority intronic or exonic variations, and include “missense”, “silent” variations or small in frame insertions or deletions (Figure 1). Any of these variants could be acting by altering the splicing process and thus change the translated product, whereas missense and in-frame rearrangements can alter the protein with unchanged splicing. When relevant, the two types of alterations have to be assessed, i.e. missense variants should be checked for mis-splicing.

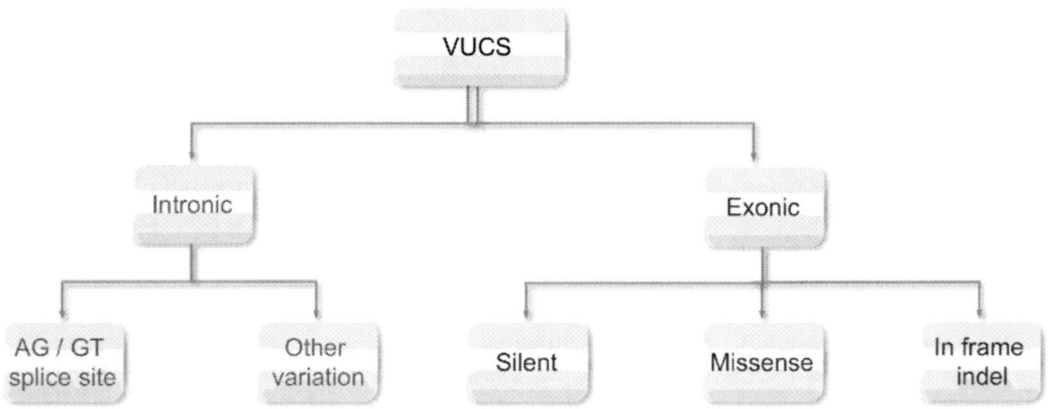

Figure 1. Definition of the VUCS.

Range of Clinical and Genetic Heterogeneity of Usher Syndrome

The three clinical types of Usher syndrome are defined and distinguished mainly based on the degree of hearing loss (HL) and the presence or not of a damaged vestibular function. HL is congenital, profound in type I, mild to severe with a down-sloping audiometric configuration in type 2 and progressive in the type 3. Retinitis pigmentosa (RP) will develop in the three subtypes, and onset of the night blindness, the first visual symptom can be noted before the age of 10 [2].

As shown in Table 1, five genes are known to cause USH1: *MYO7A*, *CDH23*, *PCDH15*, *USHIC* and *USH1G*. Three genes are involved in USH2: *USH2A*, *GPR98* and *DFNB31*. Only one gene has been cloned for USH3: *CLRN-1* [2]. Recently, the *PDZD7* gene has been involved as a modifier of the retinal phenotype on a *USH2A* background and a contributor for digenism together with *GPR98* [3].

Table 1. Usher syndrome molecular references

Gene/ USH Locus	Protein	OMIM	NCBI RefSeq ID	Exons[$]	NS form
Usher type I		#276900			
MYO7A / USH1B	Myosin VIIa	*276903	4647	49	DFNA11 DFNB2
USH1C / USH1C	Hamonin	*605242	10083	27	DFNB18
CDH23 / USH1D	Cadherin 23	*605516	64072	69	DFNB12
PCDH15 / USH1F	Protocadherin 15	*605514	65217	35	DFNB23
USH1G / USH1G	Sans	*607696	124590	3	
Usher type II		#276901			
USH2A / USH2A	Usherin	*608400	7399	72	RP39
GPR98 / USH2C	G-coupled receptor 98	*602851	84059	90	FEB4
DFNB31 / USH2D	Whirlin	*607696	25861	12	DFNB31
Usher type III		#276902			
CLRN-1 / USH3A	Clarin-1	*606397	7401	3	RP61
Digenism / Modifier					
PDZD7 / -	PDZ Domain containing 7	*612971	79955	16	

[$] Refers to the number of exons classically analysed.

Atypical Genotype/phenotype Relationships and Atypical Usher

The three clinical types accurately describe the majority of the molecular diagnosed cases (Figure 2) [4]. However, several cases have been described with unusual genotype/phenotype relationships. Astuto et al., presented USH1 patients with unusual retinal phenotypes (mild and late onset RP) linked to mutations in *CDH23* (e.g. p.(Arg1746Gln)) [5]. Garcia-Garcia et al., recently reported one case carrying two pathogenic mutations in *USH2A* but presenting with profound deafness, vestibular dysfunction and early onset of RP [6]. Kalay et al., described two consanguineous Turkish families with atypical clinical features related to a Usher type II phenotype and who carried a homozygous missense mutation in *USH1G* [7].

More recently, Bashir et al., reported a consanguineous family who presented with a typical USH2 phenotype carrying a homozygous single nucleotide deletion in *USH1G*, that was further shown to abolish the natural donor splice site of exon 1 [8]. The two latter descriptions support the fact that some *USH1G* alleles cause USH2. Thus, as shown in Figure 2, some mutations appearing in genes of a given type can be responsible for another phenotype. Patients presenting these discrepancies should be labelled (as often done) as Atypical Usher in the sense of atypical genotype/phenotype relationships.

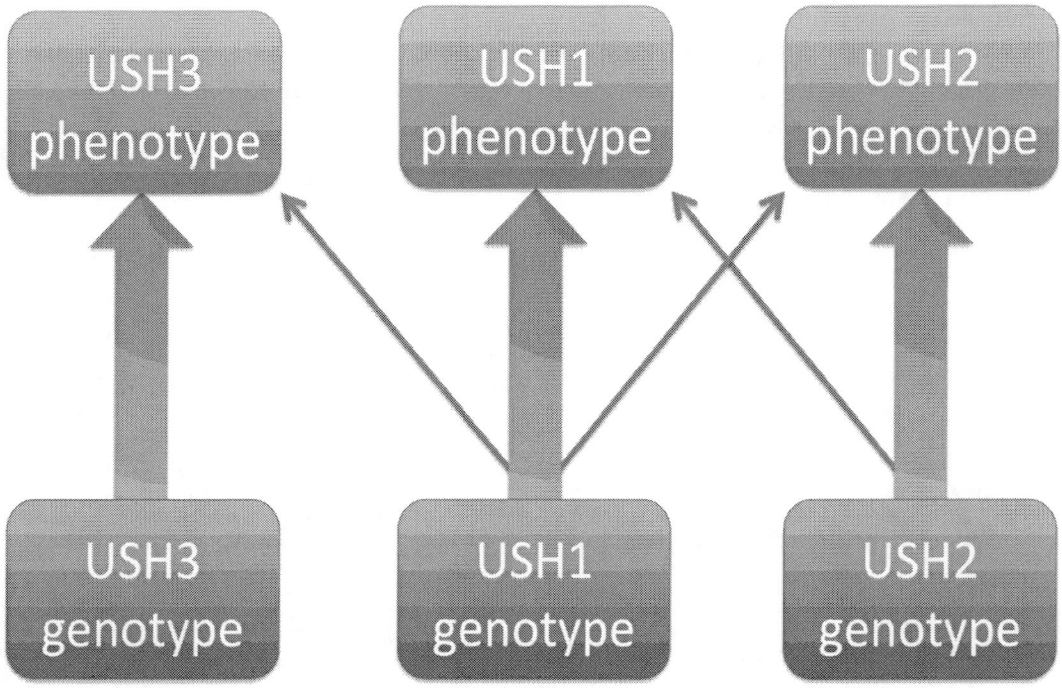

Figure 2. Genotype/ phenotype relationships.

Molecular Diagnosis/prevalence of the Usher Genes

It is not possible, at this date, to predict, within a clinical type which of the potential responsible genes is mutated. A recent audiological study of a 100 Usher type 2 patients genotyped in *USH2A*, *GPR98* and *DFNB31*, found no evidence of any statistical differences in the degree or configuration of the HL, although a trend towards more severe HL was noted in *GPR98* patients [9].

The most robust way to carry out molecular diagnosis of Usher is sequencing (but, as discussed below, this is not sufficient in some cases) because i) there are few founder mutations (such as *USH2A* c.2299delG [10, 11]), ii) the frequency of private mutations is high, iii) the high proportion of neutral variants identified in the USH genes that makes the scanning methods based on formation of heteroduplexes laborious and inefficient.

Two large recent studies involving USH1 patients from France [12] and UK [4], n=90 and n=47, respectively, give the most accurate prevalence of each USH1 gene in mixed populations with some slight differences (Table 2). Although *MYO7A* is the most frequently involved gene in USH1 with more than 50 % of the cases some discrepancy are observed for *CDH23* and for *USH1C* which represents the 2nd most common gene in USH1 patients from UK.

Concerning USH2 (Table 3), *USH2A* is the gene involved in at least 75% of cases overall Europe [4, 6, 13, 14]. *GPR98* is quite rarely involved, and this result raises the question of the relevance of the Sanger analysis of such a huge gene (18kb of coding sequence). *DFNB31* seems definitely rare as a gene responsible for Usher syndrome [4, 14].

Table 2. Prevalence of each USH1 gene in two USH1 cohorts from France (n=90) and UK (n=47)

	MYO7A	*CDH23*	*PCDH15*	*USH1C*	*USH1G*	Overall mutation detection rate
France	63.3	20	12.2	4.5	0	>90
UK	53.2	10.6	8.5	14.9	0	78.7

Table 3. Prevalence of each USH2 gene in four USH2 cohorts from Scandinavia (n=118), Spain (n=88), UK (n=121) and France (n=176)

	USH2A	*GPR98*	*DFNB31*	Overall mutation detection rate
Scandinavia	75.4	?	?	75.4
Spain	76.1	?	?	76.1
UK	79.3	6.6	0.0?	85.9
France	82.3	6.4	1.3	90

DIGENISM

Digenic inheritance of Usher syndrome has been discussed in numerous studies [3, 15, 16]. In only one case, has digenism been reported with proven deleterious mutations in two different genes (*GPR98* and *PDZD7* [3]). The highly polymorphic nature of each of the USH genes is well recorded by entries in the USHbases where 2000 variants are recorded (including the limited access section) and in the recent study of Le Quesne Stabej et al., [4]. It will, therefore, be common that missense variants will be found in more than one gene and this is where proper classification of VUCS is crucial. In fact, possible digenic cases are rare but should be seriously considered only after comprehensive study of the genes which must include sequencing of all the exons and flanking intronic sequences, study of large rearrangements (4 % of the pathogenic alleles in our cohort), and study of RNA that provides evidence of deep intronic mutations [17]. Next Generation Sequencing, which is rapidly being adopted, will also identify more VUCS than already identified and this is again where proper and extensive classification of VUCS is crucial.

That alterations identified in additional genes in a single patient could modify the phenotype is not impossible and oligogenism has been suggested in several patients, with alleles in second locus acting as modifier of the USH phenotype [3, 12, 16, 18].

CLASSIFICATION OF VARIANTS

Premature Termination Codons (PTCs)

In Usher syndrome, variants predicted to lead to PTCs are considered "a priori" to be pathogenic, and thus, not considered to be VUCS. However, it has been demonstrated in several diseases, including Usher syndrome type II, that such variations can lead to splicing alterations [19]. One can easily imagine, as shown for example in *DMD* gene [20] a nucleotide substitution predicted to lead to a PTC, but actually modifying the normal splicing pattern of the exon through disruption of an exon splice enhancer, and ultimately leading to in frame exon skipping, whose effect is hard to predict. As the spectrum of mutations in Usher genes is so wide, with a majority of private deleterious variations, not all published mutations have been analysed for this possibility, but a quick *in silico* assessment of all predicted PTC variants for their ability to alter splicing should strongly reduce this risk.

One should also keep in mind that a PTC has been described as a neutral polymorphism in *BRCA2* [21]. This variant occurring in a cancer susceptibility gene, and predicted to remove 93 amino acids from the protein, was identified with a similar frequency in both control and breast cancer populations, and was also found allelic to another variant leading to a PTC.

Variations Occurring in Regulatory Regions

To our knowledge, no variation has been described as responsible for Usher syndrome in regulatory regions such as promoters or 3'UTRs (UnTranslated Regions). However, it has been described in other pathologies, and given the number of incomplete genotypes, this is a possibility one should consider. Assessment of such variants is difficult, but should involve *in silico* tools [22-24] as well as validation with *in vitro* methods [25].

Variations at -2, -1, +1 and +2 Positions

Although an effect on RNA splicing is expected when a variation occurs at the canonical acceptor or donor splice sites AG/GT dinucleotides, the pathogenicity of this type of variant cannot be clearly established a priori especially when the open reading frame would be conserved. As a consequence, these variants usually classified as deleterious are considered as VUCS in our methodology, as shown in Figure 1, and are considered as likely to alter splicing in absence of further evidence.

VUCS in Usher Syndrome

In the context of the molecular diagnosis of Usher syndrome, it is important to design and follow a clear methodology in order to assess VUCS properly. LOVD-USHbases, a dedicated database compiling published data on the nine Usher causing genes, contains more than 800 different variants considered to have more or less uncertain pathogenic effects (including private set). In our cohort, all genes combined, we have currently encountered 1094 different variants (unpublished data). Of these, 517 (47.3%) have been classified as neutral and 214 as pathogenic (19.6%). Therefore, VUCS represent 363 unique variants, which is 33.2% and means that one unique variant out of three in Usher syndrome is a VUCS, at least in France. Each new molecular study describes new VUCS. Unfortunately, VUCS are not always assessed for pathogenicity, or, if so, there is no systematic methodology that could be used by all groups. This chapter describes a methodology, especially designed for Usher syndrome but which can be extended to similar issues, or adapted when needed.

Definition of the Classes

Our system relies on "the practice guidelines for the interpretation and reporting of unclassified variants in clinical molecular genetics", published in 2007 by the Clinical and Medical Genetics Society (CMGS), and defines 4 classes of VUCS:

Class I: certainly not pathogenic
Class II: likely not pathogenic
Class III: likely pathogenic
Class IV: certainly pathogenic

Two additional classes are Neutral and Pathogenic for well-known variants or variants leading to PTCs.

Alteration of the Splicing Process

All types of VUCS are susceptible to lead to an alteration of the splicing process; as a result all should be screened for their potential effect on splicing. As studies at RNA level cannot reasonably be carried out for each variant, predictions for splicing alterations are mandatory. Basic assessment should include destruction of natural splice sites, creation of new sites, alternative use of a natural site and branch point alterations. Unfortunately, available tools are not accurate enough to assess the pathogenicity of a modified ESE pattern. Useful *in vitro* tools have been described for Usher syndrome [19, 26-28] and when possible the effect of variants predicted to affect splicing should be confirmed at RNA level (minigenes or RNA samples).

Table 4. Decision table for potential splicing variants. The name "databases" mainly refers to dbSNP, 1000 genomes or the Exome Variant Server. *Not found in databases also means no frequency data. MAF: Minor Allele Frequency

Observation	Classification
Presence in databases and significant frequency (ex: MAF > 0.02) and negative *in silico* prediction	Neutral
Presence in databases and negative *in silico* prediction	Class I
No frequency data and negative *in silico* prediction	Class II
Positive *in silico* prediction and not found in databases*	Class III
Minigene shows alteration of splicing	Class IV
mRNA altered (nasal epithelial cells)	Pathogenic

The overall prediction should combine: the frequency of the variant in control populations matched for ethnicity when necessary (i.e. absence of the variant), *in silico* predictions obtained with at least two distinct methods and *in vitro* assays [19] (Table 4). Frequencies can be checked in general databases such as dbSNP, 1000 genomes or the Exome Variant Server.

Missense Variants not Affecting Splicing

Direct testing *in vitro* for the consequences of missense variants in Usher genes is rarely possible, and only a few studies have been published. The problem is compounded by the relatively poor understanding of the function of most of the Usher proteins and their component domains. Battacharya et al., have shown that usherin and collagen IV interact and have tested this interaction using a number of missense variants located in the identified domains of interaction (LE domains) [29]. They showed *in vitro* that p.(Gly713Arg), a variant described as pathogenic in 2000 [30], would disrupt this interaction, which would explain its pathogenic effect. However, Najera et al., have identified this variant with a significant frequency in a cohort of control Spanish patients (0.02), [31]. Moreover, this variant was found allelic to a splicing alteration [27] or a mutation predicting a PTC (unpublished data) and its allelic frequency in controls was established to 7/184 = 0.04 (unpublished data). Finally, Dreyer et al., who originally characterized the mutation, considered it as "benign" in a more recent work [13]. Therefore, if functional tests are conducted for variants in Usher genes, they must be part of an integrated approach, i.e. results must be combined with other observations or predictions and in any case are not practicable in a diagnostic context.

The following method focuses on two main approaches, a conventional part including literature analysis, molecular epidemiology and familial segregation of the variant, and a second part, namely *in silico* analysis, dealing with conservation throughout evolution of amino-acids, in similar proteins and domains, based on the theory that a stable amino acid through time is likely to be deleterious if replaced (functional constraint), and also including 3D molecular predictions.

Basic Methodology

Six criteria should be considered. Each criteria is rated a number with a numerator (a) and denominator (b) using empirical rules, as shown in Table 5. Scores can be either negative if the criteria is against pathogenicity, or positive, or even neutral if the information is not sufficient. Criteria considered as strongly informative with regard to pathogenicity (i.e. the position in cis or trans of a deleterious mutation) can be strongly positive (e.g. rate 2/2 for a variant described in trans of a PTC) or negative (e.g. -2/2 for a variant described in cis of a PTC), whereas some other criteria, either less informative or resulting from a mostly predictive (i.e. 3D modelling) method will be assigned moderate rates (basically from -1/1 to 1/1). Each rate is finally summed and the final score gives a number A/B ($A/B = \sum a/\sum b$), which directly allows the decision (Table 6).

Table 5. Possible rates of each item used to assess the pathogenic potential of missense VUCS. NA : Non Available (i.e. the residue does not belong to a defined domain, or is not present in the alignment); (+), (++) and (–) signs refer to each criteria paragraph, basically (+) and (++) mean strong conservation for alignments and strong prediction for 3D, while (–) means poor conservation for alignments and poor prediction for 3D

Subtotal (a/b) / Criteria	-2/2	-1/1	0/0	0/1	0/2	1/1	1/2	2/2
Literature			Not described	As non pathogenic (same aa position)	As non pathogenic		As pathogenic (same aa position)	As pathogenic
Allelic position	In cis (patho-genic variant)		Unknown	2 pathogenic in other USH gene	In cis (Class III-IV)		In trans (Class III-IV) - homozygote	In trans (pathogenic variant)
Control DNAs		> 0		Not tested		0		
Orthologous conservation					(-)		(+)	(++)
Domain conservation					(-) or NA		(+)	(++)
3D predictions			NA	(-)		(+)		

Biological Observations

Three criteria are considered to be biological criteria and are listed below.

Presence in Literature

Firstly, databases (LOVD-USHbases or equivalent) and literature are analysed in order to determine whether the variant has previously been described, and, if so, in which conditions and how it has been considered in the publication(s). A variant already described as pathogenic will be rated 2/2, whereas a variant described as non pathogenic will be penalized.

Allelic Position

In recessive diseases, the situation of the other allele considerably affects the argument in favour or against pathogenicity. The range of scores is large, depending on the classification of a second mutation either in cis or in trans, rates being different whether the second mutation is a proven deleterious variant or a VUCS itself.

Control DNAs

Control DNA is considered a less significant criteria, as frequent pathogenic mutations (e.g. c.2299delG or p.(Cys759Phe), in *USH2A*) can be found at relatively high (> 0.01) frequencies in controls. In particular, VUCS are often rare variants, and rarely found in controls, so the failure to find them in controls is very much less convincing (false negative) than finding them frequently. Therefore this category is not considered as strongly as the previous two.

In Silico Predictions

Three different *in silico* approaches are used. All these assessments can be performed using Usher Syndrome Missense Analysis (USMA), the web based tool we have developed to achieve this specific goal. Standard scores given by Pathogenic-or-Not-Predictors (PONPs, software that predicts pathogenicity for missense variants) are not combined as most of them are based on the same criteria, i.e. orthologous conservation. However, alternatively, these three criteria can be replaced by a combination of the output of different PONPs, e.g. SIFT [32], Polyphen 2 [33] and MAPP [34] or Align GVGD [35]. But "manual" assessment, rather than the automation involved in applying the programs, of protein multiple sequence alignments (PMSA) has several advantages. First of all, errors in alignments are more easily detected and the PMSA can be corrected accordingly. Visualizing the alignment is important to incorporate the amino acids surrounding the residue of interest. A strongly conserved region can denote a potential active site or a particular region, which could be missed by PONPs. Two types of alignments are assessed in this method: classical orthologous alignments and domain alignments.

Orthologous Alignments

Basic assessments and rates are shown in table 5. Orthologous alignments should include as many species as available. Several groups should be present, representing several evolutionary distances from *Homo sapiens*, including monkeys, some other mammals, birds/lizards, and fish/insects/others. In other words, the depth of the alignment is crucial [36].

Orthologue alignments can be assessed using the following rules:

(-) poor conservation (<50%) of the wild-type residue or conservation >50% and occurrence of the mutant residue

(+) conservation >50% and conservation of a common property (size, charge, polarity) in other residues or no occurrence of mutant residue

(++)invariant position (even better if localized in a strongly conserved region)

Domain Alignments

Most of the identified domains in Usher proteins can be studied in the light of independent domain evolution, i.e. similar domains can be aligned to highlight crucial conserved residues. These alignments can also contain repetitions of the domain of interest within the same protein (i.e. cadherin repeats in cadherin 23 or protocadherin 15, fibronectin type III domains in usherin…). Pre-computed alignments of domains present in Usher proteins can be downloaded from Prosite or Pfam. These alignments can contain hundreds of sequences in which case interpretation slightly differs from orthologue alignments.

Domain alignments can be assessed using the following rules:

(-) poor conservation (<25%)

(+) conservation >25% and conservation of a common property (size, charge, polarity) in other residues or no significant occurrence of mutant residue (<5%)

(++)conservation >50%

3D Predictions

Some structures of a portion of Usher proteins have been elucidated, using either crystallography [37-39] or Nuclear Magnetic Resonance (Protein Data Bank IDs 1UEZ, 1UF1, 1UFX for whirlin structures). Moreover, the structure of a significant part of these proteins can be predicted using classical homology modelling. This has been done by several groups [7, 29, 40, 41] and can provide useful clues in terms of determining a molecular mechanism for pathogenicity.

3D models can be assessed using the following rules:

(-) no particular role or minor role identified for wild-type residue and no alteration of the region resulting from the introduction of the mutant residue.

(+) identified role of wild type residue altered by mutant residue, or probable disruption of the region by introduction of the mutant residue (e.g. introduction of a large polar residue in an hydrophobic pocket).

Several authors have extensively described the different alterations likely to destabilize a peptide structure [42, 43].

Table 6. Decision table for missense VUCS A/B = $\sum a/\sum b$

Class	Effect	Decision thresholds
I	Certainly benign	$A/B < 0.25$
II	Likely benign	$0.25 < A/B < 0.5$
III	Likely pathogenic	$0.5 < A/B < 0.75$ OR ($0.5 < A/B$ AND $B < 8$)
IV	Certainly pathogenic	$0.75 < A/B$ AND $B >= 8$

Final Assessment

The sum of the scores obtained for each criteria is made, giving a result in the form of a ratio A/B (putatively negative). Table 6 describes the assignment that can be used using this ration.

The global work flow to classify VUCS in Usher syndrome has been recently published in Roux et al., [12]. First, each variant is clearly identified as a type of VUCS (intronic, exonic…) as the different steps will differ between missense variants and the others. It should also be noted that *in vitro* testing of splicing, either directly on RNA samples or using minigene constructs are conducted only when an effect is expected. This multi-step analysis has been applied on more than 350 different DNA variations, and lead to the classification of more than 120 as likely/certainly pathogenic. Finally, such classifications are susceptible to evolve with time with acquisition of new data (e.g. the arrival of new familial samples), and although quite rarely (3/363, <0.01) a variant can change of pathogenic class (i.e. Class II to III or vice versa). It is important to note, that close specific analysis should be applied to each variant and routine automated analysis is likely to be superficial and probably often misleading.

Conclusion

This chapter has shown the importance of using a validated approach to assess VUCS in Usher syndrome. The method combines several types of criteria chosen in order to be complementary and as little redundant as possible. The criteria can be classified into two major categories, namely biological observations and *in silico* predictions. Once the criteria are analysed, a simple score is established which allows the classification into 4 classes from the least likely to be pathogenic to the most. This methodology can easily be used in other recessive disorders, and adapted to all types of assessment of genetic variants in human diseases.

Cited URLs

LOVD-USHbases: https://grenada.lumc.nl/LOVD2/Usher_montpellier/
CMGS guidelines for VUCS: http://www.cmgs.org/BPGs/Best_Practice_ Guidelines.htm
dbSNP: http://www.ncbi.nlm.nih.gov/projects/SNP/
1000 genomes: http://www.1000genomes.org/
Exome Variant Server: http://evs.gs.washington.edu/EVS/
USMA: https://neuro-2.montp.inserm.fr/USMA/
Prosite: http://prosite.expasy.org/
Pfam: http://pfam.sanger.ac.uk/

References

[1] Kimberling WJ, Hildebrand MS, Shearer AE, Jensen ML, Halder JA, Trzupek K, Cohn ES, Weleber RG, Stone EM, Smith RJ: Frequency of Usher syndrome in two pediatric populations: Implications for genetic screening of deaf and hard of hearing children. *Genet Med* 2010, 12(8):512-516.

[2] Saihan Z, Webster AR, Luxon L, Bitner-Glindzicz M: Update on Usher syndrome. *Curr Opin Neurol* 2009, 22(1):19-27.

[3] Ebermann I, Phillips JB, Liebau MC, Koenekoop RK, Schermer B, Lopez I, Schafer E, Roux AF, Dafinger C, Bernd A *et al*: PDZD7 is a modifier of retinal disease and a contributor to digenic Usher syndrome. *J Clin Invest* 2010, 120(6):1812-1823.

[4] Le Quesne Stabej P, Saihan Z, Rangesh N, Steele-Stallard HB, Ambrose J, Coffey A, Emmerson J, Haralambous E, Hughes Y, Steel KP *et al*: Comprehensive sequence analysis of nine Usher syndrome genes in the UK National Collaborative Usher Study. *Journal of medical genetics* 2012, 49(1):27-36.

[5] Astuto LM, Bork JM, Weston MD, Askew JW, Fields RR, Orten DJ, Ohliger SJ, Riazuddin S, Morell RJ, Khan S *et al*: CDH23 mutation and phenotype heterogeneity: a profile of 107 diverse families with Usher syndrome and nonsyndromic deafness. *Am J Hum Genet* 2002, 71(2):262-275.

[6] Garcia-Garcia G, Aparisi MJ, Jaijo T, Rodrigo R, Leon AM, Avila-Fernandez A, Blanco-Kelly F, Bernal S, Navarro R, Diaz-Llopis M *et al*: Mutational screening of the USH2A gene in Spanish USH patients reveals 23 novel pathogenic mutations. *Orphanet J Rare Dis* 2011, 6:65.

[7] Kalay E, de Brouwer AP, Caylan R, Nabuurs SB, Wollnik B, Karaguzel A, Heister JG, Erdol H, Cremers FP, Cremers CW *et al*: A novel D458V mutation in the SANS PDZ binding motif causes atypical Usher syndrome. *J Mol Med* 2005, 83(12):1025-1032.

[8] Bashir R, Fatima A, Naz S: A frameshift mutation in SANS results in atypical Usher syndrome. *Clinical genetics* 2010, 78(6):601-603.

[9] Abadie C, Blanchet C, Baux D, Larrieu L, Besnard T, Ravel P, Biboulet R, Hamel C, Malcolm S, Mondain M *et al*: Audiological findings in 100 USH2 patients. *Clinical genetics* 2011.

[10] Dreyer B, Tranebjaerg L, Brox V, Rosenberg T, Moller C, Beneyto M, Weston MD, Kimberling WJ, Cremers CW, Liu XZ *et al*: A common ancestral origin of the frequent and widespread 2299delG USH2A mutation. *Am J Hum Genet* 2001, 69(1):228-234.

[11] Aller E, Larrieu L, Jaijo T, Baux D, Espinos C, Gonzalez-Candelas F, Najera C, Palau F, Claustres M, Roux AF *et al*: The USH2A c.2299delG mutation: dating its common origin in a Southern European population. *Eur J Hum Genet* 2010, 18(7):788-793.

[12] Roux AF, Faugere V, Vache C, Baux D, Besnard T, Leonard S, Blanchet C, Hamel C, Mondain M, Gilbert-Dussardier B *et al*: Four year follow-up of diagnostic service in USH1 patients. *Invest Ophthalmol Vis Sci* 2011, 52(7):4063-4071.

[13] Dreyer B, Brox V, Tranebjaerg L, Rosenberg T, Sadeghi AM, Moller C, Nilssen O: Spectrum of USH2A mutations in Scandinavian patients with Usher syndrome type II. *Hum Mutat* 2008, 29(3):451.

[14] Besnard T, Vache C, Baux D, Larrieu L, Abadie C, Blanchet C, Odent S, Blanchet P, Calvas P, Hamel C *et al*: Non-USH2A Mutations in USH2 Patients. *Human mutation* 2012, 33(3):504-510.

[15] Zheng QY, Yan D, Ouyang XM, Du LL, Yu H, Chang B, Johnson KR, Liu XZ: Digenic inheritance of deafness caused by mutations in the genes encoding cadherin 23 and protocadherin 15 in mice and humans. *Hum Mol Genet* 2005, 14:103-111.

[16] Bonnet C, Grati M, Marlin S, Levilliers J, Hardelin JP, Parodi M, Niasme-Grare M, Zelenika D, Delepine M, Feldmann D *et al*: Complete exon sequencing of all known

Usher syndrome genes greatly improves molecular diagnosis. *Orphanet J Rare Dis* 2011, 6(1):21.

[17] Vaché C, Besnard T, le Berre P, Garcia-Garcia G, Baux D, Larrieu L, Abadie C, Blanchet C, Bolz HJ, Millan J *et al*: Usher syndrome type 2 caused by activation of an USH2A pseudoexon: Implications for diagnosis and therapy. *Human mutation* 2012, 33(1):104-108.

[18] Adato A, Kalinski H, Weil D, Chaib H, Korostishevsky M, Bonne-Tamir B: Possible interaction between USH1B and USH3 gene products as implied by apparent digenic deafness inheritance [letter]. *Am J Hum Genet* 1999, 65(1):261-265.

[19] Vaché C, Besnard T, Blanchet C, Baux D, Larrieu L, Faugère V, Mondain M, Hamel C, Malcolm S, Claustres M *et al*: Nasal epithelial cells are a reliable source to study splicing variants in Usher syndrome. *Hum Mutat* 2010, 31(6):734-741.

[20] Flanigan KM, Dunn DM, von Niederhausern A, Soltanzadeh P, Howard MT, Sampson JB, Swoboda KJ, Bromberg MB, Mendell JR, Taylor LE *et al*: Nonsense mutation-associated Becker muscular dystrophy: interplay between exon definition and splicing regulatory elements within the DMD gene. *Human mutation* 2011, 32(3):299-308.

[21] Mazoyer S, Dunning AM, Serova O, Dearden J, Puget N, Healey CS, Gayther SA, Mangion J, Stratton MR, Lynch HT *et al*: A polymorphic stop codon in BRCA2. *Nature genetics* 1996, 14(3):253-254.

[22] Sandelin A, Wasserman WW, Lenhard B: ConSite: web-based prediction of regulatory elements using cross-species comparison. *Nucleic acids research* 2004, 32(Web Server issue):W249-252.

[23] Schug J: Using TESS to predict transcription factor binding sites in DNA sequence. *Curr Protoc Bioinformatics* 2008, Chapter 2:Unit 2 6.

[24] Lewis BP, Burge CB, Bartel DP: Conserved seed pairing, often flanked by adenosines, indicates that thousands of human genes are microRNA targets. *Cell* 2005, 120(1):15-20.

[25] Lopez E, Viart V, Guittard C, Templin C, Rene C, Mechin D, Des Georges M, Claustres M, Romey-Chatelain MC, Taulan M: Variants in CFTR untranslated regions are associated with congenital bilateral absence of the vas deferens. *Journal of Medical Genetics* 2011, 48(3):152-159.

[26] von Brederlow B, Bolz H, Janecke A, La OCA, Rudolph G, Lorenz B, Schwinger E, Gal A: Identification and in vitro expression of novel CDH23 mutations of patients with Usher syndrome type 1D. *Hum Mutat* 2002, 19(3):268-273.

[27] Le Guédard-Mereuze S, Vaché C, Baux D, Faugère V, Larrieu L, Abadie C, Janecke A, Claustres M, Roux AF, Tuffery-Giraud S: Ex vivo splicing assays of mutations at non-canonical positions of splice sites in USHER genes. *Hum Mutat* 2010, 31:347-355.

[28] Nakanishi H, Ohtsubo M, Iwasaki S, Hotta Y, Mizuta K, Mineta H, Minoshima S: Hair roots as an mRNA source for mutation analysis of Usher syndrome-causing genes. *J Hum Genet* 2010, 55(10):701-703.

[29] Bhattacharya G, Kalluri R, Orten DJ, Kimberling WJ, Cosgrove D: A domain-specific usherin/collagen IV interaction may be required for stable integration into the basement membrane superstructure. *Journal of cell science* 2004, 117(Pt 2):233-242.

[30] Dreyer B, Tranebjaerg L, Rosenberg T, Weston MD, Kimberling WJ, Nilssen O: Identification of novel USH2A mutations: implications for the structure of USH2A protein. *Eur J Hum Genet* 2000, 8(7):500-506.

[31] Najera C, Beneyto M, Blanca J, Aller E, Fontcuberta A, Millan JM, Ayuso C: Mutations in myosin VIIA (MYO7A) and usherin (USH2A) in Spanish patients with Usher syndrome types I and II, respectively. *Hum Mutat* 2002, 20(1):76-77.

[32] Kumar P, Henikoff S, Ng PC: Predicting the effects of coding non-synonymous variants on protein function using the SIFT algorithm. *Nat Protoc* 2009, 4(7):1073-1081.

[33] Adzhubei IA, Schmidt S, Peshkin L, Ramensky VE, Gerasimova A, Bork P, Kondrashov AS, Sunyaev SR: A method and server for predicting damaging missense mutations. *Nat Methods* 2010, 7(4):248-249.

[34] Stone EA, Sidow A: Physicochemical constraint violation by missense substitutions mediates impairment of protein function and disease severity. *Genome research* 2005, 15(7):978-986.

[35] Tavtigian SV, Deffenbaugh AM, Yin L, Judkins T, Scholl T, Samollow PB, de Silva D, Zharkikh A, Thomas A: Comprehensive statistical study of 452 BRCA1 missense substitutions with classification of eight recurrent substitutions as neutral. *Journal of Medical Genetics* 2005, 43:295-305.

[36] Tavtigian SV, Greenblatt MS, Lesueur F, Byrnes GB: In silico analysis of missense substitutions using sequence-alignment based methods. *Human mutation* 2008, 29(11):1327-1336.

[37] Elledge HM, Kazmierczak P, Clark P, Joseph JS, Kolatkar A, Kuhn P, Muller U: Structure of the N terminus of cadherin 23 reveals a new adhesion mechanism for a subset of cadherin superfamily members. *Proceedings of the National Academy of Sciences of the United States of America* 2010, 107(23):10708-10712.

[38] Yan J, Pan L, Chen X, Wu L, Zhang M: The structure of the harmonin/sans complex reveals an unexpected interaction mode of the two Usher syndrome proteins. *Proceedings of the National Academy of Sciences of the United States of America* 2010, 107(9):4040-4045.

[39] Wu L, Pan L, Wei Z, Zhang M: Structure of MyTH4-FERM domains in myosin VIIa tail bound to cargo. *Science* 2011, 331(6018):757-760.

[40] Baux D, Larrieu L, Blanchet C, Hamel C, Ben Salah S, Vielle A, Gilbert-Dussardier B, Holder M, Calvas P, Philip N *et al*: Molecular and in silico analyses of the full-length isoform of usherin identify new pathogenic alleles in Usher type II patients. *Hum Mutat* 2007, 28(8):781-789.

[41] Watanabe S, Umeki N, Ikebe R, Ikebe M: Impacts of Usher syndrome type IB mutations on human myosin VIIa motor function. *Biochemistry* 2008, 47(36):9505-9513.

[42] Villoutreix BO: Structural bioinformatics: methods, concepts and applications to blood coagulation proteins. *Curr Protein Pept Sci* 2002, 3(3):341-364.

[43] Thusberg J, Vihinen M: Pathogenic or not? And if so, then how? Studying the effects of missense mutations using bioinformatics methods. *Hum Mutat* 2009, 30(5):703-714.

In: Inner Ear Development and Hearing Loss
Editors: Saima Riazuddin and Zubair Ahmed
ISBN: 978-1-62417-011-9

Chapter 11

MOLECULAR GENETIC STUDIES ON THE *GJB2* GENE IN THE KOREAN POPULATION

***Soo-Young Choi*[1], *Kyu Yup Lee*[2] *and Un-Kyung Kim*[1,*]**
[1]Department of Biology, College of Natural Sciences,
Kyungpook National University,
Daegu, Korea
[2]Department of Otolaryngology, College of Medicine,
Kyungpook National University, Daegu, Korea

ABSTRACT

Gap junction beta 2 (*GJB2*) gene, encoding the connexin26 (Cx26) protein, is one of the main causative genes of nonsyndromic hearing loss (HL) in many populations, and a number of different mutations in the *GJB2* gene has been reported from diverse ethnic groups. The *GJB2* gene has been analyzed for the spectrum and prevalence of the mutations from 324 subjects with nonsyndromic HL in the Korean population. A total of nine different mutations were found in 28 unrelated patients (8.6%). In addition, four previously reported as polymorphisms, p.V27I, p.E114G, p.T123N, and p.I203T, were found in patients and controls. The c.235delC was the most prevalent mutation which accounts for 61.5% of all pathogenic mutant alleles in the Korean NSHI population with a total of 24 alleles. This study further supports the view that mutations in the *GJB2* gene are a less common cause of hearing loss in East Asian populations when compared to Caucasian populations.

INTRODUCTION

Gap junctions (GJs) are a specialized intercellular connection mediating direct cell-to-cell communication and tissue homeostasis, which allow small molecules with molecular weights of below 1 kDa and inorganic ion to pass between adjacent cells by nonspecific and passive

---

[*] E-mail address: kimuk@knu.ac.kr

diffusion [1]. A complete GJ channel consists of two hemichannels, which are also called connexins. Each hemichannel is comprised of six connexin (Cx) subunits [2], which all share a common topology consisting of four transmembrane domains (TM1-TM4), two extracellular loops (EC1 and EC2), a single intracellular loop (IC), and cytoplasmic amino- and carboxy-terminal domains. GJs assembled from the same Cxs are called homomeric GJs, while GJs assembled from different Cx subtypes form heteromeric hemichannels and hybrid GJs [3]. The exact biochemical assembly of mixed types of compatible Cxs determines the specific permeability of the GJ channels [4].

Mutations in Cx genes are associated with human disorders, mostly hearing loss and skin diseases [5-6]. Mutations in three Cx genes, Cx26 (MIM# 1221011), Cx30 (MIM# 604418), and Cx31 (MIM# 603324), are associated with hearing loss. Cx26 and Cx30 are expressed in the fibrocytes of the spiral ligament and spiral limbus, basal cells of stria vascularis, and all types of supporting cells in the organ of Corti. These proteins have been suggested to play an important role in the recycling of the K^+ ion between the endolymph and perilymph [7].

GJB2 Gene

The *Gap junction protein beta2* (*GJB2*) gene encodes a gap junction protein connexin 26, and is one of the most common causes of nonsyndromic hearing loss in humans. Mutations in the gene encoding Cx26 (*GJB2*) are the most common cause of non-syndromic autosomal recessive hearing loss in humans [8]. A number of *GJB2* mutations have also been associated with autosomal dominant hearing loss (Connexin Deafness Homepage: http://davinci.crg.es /deafness/). The spectrum and prevalence of the mutations and polymorphisms in *GJB2* gene vary significantly among different ethnic groups. The most frequent pathogenic mutations, c.35delG and c.167delT, account for 70% and 40% of *GJB2*-related HL in Caucasians and Ashkenazi Jews, respectively [9-12]. In contrast, East Asian HL patients rarely display these mutations, however, another single base pair deletion, c.235delC, is present [13]. In addition to these mutations, more than 150 different variants have been reported in the *GJB2* gene (http://davinci.crg.es/deafness/). These variants were predicted to be pathogenic since the mutations were only found in patients and the residues were highly conserved among different species. The effects of these mutations on Cx26 function have been shown to be different depending on the position and type of amino acid substitution. Furthermore, the same mutation can cause different phenotypes in different individuals. For example, a p.V37I mutation in Cx26 causes various phenotypes from mild to severe hearing loss.

We performed in molecular analysis of the entire *GJB2* gene, including non-coding exon 1 from 324 unrelated patients with nonsyndromic hearing loss (NSHL) in the Korean population. Nine different mutations were identified in the coding region (Table 1). Among the variations, 8 types (p.V37I, p.G45E, p.E47K, c.176-191del16, c.235delC, p.T86R, p.R143W, and p.S199F) were identified and 1 novel mutation, p.D46E, was observed in a highly conserved region of the *GJB2* gene [14-21].

Table 1. The frequency of *GJB2* mutations detected in Koreans

Codon location	Nucleotide change	Heterozygous individuals (N)		Homozygous individuals (N)		Allele Frequency (%)		Type of mutation	Protein domain	References
		Controls (N=110)	Patients (N=324)	Controls (N=110)	Patients (N=324)	Controls (n=220)	Patients (n=648)			
p.V37I	c.109G>A	-	4	-	-	0	0.6	Missense	TM1	[14]
p.G45E	c.134G>A	-	1	-	-	0	0.2	Missense	EC1	[15]
p.D46E	c.138T>G	-	1	-	-	0	0.2	Missense	EC1	[25]
p.E47K	c.139G>A	-	2	-	-	0	0.3	Missense	EC1	[16]
59	c.176 - 191del16	-	2	-	-	0	0.3	Deletion	EC1	[17]
79	c.235delC	2	10	-	7	0.9	3.7	Deletion	TM2	[18l]
p.T86R	c.257C>G	-	-	-	1	0	0.3	Missense	TM2	[19]
p.R143W	c.426C>T	-	2	-	-	0	0.3	Missense	TM3	[20]
p.S199F	c.596C>T	-	1	-	-	0	0.2	Missense	TM4	[21]

IC1-3; intracellular domains, TM1-4; transmembrane domains, EC1-2; extracellular domains

The 235delC was the most prevalent mutation, with an allele frequency of 3.7% (24/648), followed by p.V37I (0.6%, 4/648). The p.V37I was originally described as a non-pathogenic polymorphism in Hispanics and Asians, but recently this variant was proposed to be pathogenic and associated with mild HL [22-23]. Recent electrophysiological studies using *Xenopus* oocytes of p.V37I showed defects in hemichannel activity [24].

The novel mutation p.D46E was associated with dominantly inherited non-syndromic hearing loss and was not found in normal hearing controls from the Korean population, indicating that this mutation is a pathogenic variant. The functional analysis of the p.D46E mutant showed the normal localization into the membrane but exhibited defective gap junction channel activity. Also, heterologous gap junctions reconstituted with Cx26-WT and Cx26-p.D46E demonstrated a dominant-negative effect which is consistent in agreement with its inheritance pattern [25]. The p.D46E mutation is located in the first extracellular domain (EC1), which is critical for hemichannel docking to form GJ channels, voltage gating, and connexin-connexin interactions [26-27]. Therefore, the dominant-negative effect of the p.D46E mutation may be due to defective docking of the two opposing connexin hemichannels. In many cases, mutations in extracellular domains are associated with dominant inheritance and syndromic phenotype, such as skin disorders and other ectodermal abnormalities [28-30]. The p.W44C and p.W44S mutations in the EC1 have been also reported to be associated with dominantly inherited non-syndromic hearing loss and to exert a dominant-negative effect on GJ permeability [29, 31].

Three mutations p.E47K, p.T86R, and p.S199F, have been reported previously in other ethnic groups, but were reported in Koreans for the first time in this study [16, 19, 21]. The p.E47K mutation was located in the first extracellular domain (EC1) of the connexin 26 protein. The extracellular loops contain a set of three cysteine residues, which help maintain the rigid tertiary structure that enables two opposing connexon to dock with each other [32]. Functional analysis of the p.E47K mutant Cx26 *in vitro* demonstrated that this mutation completely disrupts the ionic and biochemical permeability of hemichannels and gap junctions [33]. The p.T86R mutation has been reported previously in Japanese hearing loss patients, and the cell biological function of this mutation has been reported recently [19]. The functional analysis of p.T86R in HEK293 cell line showed a functionally null protein that does not interfere with normal GJ function in the presence of wild-type Cx26 which is consistent with autosomal recessive inheritance [25]. The p.S199F has been reported to be a recessive mutation and this mutation was shown to disrupt normal GJ functions by affecting oligormerization, assembly, transport, or membrane targeting in a previous *in vitro* study [34]

Two mutations, p.G45E and p.R143W, have been reported previously in several genetic and functional studies [15, 20, 33]. The p.G45E mutant was detected compound heterozygous form with c.235delC in this study. However, the p.G45E variant was first reported as an autosomal recessive hearing loss mutation in Caucasian. In addition, the p.G45E was shown to cause cell deaths by making the hemichannels leaky under normal physiological conditions [33, 35]. In this study, the p.R143W was detected in two patients - one contained only a heterozygous allele and the other was compound heterozygous with c.235delC. This mutation has been reported to result in autosomal recessive hearing loss in the Africa population [20, 36]. The p.R143W mutation was shown to prevent the formation of functional channels, which altered the voltage gating properties and biochemical coupling [37-38].

Twenty-eight patients (8.6%) had at least one pathogenic *GJB2* mutant allele. The c.235delC was the most prevalent mutation (61.5% of all pathogenic mutant allele) in the

Korean NSHI population with a total of 24 alleles (7 homozygous, 3 compound heterozygous with other pathogenic mutant alleles, and 7 one heterozygous allele only). In 10 patients with the c.235delC heterozygous allele, 7 patients had one heterozygous allele and 3 patients had compound heterozygous with other pathogenic mutant alleles. In addition, Four patients were heterozygous for a valine to isoleucine change at position 37 (p.V37I). A heterozygote for a glutamic acid to lysine substitution at position 47 (p.E47K) was observed in two patients. A 16 bp deletion, 176-191del16, was found in two patients – one contained only a heterozygous allele and the other was compound heterozygous with c.235delC. A mutation from arginine to tryptophan at the amino acid position 143 (p.R143W) was detected in two patients - one had only a heterozygous allele and the other was compound heterozygous with c.235delC. One patient had compound heterozygous glycine to glutamic acid at the amino acid position 45 (p.G45E) with c.235delC. A heterozygote for an aspartic acid to glutamic acid at the codon 46 (p.D46E), a threonine to arginine change at codon 86 (p.T86R), and a serine to phenylalanine at codon 199 (p.S199F), were found in one patient, respectively.

Four previously described polymorphisms, a valine to isoleucine change at codon 27 (p.V27I), a glutamic acid to glycine at codon 114 (p.E114G), a threonine to asparagines at codon 123 (p.T123N), and isoleucine to threonine at codon 203 (p.I203T), were also found in both patients and in the controls (Table 2). The minor allele frequencies of p.V27I and p.E114G variants were 34.7 and 16.5% respectively. However, p.T123N and p.I203T were found only in 5 and the 14 heterozygotes, respectively, suggesting these variants are rare in Koreans.

Table 2. The frequency of *GJB2* polymorphisms detected in Korean hearing loss patients

Codon location	Nucleotide change	Heterozygous individuals (n)	Homozygous individuals (n)	Allele frequency (%)	Protein domain	References
p.V27I	79G>A	111	57	34.7	TM1	[14]
p.E114G	341A>G	73	17	16.5	IC2	[18]
p.T123N	367A>C	5	-	0.8	IC2	[13]
p.I203T	608T>C	14	-	2.2	TM4	[17]

IC1-3; intracellular domains, TM1-4; transmembrane domains

CONCLUSION

Genetic study of the *GJB2* gene indicates that mutations in the *GJB2* gene are a less common cause of hearing loss in East Asian populations when compared to Caucasian populations, and the c.235delC mutation accounts for more than half of the mutations in the Korean population.

REFERENCES

[1] R. Bruzzone, T. W. WhiteandD. L. Paul, *Eur J Biochem* 238, 1 (1996).

[2] G. E. SosinskyandB. J. Nicholson, *Biochim Biophys Acta* 1711, 99 (2005).

[3] G. Sosinsky, *Proc Natl Acad Sci U S A* 92, 9210 (1995).

[4] F. Cao, R. Eckert, C. Elfgang, J. M. Nitsche, S. A. Snyder, H. u. DF, K. WilleckeandB. J. Nicholson, *J Cell Sci* 111 (Pt 1), 31 (1998).

[5] K. Arita, M. Akiyama, T. Aizawa, Y. Umetsu, I. Segawa, M. Goto, D. Sawamura, M. Demura, K. KawanoandH. Shimizu, *Am J Pathol* 169, 416 (2006).

[6] D. W. Laird, *Biochem J* 394, 527 (2006).

[7] T. Kikuchi, R. S. Kimura, D. L. PaulandJ. C. Adams, *Anat Embryol (Berl)* 191, 101 (1995).

[8] L. Zelante, P. Gasparini, X. Estivill, S. Melchionda, L. D'Agruma, N. Govea, M. Mila, M. D. Monica, J. Lutfi, M. Shohat, E. Mansfield, K. Delgrosso, E. Rappaport, S. SurreyandP. Fortina, *Hum Mol Genet* 6, 1605 (1997).

[9] X. Estivill, P. Fortina, S. Surrey, R. Rabionet, S. Melchionda, L. D'Agruma, E. Mansfield, E. Rappaport, N. Govea, M. Mila, L. ZelanteandP. Gasparini, *Lancet* 351, 394 (1998).

[10] R. Rabionet, L. Zelante, N. Lopez-Bigas, L. D'Agruma, S. Melchionda, G. Restagno, M. L. Arbones, P. GaspariniandX. Estivill, *Hum Genet* 106, 40 (2000).

[11] T. Sobe, S. Vreugde, H. Shahin, M. Berlin, N. Davis, M. Kanaan, Y. Yaron, A. Orr-Urtreger, M. Frydman, M. ShohatandK. B. Avraham, *Hum Genet* 106, 50 (2000).

[12] O. Bartsch, A. Vatter, U. Zechner, N. Kohlschmidt, C. Wetzig, A. Baumgart, S. Nospes, T. HaafandA. Keilmann, *Audiol Neurootol* 15, 375 (2010).

[13] H. J. Park, S. H. Hahn, Y. M. Chun, K. ParkandH. N. Kim, *Laryngoscope* 110, 1535 (2000).

[14] P. M. Kelley, D. J. Harris, B. C. Comer, J. W. Askew, T. Fowler, S. D. SmithandW. J. Kimberling, *Am J Hum Genet* 62, 792 (1998).

[15] S. Abe, S. Usami, H. Shinkawa, P. M. KelleyandW. J. Kimberling, *J Med Genet* 37, 41 (2000).

[16] S. Prasad, R. A. Cucci, G. E. GreenandR. J. Smith, *Hum Mutat* 16, 502 (2000).

[17] T. Kudo, K. Ikeda, S. Kure, Y. Matsubara, T. Oshima, K. Watanabe, T. Kawase, K. NarisawaandT. Takasaka, *Am J Med Genet* 90, 141 (2000).

[18] Y. Fuse, K. Doi, T. Hasegawa, A. Sugii, H. HibinoandT. Kubo, *Neuroreport* 10, 1853 (1999).

[19] A. Ohtsuka, I. Yuge, S. Kimura, A. Namba, S. Abe, L. Van Laer, G. Van CampandS. Usami, *Hum Genet* 112, 329 (2003).

[20] G. W. Brobby, B. Muller-MyhsokandR. D. Horstmann, *N Engl J Med* 338, 548 (1998).

[21] G. E. Green, D. A. Scott, J. M. McDonald, G. G. Woodworth, V. C. SheffieldandR. J. Smith, *JAMA* 281, 2211 (1999).

[22] H. H. Dahl, S. E. Tobin, Z. Poulakis, F. W. Rickards, X. Xu, L. Gillam, J. Williams, K. Saunders, B. Cone-WessonandM. Wake, *J Med Genet* 43, 850 (2006).

[23] C. Huculak, H. Bruyere, T. N. Nelson, F. K. KozakandS. Langlois, *Am J Med Genet A* 140, 2394 (2006).
[24] M. Palmada, K. Schmalisch, C. Bohmer, N. Schug, M. Pfister, F. LangandN. Blin, *Neurobiol Dis* 22, 112 (2006).
[25] S. Y. Choi, H. J. Park, K. Y. Lee, E. H. Dinh, Q. Chang, S. Ahmad, S. H. Lee, J. Bok, X. LinandU. K. Kim, *Hum Mutat* 30, E716 (2009).
[26] C. I. Foote, L. Zhou, X. ZhuandB. J. Nicholson, *J Cell Biol* 140, 1187 (1998).
[27] V. B. Hua, A. B. Chang, J. H. Tchieu, N. M. Kumar, P. A. NielsenandM. H. Saier, Jr., *J Membr Biol* 194, 59 (2003).
[28] Y. Deng, Y. Chen, L. ReussandG. A. Altenberg, *Hear Res* 220, 87 (2006).
[29] N. K. Marziano, S. O. Casalotti, A. E. Portelli, D. L. BeckerandA. Forge, *Hum Mol Genet* 12, 805 (2003).
[30] T. D. Matos, H. Caria, H. Simoes-Teixeira, T. Aasen, O. Dias, M. Andrea, D. P. KelsellandG. Fialho, *Hear Res* 240, 87 (2008).
[31] P. E. Martin, S. L. Coleman, S. O. Casalotti, A. ForgeandW. H. Evans, *Hum Mol Genet* 8, 2369 (1999).
[32] N. M. KumarandN. B. Gilula, *Cell* 84, 381 (1996).
[33] B. C. Stong, Q. Chang, S. AhmadandX. Lin, *Laryngoscope* 116, 2205 (2006).
[34] Z. Xiao, Z. Yang, X. LiuandD. Xie, *Acta Otolaryngol* 131, 59 (2011).
[35] H. A. Sanchez, G. Mese, M. Srinivas, T. W. WhiteandV. K. Verselis, *J Gen Physiol* 136, 47 (2010).
[36] C. Hamelmann, G. K. Amedofu, K. Albrecht, B. Muntau, A. Gelhaus, G. W. BrobbyandR. D. Horstmann, *Hum Mutat* 18, 84 (2001).
[37] Y. K. Man, C. Trolove, D. Tattersall, A. C. Thomas, A. Papakonstantinopoulou, D. Patel, C. Scott, J. Chong, D. J. Jagger, E. A. O'Toole, H. Navsaria, M. A. CurtisandD. P. Kelsell, *J Membr Biol* 218, 29 (2007).
[38] G. Mese, E. Londin, R. Mui, P. R. BrinkandT. W. White, *Hum Genet* 115, 191 (2004).

In: Inner Ear Development and Hearing Loss
Editors: Saima Riazuddin and Zubair Ahmed
ISBN: 978-1-62417-011-9

Chapter 12

HEREDITARY HEARING LOSS AND ITS MANAGEMENT IN THE JAPANESE POPULATION

Koji Nishimura and Shin-ichiro Kitajiri
Department of Otolaryngology, Head and Neck Surgery,
Graduate School of Medicine, Kyoto University, Japan

ABSTRACT

In this short communication, we summarized the genetic background of hereditary hearing loss in Japan, focusing on the *GJB2*, *SLC26A4*, *CDH23* and mitochondrial mutations that are common in the Japanese population. Some mutations that are common in the Japanese population differ from those in the western populations, suggesting the existence of a founder effect for deafness in each population group. Furthermore, we introduced what the medical society in Japan has done in the past decades for children with congenital hearing loss and their parents. Newborn hearing screening, hearing checkups for both one-and-a-half-year-old and three-year-old toddlers, and genetic diagnosis of congenital hearing loss are presented.

INTRODUCTION

At least 50 % of childhood hearing loss has been estimated to be of genetic etiology from several etiological studies [1]. Nearly 100 genes have been found to cause hereditary hearing loss and an overview of the genetics of hereditary hearing impairment is updated at the Hereditary Hearing Loss Homepage (http://hereditaryhearingloss.org/). Usami *et al.* compared the difference in mutation spectrum between the Japanese population and populations with European ancestry using an Invader assay and reported that the alleles of *GJB2*, *SLC26A4* and *CDH23* mutations in Japanese were quite different from those in Europeans [2]. We will summarize the mutations of *GJB2*, *SLC26A4*, *CDH23* and the mutations in the mitochondrial genes that are particular to the Japanese population.

GJB2

Connexin 26 (*GJB2*) was first reported as the gene responsible for hearing loss in DFNB1 by Kelsell *et al* in 1997 [3]. Although one mutation, namely 35delG, accounts for the majority of cases in Caucacians [4], it is rarely found in the Japanese population. This difference may be due to a founder effect for deafness in each population group, because significant differences between the genotypes of patients and controls for the five single nucleotide polymorphisms (SNPs) closest to *GJB* were found, with nearly complete association of one SNP allele with the 35delG mutation [5]. Table 1 summarizes the reported mutations in the *GJB2* gene in the Japanese population. Of those mutations, 235delC is the most prevalent [12]. Within the spectrum of *GJB2* mutations found in the Japanese population, 235delC shows a more severe form of hearing impairment than that of V37I, which is the second most frequent mutation [13].

Table 1. *GJB2* mutations reported in Japanese patients with hearing loss

Mutations	Mutation type	References
R143W	Missense	Brobby et al., 1998 [6]
Y136X	Nonsense	Fuse et al., 1999 [7]
235delC	Frameshift	Fuse et al., 1999 [7]
V37I	Missense	Abe et al., 2000 [8]
605ins46	Frameshift	Yuge et al., 2002 [9]
*D50Y	Missense	Yotsumoto et al., 2003 [10]
*D50N	Missense	Yotsumoto et al., 2003 [10]
P225L	Missense	Hayashi et al., 2011[11]
R32S	Missense	Hayashi et al., 2011[11]

*Patients demonstrated with keratitis-ichthyosis-deafness syndrome

SLC26A4

PDS (*SLC26A4*) gene is a responsible for both Pendred syndrome and nonsyndromic hearing loss associated with an enlargement of the vestibular aqueduct. Tsukamoto *et al*, investigated the *PDS* mutational spectrum in Japan and reported that 53% had the H723R mutation, suggesting a possible founder effect [14]. However, no genotype-phenotype correlations with *SLC26A4* mutations were found, unlike in the case of *GJB2* [15].

CDH23

Cadherin 23 forms the tip links between the stereocilia and mutations in the *CDH23* gene are responsible for Usher syndrome type ID (USH1D) and non-syndromic hearing loss (DFNB12). Wagatsuma *et al.* reported 51 *CDH23* sequence variants in Japanese patients with non-syndromic hearing loss and listed P240L, R301Q, Q1716P and R2029W as possible pathologic variants [16].

Mitochondrial Mutations

Mitochondria generate energy in the form of adenosine triphosphate (ATP) by means of the electron transport chain and the oxidative phosphorylation system. Several mitochondrial mutations are known to cause syndromic and non-syndromic hearing loss in the Japanese population. Tsuiki reported on the first Japanese cases of mitochondrial hearing loss that appeared in brothers who received streptomycin therapy [17] and then Tsuiki and Murai reported on a family with several members that developed hearing loss after receiving dihydrostreptomycin [18]. At the time of those reports, causes of the vulnerability of the inner ear were not fully understood, although familial streptomycin hearing loss occurring by maternal transmission suggested mitochondrial inheritance to be the most probable source [19]. In 1993, Prezant *et al* [20] and Hutchin *et al* [21] reported that it had been caused by a nucleotide 1555 mutation of mitochondrial DNA. Tsuiki *et al* described audiologic features of Japanese hearing loss patients due to the 1555 mutation of mitochondrial DNA as sensorineural, bilateral, and symmetric, while also showing a high-tone loss or a profound loss particularly in the high-tone range [22]. Further studies have shown that the A1555G mutation is the most prevalent mitochondrial mutation in the Japanese population [23]. Goto *et al.* found the A3243G mutation in the tRNALeu(UUR) gene causes mitochondrial encephalopathy, lactic acidosis, and stroke-like episodes (MELAS [24] and 30 to 70% of patients with MELAS have sensorineural hearing loss.. Ishikawa *et al.* reported the severe loss of spiral ganglion neurons in all turns of the cochlea in a 60-year-old Japanese male subject with non-syndromic hearing loss due to the T7551C mutation in the tRNASer(UCN) gene [25].

Management for Patients with Hereditary Hearing Loss in Japan

The first Japanese trial of newborn hearing screening was performed in 1998 by administrating automated auditory brainstem response (AABR) and otoacoustic emissions (OAEs) tests for 10,000 newborns. Today newborn hearing screening is done throughout Japan and is partially sponsored by cities and towns, not by the Japanese central government. If a newborn does not pass the screening, he/she is referred to another hospital where he/she will undergo several kinds of hearing tests (e.g. ABR and/or auditory steady-state response; ASSR). The Oto-Rhino-Laryngological Society of Japan, Inc. has approved 163 hospitals where newborns can be referred to for these examinations.

Although newborn hearing screening is effective for detecting toddlers with congenital hearing loss, it could fail to identify newborns that will present with progressive hearing loss later in life. The Oto-Rhino-Laryngological Society of Japan, Inc. issued leaflets in order to raise awareness about hearing loss amongst pediatricians. The society maintains the importance of hearing checkup for both one-and-a-half-year-old and three-year-old toddlers. Hearing examinations for one-and-a-half-year-old children aims to detect children with severe to profound hearing loss using objective hearing tests (e.g. ABR, ASSR, OAEs) and for three-year-old children that have moderate hearing loss, using several development tests to evaluate verbal abilities.

In 2008, Japanese Ministry of Health, Labor and Welfare approved genetic diagnosis of congenital hearing loss as a form of highly advanced medical treatment at Shinsyu Univerisity Hospital. It is now being performed in several other hospitals in Japan, including Kyoto University Hospital and the Japanese National Health Insurance began to cover its costs from April, 2012. In addition to a clinical diagnosis, the parents of affected children are also offered genetic counseling, which is done by specialists certified by Japanese board of medical genetics.

CONCLUSION

Recent studies have revealed that some of the mutations that cause hereditary hearing loss in the Asian population are different from those found in the Caucasian population group. The 235delC (*GJB2*), H723R (*SLC26A4*) and A1555G (mitochondrial gene) mutations are the most prevalent pathogenic alleles in the Japanese population. Because early diagnosis and medical interventions are important for children with congenital or progressive hearing loss, Japanese society has implemented newborn hearing screening and hearing checkups for one-and-a-half-year-old and three-year-old children. Also, genetic diagnosis of children with sensorineural hearing loss followed counseling for parents is routinely performed all over Japan as a form of highly advanced medical treatment approved by Japanese Ministry of Health, Labor and Welfare.

REFERENCES

[1] R. J. Smith, J. F. Bale Jr., K. R. White, *Lancet*, 365, 879-90 (2005).

[2] S. Usami, M. Wagatsuma, H. Fukuoka, H. Suzuki, K. Tsukada, S. Nishio, Y. Takumi and S. Abe, *Acta Otolaryngol.*, 128, 446-54 (2008).

[3] D. P. Kelsell, J. Dunlop, H. P. Stevens, N. J. Lench, J. N. Liang, G. Parry, R. F. Mueller and I. M. Leigh, *Nature*, 387, 80-83 (1997).

[4] P. M. Kelley, D. J. Harris, B. C. Comer, J. W. Askew, T. Fowler, S. D. Smith, W. J. Kimberling, *Am. J. Hum. Genet.*, 62, 792-9 (1998).

[5] L. Van Laer, P. Coucke, R. F. Mueller, G. Caethoven, K. Flothmann, S. D. Prasad, G. P. Chamberlin, M. Houseman, G. R. Taylor, C. M. Van de Heyning, E. Fransen, J. Rowland, R. A. Cucci, R. J. Smith and G. Van Camp, *J. Med. Genet.*, 38, 515-8 (2001).

[6] G. W. Brobby, B. Müller-Myhsok and R. D. Horstmann, *N. Engl. J. Med.*, 338, 548-50 (1998).

[7] Y. Fuse, K. Doi, T. Hasegawa, A. Sugii, H. Hibino and T. Kubo, *Neuroreport*, 10, 1853-7 (1999).

[8] S. Abe, S. Usami, H. Shinkawa, P. M. Kelley and W. J. Kimberling, *J. Med. Genet.*, 37, 41-43 (2000).

[9] I. Yuge, A. Ohtsuka, T. Matsunaga and S. Usami, *Auris Nasus Larynx*, 29, 379-82 (2002).

[10] A. Yotsumoto, T. Hashiguchi, X. Chen, N. Ohtake, A. Tomitaka, H. Akamatsu, K. Matsunaga, S. Shiraishi, H. Miura, J. Adachi and T. Kanzaki, *Br. J. Dermatol*, 148, 649-53 (2003).

[11] A. Hayashi, M. Funayama, Y. Li, K. Kamiya, A. Kawano, M. Suzuki, N. Hattori and K. Ikeda, *Int. J. Pediatr. Otorhinolaryngol.*, 75, 211-214 (2011).

[12] Ohtsuka, I. Yuge, S. Kimura, A. Namba, S. Abe, L. Van Laer, G. Van Camp and S. Usami, *Hum. Genet.*, 112, 329-33 (2003).

[13] T. Oguchi, A. Ohtsuka, S. Hashimoto, A. Oshima, S. Abe, Y. Kobayashi, K. Nagai, T. Matsunaga, *J. Hum. Genet.*, 50, 76-83 (2005).

[14] K. Tsukamoto, H. Suzuki, D. Harada, A. Namba, S. Abe and S. Usami, *Eur. J. Hum. Genet*, 11, 916-22 (2003).

[15] H. Suzuki, A. Oshima, K. Tsukamoto, S. Abe, K. Kumakawa, K. Nagai, H. Satoh, Y. Kanda, S. Iwasaki and S. Usami, *Acta Otolaryngol.*, 127, 1292-7 (2007).

[16] M. Wagatsuma, R. Kitoh, H. Suzuki, H. Fukuoka, Y. Takumi, S. Usami, *Clin. Genet.*, 72, 339-44 (2007).

[17] T. Tsuiki, *Otolaryngology (Tokyo)*, 28, 230-4 (1956).

[18] T. Tsuiki and S. Murai, *Audiology*, 10, 315-22 (1971).

[19] D. N. Hu, W. Q. Qui, B.T. Wu, L. Z. Fang, F. Zhou, Y. P. Gu, Q.H. Zhang, J.H. Yan, Y. Q. Ding and H. Wong, *J. Med. Genet.*, 28, 79-83 (1991).

[20] T. R. Prezant, J. V. Agapian, M. C. Bohlman, X. Bu, S. Oztas, W.Q. Qiu, K. S. Arnos, G. A. Cortopassi, L. Jaber, J. I. Rotter, M. Shohat and N. Fischel-Ghodsian, *Nat. Genet.*, 4, 289-94 (1993).

[21] T. P. Hutchin, M. Stoneking, W. O. Qiu, N. Fischel-Ghodsian and G. A. Cortopassi, *Am. J. Hum. Genet.*, 53(suppl): session 19, No. 20 (1993).

[22] T. Tsuiki, K. Murai, S. Murai, K. Kitamura and Y. Tamagawa, *Ann. Otol. Rhinol. Laryngol.*, 106, 643-8 (1997).

[23] S. Usami, S. Abe, J. Akita, A. Namba, H. Shinkawa, M. Ishii, S. Iwasaki, T. Hoshino, J. Ito, K. Doi, T. Kubo, T. Nakagawa, S. Komiyama, T. Tono and S. Komune, *J. Med. Genet.*, 37, 38-40 (2000).

[24] Y. Goto, I. Nonaka and S. Horai, *Nature*, 348, 651-3 (1990).

[25] K. Ishikawa, Y. Tamasawa, K. Takahashi, Y. Iino, Y. Murakami, K. Kakizaki, H. Kimura, J. Kusakari, A. Hara and K. Ichimura, *Laryngoscope*, 116, 1982-6 (2006).

INDEX

L

M

N

O

P

X

Y

Z

Α

Γ